GENETICS *and*
GENOMICS
in NURSING *and*
HEALTH CARE

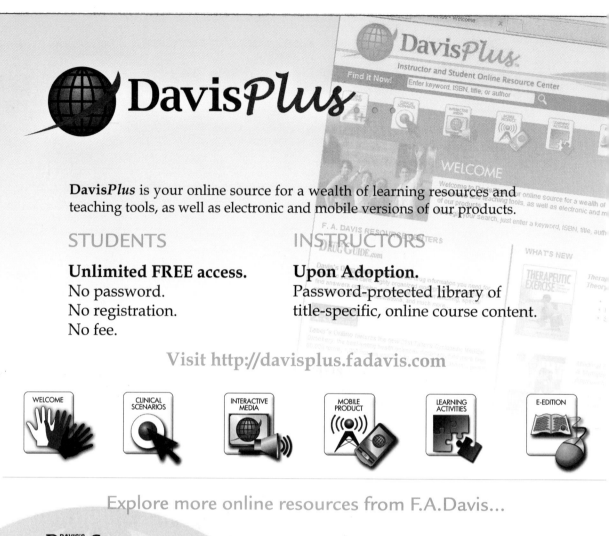
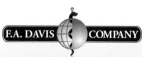

GENETICS *and* GENOMICS
in NURSING *and* HEALTH CARE

Theresa A. Beery,
PhD, RN, ACNP-BC, CNE
Professor
Director of the Center for Educational Research,
Scholarship, and Innovation
Institute for Nursing Research and Scholarship
University of Cincinnati College of Nursing
Cincinnati, Ohio

M. Linda Workman, PhD, RN
Senior Volunteer Faculty
University of Cincinnati College of Nursing
Cincinnati, Ohio

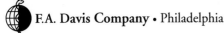
F.A. Davis Company • Philadelphia

F. A. Davis Company
1915 Arch Street
Philadelphia, PA 19103
www.fadavis.com

Printed in the United States of America

Last digit indicates print number: 10 9 8 7 6 5 4 3 2 1

Publisher, Nursing: Joanne P. DaCunha, RN, MSN
Director of Content Development: Darlene D. Pedersen
Project Editor: Elizabeth Hart
Manager of Art and Design: Carolyn O'Brien

As new scientific information becomes available through basic and clinical research, recommended treatments and drug therapies undergo changes. The author(s) and publisher have done everything possible to make this book accurate, up to date, and in accord with accepted standards at the time of publication. The author(s), editors, and publisher are not responsible for errors or omissions or for consequences from application of the book, and make no warranty, expressed or implied, in regard to the contents of the book. Any practice described in this book should be applied by the reader in accordance with professional standards of care used in regard to the unique circumstances that may apply in each situation. The reader is advised always to check product information (package inserts) for changes and new information regarding dose and contraindications before administering any drug. Caution is especially urged when using new or infrequently ordered drugs.

Library of Congress Cataloging-in-Publication Data

Beery, Theresa A.
  Genetics and genomics in nursing and health care / Theresa A. Beery, M. Linda Workman.
  p. ; cm.
  Includes bibliographical references and index.
  ISBN 978-0-8036-2488-7 (pbk. : alk. paper)
  I. Workman, M. Linda. II. Title.
  [DNLM: 1. Genomics. 2. Genetic Diseases, Inborn—nursing. 3. Genetic Techniques—nursing. QU 58.5]
  LC-classification not assigned
  576.5—dc23

                                                                                    2011025932

To our genetics mentors, those scientific giants upon whose shoulders we stand to reach greater heights. Their vision, patience, and dedicated service to others were instrumental in shaping our genetics worldview as well as the format and content of this textbook.

Dr. D. Woodrow Benson
Dr. Mary M. Haag
Ms. Cynthia Prows
Dr. Shirley Soukup
Dr. Josef Warkany

To our families and loved ones who made the difficult times better and the good times great, especially:

Dennis C. Beery
John B. Workman

About the Authors

Theresa (Terry) A. Beery received her BSN from Miami University, her MS in Nursing from Wright State University, and her PhD in Nursing Science from the University of Cincinnati. She completed a post-master's certificate and is certified as an acute care nurse practitioner (ACNP-BC) and a certified nurse educator (CNE). Her genetics training included the Summer Genetics Institute at the National Institute for Nursing Research. In 2002 she received a career award from the National Institutes of Health, which supported her development in molecular genetics. This enabled her to spend 3 years working in the cardiovascular genetics laboratory at Cincinnati Children's Hospital Medical Center under the mentorship of Dr. D. Woodrow Benson. Terry is a Professor at the University of Cincinnati (UC) College of Nursing, where she teaches undergraduate and graduate genetics. She is the recipient of the College of Nursing's Excellence in Teaching Award and is a member of the UC Academy of Fellows for Teaching and Learning. Terry is also the Director of the Center for Educational Research, Scholarship, and Innovation at the UC College of Nursing.

M. Linda Workman received her BSN from the University of Cincinnati (UC) College of Nursing. She later earned her MSN and a PhD in Developmental Biology from the UC. The Developmental Biology education provided Linda with extensive formal education in genetics. In addition, she worked for more than 5 years in a cytogenetics laboratory, where she conducted basic genetic research on human tumors. Linda has taught genetics to undergraduate and graduate nursing students, practicing nurses, advanced practice nurses, and physicians. She has been recognized nationally for her ability to present genetics/genomics and other complex physiologic concepts in a manner that promotes student retention of the information. In addition, she received Excellence in Teaching awards from Raymond Walters College, the UC, and Case Western Reserve University. Over the past 30 years she has presented numerous seminars and authored many journal articles and book chapters on the topic of genetics. Currently, she is Senior Volunteer Faculty at the UC College of Nursing.

Genetics and Genomics in Nursing and Health Care is focused for nurses and other health-care professionals who are not basic science majors. This text was derived from our desire, both as nurses and educators, to create a book that would help students identify the most important content areas for incorporating genetic information into their practices and interactions with patients, families, and the general public. Part of making this information accessible is the use of second-person writing ("you") format rather than the more "scholarly" third-person style. With the goal of clarity and understanding in mind, we developed a unique format based on six focus areas:

1. *Basic concepts from molecular genetics*
2. *Gene expression*

These first two focus areas present foundational information on the biological basis of genetic inheritance as well as how environmental factors influence the actual risk or resistance for a developing disorder. Although genetic terminology is used throughout this section, it is tempered with "everyday" language to help students learn, retain, and use this conceptual information. Complex concepts are reduced to basic components and presented in a style that makes them logical to the learner. Essential to this process is the use of clear, concise explanations that are free from jargon and academic pretension. Information critical for individual and family assessment of genetic risk and variation from normal is presented in a manner that enables it to be incorporated into general assessment techniques and data management.

3. *Genomic health problems across the life span*

The three chapters in this focus area explain genetic factors influencing *common* health problems rather than rare syndromes. In addition to genetic disorders that are identified in childhood, this section also discusses those genetic disorders that may not manifest until adulthood and older adulthood. Clinical examples abound, and case studies help personalize the information. It presents what every nurse or other health-care professional needs to know about applying genetic information when caring for patients and families.

4. *Genomic influences on selected complex health problems*

The issues presented in the three chapters of this focus area include disorders that have both a strong genetic influence coupled with strong environmental influences on disease expression. This focus area brings common disorders to the forefront that are the result of the input of more than one gene and that may respond to personal changes to alter the severity of the problem. Again, clinical examples abound, and case studies help personalize the information.

5. *Genomics and disease management*

The three chapters in this focus area include thought-provoking issues regarding the benefits and risks of genetic testing and the roles of various professionals in the genetic counseling process. Additionally, personalized health care, especially the variation in responses to drug therapy, is explored and explained.

6. *Global genomic issues*

The two chapters in this focus area concern the questions "How did we get here?" and "Where are we going?" They explain the reasons why the predisposition and expression of some genetic disorders are greater for some ethnic groups than for others. They also present issues and potential problems people are likely to face as they rush into the genomic era of health care.

The style of presentation for the content of this textbook is direct, active, and clear. Healthcare terms and related physiological mechanisms are explained in common, everyday language to promote better student understanding and continuuous application of the content. **Illustrations** and **tables** were selected and developed to enhance student understanding about cellular activities, inheritance patterns, and genetic risks.

We have included key features in each chapter. Each chapter opens with a list of **learning outcomes** followed by a list of **key terms**. Each key term is also presented in the chapter text and highlighted in boldface when first used. A full alphabetical listing of key terms with definitions can be found in the **glossary** at the end of the text. At the end of each chapter, there is a list of **Gene Gems** highlighting essential key points for the student to take away from the reading. Students will also find **self-assessment questions** keyed to the learning outcomes of the chapter. The answers for these can be found at the end of each chapter. Finally, critical-thinking **case studies** are located at the end of every clinical chapter. These realistic cases present issues and problems that require clinical decision making about individual patients and families who are at increased genetic risk for health problems.

Additional materials and study tools can be found on *DavisPlus*, including activities for critical thinking and learning key terms, links to online genetics resources, and extensive teaching resources for instructors.

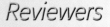

Janet Adams, MSN, RT (ARRT), RN
Instructor
Southeast Missouri State University
Cape Girardeau, Missouri

Julie Baldwin, RN, MSN
Assistant Professor of Nursing
Missouri Western State University
St. Joseph, Missouri

Laurie Brooks, MSN, MBA, RN
Assistant Professor
Saint Luke's College of Health Sciences
Kansas City, Missouri

Julia A. Eggert, PhD, APRN-BC, GNP AOCN
Associate Professor and Healthcare Genetics
    Doctoral Program Coordinator
Clemson University School of Nursing
Clemson, South Carolina

Deborah Ellis, RN, MSN, NP-C
Assistant Professor
Missouri Western State University
St. Joseph, Missouri

Kathleen T. Hickey, EdD, FNP-BC, ANP-BC
Assistant Professor of Nursing
Columbia University
New York, New York

Anita H. King, DNP, MA, FNP-BC, CDE, FAADE
Clinical Associate Professor, College of Nursing
University of South Alabama
Fairhope, Alabama

Judith A. Lewis, PhD, RN, WNP-BC, FAAN
Professor *Emerita*
Virginia Commonwealth University
Richmond, Virginia

Carrie J. Merkle, PhD, RN, FAAN
Associate Professor
University of Arizona College of Nursing
Tucson, Arizona

Elizabeth Louise Pestka, MS, RN,
PMHCNS-BC, APNG
Assistant Professor of Nursing & Clinical Nurse
    Specialist
Mayo Clinic
Rochester, Minnesota

Michael A. Rackover, PA-C, MS
PA Program Director & Associate Professor
Philadelphia University
Philadelphia, Pennsylvania

Catherine Read, PhD, RN
Associate Dean/Associate Professor
Connell School of Nursing, Boston College
Chestnut Hill, Massachusetts

Jackie Shrock, RN, BSN, MEd
Nursing Program Coordinator/Teacher
Wayne County Schools Career Center
Orrville, Ohio

Yona D. Victor, MD
Full-Time Faculty
The School of Nursing at Platt College
Aurora, Colorado

Lottchen Wider, RN, PhD
Associate Professor
Maryville University
St. Louis, Missouri

Acknowledgments

Many talented people are needed to make any textbook a success. The authors wish to acknowledge the following individuals and groups for their guidance, dedication, hard work, constructive criticism, and creative input that were so important to this project: Julie Scardiglia, Elizabeth Hart, and Joanne DaCunha.

Table of Contents

Basic Concepts From Molecular Genetics

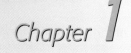

Chapter 1

DNA Structure and Function

Learning Outcomes

1. Use the genetic terminology associated with DNA structure and function.
2. Compare the components, structures, and forms of DNA.
3. Explain how and why double-stranded DNA has complementary strands.
4. Describe the events and processes involved in DNA replication.
5. Explain the formation and purpose of chromosomes.
6. Determine the gender and ploidy of a person based on his or her karyotype.
7. Distinguish genotype from phenotype.
8. Explain how dominant gene alleles and recessive gene alleles determine expression of single-gene traits.

KEY TERMS

Allele	Dominant trait	Mitosis
Aneuploid	Euploid	Nucleoside
Autosomes	Gene	Nucleotide
Base pairs	Gene locus	P arm
Bases	Genetics	Phenotype
Centromere	Genome	Ploidy
Chromatid	Genomics	Polyploidy
Chromosome	Genotype	Proteome
Codominant trait	Haploid chromosome number	Proteomics
Complementary pairs	Heterozygous	q arm
Deoxyribonucleic acid (DNA)	Histones	Recessive trait
Diploid chromosome number	Homozygous	Sex chromosomes
DNA replication	Karyotype	Single-gene trait

Introduction

The recent vast increase in information about how genetic factors influence the development of health problems has led to recognition by many professional organizations of the need to ensure that all health-care professionals have a basic understanding of genetics and genomics. People who are neither scientists nor in the health professions may mistakenly believe that with today's level of genetic understanding, we can know everything there is to know about a person. Although this is not true, the use of genetics and genomics can assist in developing health-problem prevention strategies and therapies that take into account each person's genetic differences. The purpose of this chapter is to present information about basic genetics to help in your understanding of how this information can have an impact in your care of all patients and their families. All health-care professionals should be familiar with basic genetic terminology and should be able to recognize when a patient or family has a possible genetic risk for a health problem.

Many people use the terms *genetics* and *genomics* interchangeably. Although they are similar, there is some difference. **Genetics** is the study of the general mechanisms of heredity and the variation of inherited traits. **Genomics** is the study of the function of all the nucleotide sequences present within the entire genome of a species, including genes in **DNA (deoxyribonucleic acid)** coding regions and in DNA noncoding regions (per the National Cancer Institute; National Human Genome Research Institute). DNA coding regions and noncoding regions are discussed in Chapter 2. These definitions indicate that genomics includes genetics but has a broader scope.

Genetic Biology

All living cells, even bacteria and other lower organisms, have genes. A **gene** is a specific set of instructions cells use to produce a specific protein. Consider all the hormones, enzymes, and other proteins your body makes, both those that exist as individual identifiable substances and those that are parts of larger components. Some genes tell each cell what protein to make and how to make it, whereas other genes control a cell's protein-making activity by telling it when to make a specific protein and how much to make. Thus, a gene acts as a specific "recipe" for making a protein.

Most genes are part of the DNA located in the nucleus of body cells. Figure 1–1 shows a cell nucleus with DNA in the form of chromosomes. Figure 1–2 depicts an enlargement of one chromosome to show that a chromosome is composed of DNA and contains segments that are genes.

All human cells with a nucleus contain two sets of every gene that humans possess. This complete set of genes for our species is called the **human genome** and contains between 20,000 and 25,000 individual genes. (Mature germ cells—sperm and ova—contain only one set of every human gene.) The fact that all nucleated cells contain all the human genes can be a confusing concept, because no cell produces all the proteins coded for by these genes. For example, only the ovary and the adrenal gland normally produce estrogen, even though all cells have the gene for estrogen. Although the structural gene for estrogen is present in all cells, only in the ovary and adrenal gland is this gene selectively activated, resulting in the production of estrogen. The activation of a gene allowing its product to be made by the cell is called *gene expression*. In all other cell types, regulator genes prevent the structural gene for estrogen from being expressed.

The DNA that codes for the complete set of all *proteins* that a person can make at a given time under certain conditions is called the **proteome**. This term combines the words *protein* and *genome* to indicate the gene sequences that are critical in programming the instructions for each protein. The study of how protein genes are selectively expressed, are modified after expression, and interact with each other

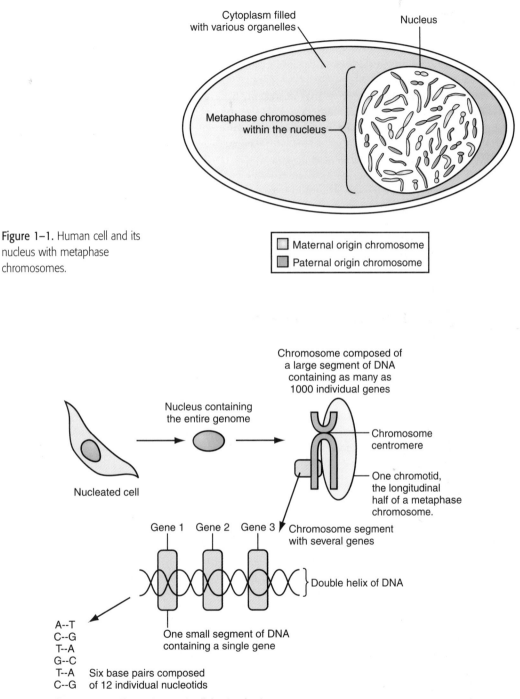

Cytoplasm filled
with various organelles

Nucleus

Metaphase chromosomes
within the nucleus

Figure 1–1. Human cell and its
nucleus with metaphase
chromosomes.

☐ Maternal origin chromosome
■ Paternal origin chromosome

Chromosome composed of
a large segment of DNA
containing as many as
1000 individual genes

Nucleus containing
the entire genome

Chromosome
centromere

One chromotid,
the longitudinal
half of a metaphase
chromosome.

Nucleated cell

Gene 1   Gene 2   Gene 3   Chromosome segment
with several genes

Double helix of DNA

A--T
C--G
T--A
G--C
T--A   Six base pairs composed
C--G   of 12 individual nucleotids

One small segment of DNA
containing a single gene

Figure 1–2. Different forms of cellular (nuclear) DNA.

is known as **proteomics.** Proteomes can be examined for one cell type or for an entire organism. The protein estrogen is part of the proteome for ovarian cells but is not part of the cardiac muscle cell (myocardial cell) proteome. When considering the entire human proteome, we are looking at the proteins produced by all the individual cellular proteomes. Issues about proteomes are discussed in Chapter 2.

Some people get confused about how DNA is different from a gene and from a chromosome. DNA is the basic genetic chemical structure, containing gene coding regions and noncoding regions, which can be compressed into a chromosome form (see Fig. 1–2). A **chromosome** is a temporary but consistent state of condensed DNA structure formed for the purpose of cell division. The nature and function of chromosomes are discussed later in this chapter. Genes and chromosomes are both parts of the DNA. Consider a sweater as a chromosome and each separate part of the sweater (right sleeve, left sleeve, pocket, collar, front, and back) as a gene. Now consider that the entire sweater (chromosome) and its parts (genes) are composed of yarn (DNA). A sweater is not a person's entire wardrobe, however, just like one chromosome and all the genes it contains are not the entire genome. Think of the genome as being the entire wardrobe (all the person's shoes, socks, underpants, undershirts, pants, shirts, sweaters, coats, hats, gloves, and scarves). Each single chromosome has many genes within it. Larger chromosomes contain thousands of genes, and smaller chromosomes may have fewer than 100 genes.

Another analogy for understanding how DNA, chromosomes, and genes are connected is to consider the DNA of the genome to be a large recipe book with all the instructions (recipes) needed to make every protein your body can produce. Each chromosome is a separate chapter, and the genes are the individual recipes. Each gene has a specific chromosome location, called a **gene locus**; think of this as the "page" of the chapter in which the recipe is located. For example, the insulin gene's locus is 11q13, which means that the gene is located on the long arm of chromosome 11 in region 13 (Fig. 1–3). When it is time to make more insulin, this is the "page" where the recipe can be found.

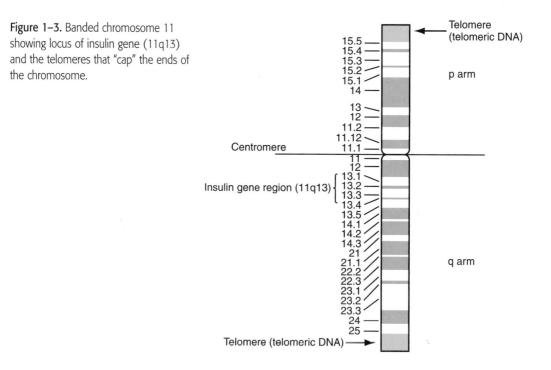

Figure 1–3. Banded chromosome 11 showing locus of insulin gene (11q13) and the telomeres that "cap" the ends of the chromosome.

Although all cells have the "recipe" for insulin on chromosome 11, it is only opened and read by the beta cells of the pancreas. Other cells normally cannot "read" the insulin recipe and do not make insulin. Protein synthesis, which is the actual making of proteins, is discussed in Chapter 2.

DNA

About 99% of the human body's DNA is in the nucleus. This DNA is termed *nuclear DNA*. Cell mitochondria also contain a small amount of DNA called *mitochondrial DNA*. This is discussed in Chapter 5.

DNA Structure

The basic structure of DNA is a set of four nucleic acids. These nucleic acids are nitrogen-containing compounds made from the individual amino acids derived from the proteins we eat. Because these elements are the basic structure of DNA, they are called **bases**. These four bases are adenine (A), cytosine (C), guanine (G), and thymine (T) (Fig. 1–4). Thymine and cytosine are single-ring structures known as *pyrimidines*. (Memory hint: the words *thymine* and *cytosine* contain a *Y*, as does the word *pyrimidine*.) Adenine and guanine are each double-ringed structures known as *purines*. (Memory hint: the words *adenine*, *guanine*, and *purine* do not contain a *Y*.) These four bases are present in any type of DNA, whether from humans and other mammals, plants, bacteria, or viruses.

Each base becomes a **nucleoside** when a five-sided sugar (known as a *deoxyribose sugar*) is attached to it (see Fig. 1–4). Each nucleoside becomes a complete **nucleotide** when phosphate groups are attached. The nucleotide is the final form of a base that is placed into the DNA strand. The nucleotides within each strand are held in position by the linked phosphate groups, which act like the string holding beads together to form a necklace.

Base pairs are the complementary bases in the two opposite strands of DNA. These DNA strands must remain perfectly parallel to each other, and the pairings of the nucleotides make this happen. For double-stranded DNA to remain parallel, the two strands stay the same distance apart down the total length of DNA. A pyrimidine with a single-ring structure always pairs up with a purine that has a double-ring structure to maintain this proper distance (see Fig. 1–4). Not only is it necessary for a

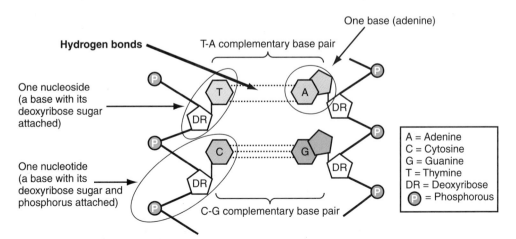

Figure 1–4. Four bases arranged as nucleotides in complementary base pairs. A = adenine, C = cytosine, G = guanine, T = thymine, DR = deoxyribose, and P = phosphorus.

purine to always pair with a pyrimidine, but the bases are also always specific, forming **complementary pairs**.

Normally, adenine and thymine always pair together, whereas cytosine and guanine always pair together (Fig. 1–5). The reason for these specific and complementary pairings of bases is related to the forces that hold the two DNA strands together. The two strands are held together loosely most of the time by weak hydrogen bonds. The fact that hydrogen bonds are weak is a good thing, because when the two strands of DNA need to separate during cell division when the DNA has to replicate, they come apart easily and do not require a lot of energy to perform this separation. Within a base pair, the hydrogen bonds form between the two nucleotides. Adenine and thymine each have a site for two hydrogen bonds to form, whereas cytosine and guanine each have three sites for hydrogen bonds to form (see Fig. 1–4). Although purines must always pair with pyrimidines, they can pair only with the base that can form the same number of hydrogen bonds. Thus, adenine can pair only with thymine, and cytosine can pair only with guanine.

DNA in humans and other mammals is a linear, double-stranded (dsDNA) structure with the nucleotides of each strand connected together by the phosphate groups as the backbone of the strand (see Fig. 1–4). These two individual strands are held together loosely by hydrogen bonds. In this way, double-stranded DNA is arranged like a long set of railroad tracks. The long steel rails of the track are the phosphate backbones, and the bases of the nucleotides are each half of the individual railroad ties (Fig. 1–6).

Complementary base pairs in DNA are specific because adenine normally always pairs with thymine, and cytosine normally always pairs with guanine. This means that if the base sequence of one strand of DNA is known, the opposite strand's sequence could be predicted accurately. For example, the left-hand strand of DNA in Figure 1–6 has the sequence T-G-G-C-A-T-T-G from top to bottom, and the corresponding (complementary) right-hand section has the sequence A-C-C-G-T-A-A-C. Most of the time, the two parallel strands of DNA are twisted into a loose helical shape (see Figs. 1–2 and 1–5). The DNA supercoils tightly into the chromosome shape (which can be seen with standard microscopes) only when a cell undergoes mitosis.

Billions of bases are found in the DNA of just one cell. In its most common shape, DNA can be seen only by using an electron microscope; however, if the DNA of one cell could be put together and

Figure 1–5. Double-stranded DNA arranged as complementary strands in a linear structure and a loose double helix. T = thymine, A = adenine, C = cytosine, G = guanine.

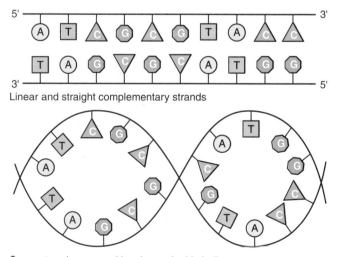

Linear and straight complementary strands

Same strands arranged in a loose double helix

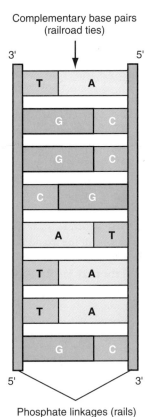

Complementary base pairs
(railroad ties)

3'   5'

5'   3'

Phosphate linkages (rails)

Figure 1–6. An 8-base pair segment of double-stranded (ds) DNA similar to a section of railroad track.

stretched out, it would be about 6 feet long. If this same piece of DNA from one cell could be made about a half-inch wide, it would stretch out more than 1000 feet. There is much more DNA in each nucleus than is needed for the 20,000 to 25,000 genes. The gene part of the DNA is only about 5% of all the total DNA in each cell's nucleus.

DNA Replication

CELL DIVISION

Every time a cell divides, the DNA undergoes **replication**, which is duplication or reproduction of itself, resulting in two *identical* sets of DNA. This is needed because every time a cell undergoes **mitosis**, a duplication division resulting in two new cells that are identical both to each other and to the original cell (parent cell) that began the mitosis, each cell must have a complete genome. For the two new cells created as a result of mitosis to be identical to the parent cell, the DNA of the parent cell must replicate exactly. Mitosis occurs in a regulated pattern known as the *cell cycle*. Figure 1–7 shows the phases of the cell cycle, which starts with one cell and ends with two new cells. When mitosis is normal and the parent cell divides correctly, each new cell has the identical (and correct) amount of DNA and genes.

   Cells not actively dividing are in a reproductive resting state known as G_0. In this state, the cell is actively performing its designated functions but is not dividing. For example, skin cells in the G_0 state produce keratin and other skin products but do not reproduce. Most normal cells are in the state of G_0 most of the time and leave it only to reproduce when generation of more cells is needed. To undergo

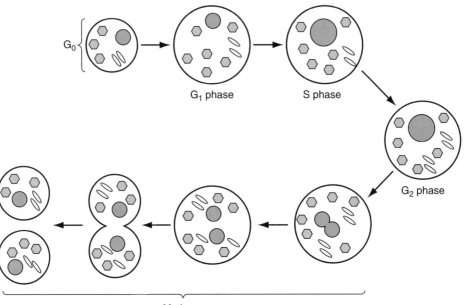

Figure 1–7. Phases of the cell cycle for a cell undergoing mitosis.

mitosis, a cell first must be a cell type capable of cell division. Some cells do not divide once organ maturation is complete. Examples of these nondividing cells include skeletal muscle cells, cardiac muscle cells, and neurons. If a cell is the type that has retained the ability to divide when needed (e.g., skin cells; bone marrow cells; liver cells; and epithelial cells that line the lungs, GI tract, bladder, uterus, and so on), it will respond to signals to leave G_0 and enter the cell cycle. The cell cycle involves four phases, and movement through these phases and to successful generation of two new cells requires selective gene input. The actions of these promitosis genes are discussed in Chapter 3. The activities occurring at each stage of the cell cycle are outlined in Table 1–1.

TABLE 1–1

Activities of the Cell Cycle

Cell Cycle Phase	Activities/Purposes
G_1	The cell is getting ready for division by taking on extra nutrients, making more energy, and growing extra membrane. The amount of cell fluid (cytoplasm) also increases.
S	DNA replication and synthesis
G_2	Production of proteins important to cell division and in normal physiological function after mitosis is complete
M	Mitosis in which the DNA in the nucleus pulls apart and creates two nuclei (nucleokinesis), followed by the cell separating into two cells, each with one nucleus (cytokinesis)

DNA SYNTHESIS

Generating two new cells from one parent cell requires twice as much DNA as originally present in the parent cell. Notice in Figure 1–7 that the nucleus during S phase is twice as large as it was during G_1 because it now has twice as much DNA. This replication of the DNA ensures that the two new cells that result from completion of mitosis will each have the same amount of DNA as the parent cell. The parent cell doubles its DNA content through DNA synthesis by DNA replication in S phase. (Memory hint: S phase stands for *synthesis* of DNA.) How are DNA replication and DNA synthesis different? Whenever DNA is made, it is called *DNA synthesis*. When the newly made DNA is identical to the original DNA in the parent cell, it is called *DNA replication*.

One point to remember about human cellular DNA is that it is present in the cell as 46 separate chunks corresponding to the 46 chromosomes. The complete genome within any one cell is not present as one very long double strand (ds) of DNA. Instead, there are 46 separate sets of dsDNA (see Fig. 1–1). Although this DNA is present in this form as 46 chromosomes that are visible only during metaphase of mitosis, these represent the 46 loosely coiled double helices. They are not visible in this form with the use of standard microscopes.

DNA replication begins when the individual sets of dsDNA separate by breaking the hydrogen bonds holding the two strands in the double helix form (Fig. 1–8). Once they separate, enzymes at each end of the strands read the sequence of the original strands and build two new strands that are complementary to the original strands. DNA must be "read" in one direction to correctly place the new nucleotides during DNA synthesis, just like written languages must be read in only one direction to make sense. These strands are read from the 5 prime (5') end of the DNA to the 3 prime (3') end (these numbers just refer to the specific carbon on the sugar molecule that connects with the phosphorous molecule). At the end

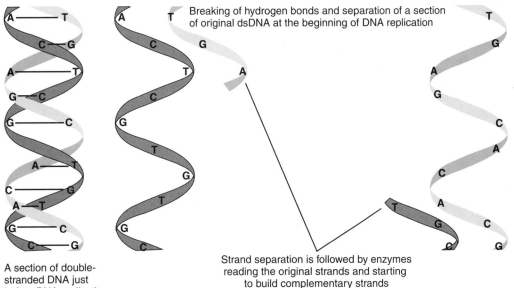

Breaking of hydrogen bonds and separation of a section of original dsDNA at the beginning of DNA replication

A section of double-stranded DNA just before DNA replication

Strand separation is followed by enzymes reading the original strands and starting to build complementary strands

Figure 1–8. A section of double-stranded DNA just before DNA replication, during breaking of hydrogen bonds and separation of the double-stranded DNA at the beginning of DNA replication and the beginning of the building of new complementary strands.

of DNA replication, two new sets of dsDNA representing each of the 46 chromosomes are present in the cell. Each new set of dsDNA contains one strand of the original dsDNA and one newly synthesized strand (Fig. 1–9). Because each of the two new sets of dsDNA contains one of the original strands, this type of DNA synthesis is known as the *semiconservative model* of DNA replication.

Thus, new complementary strands are synthesized along the old strands, using the old strands as a model or template to place each new complementary base in the proper order. We tend to think that the new strand is built in a continuous fashion, starting at one end and proceeding to the other. Instead, to make the process of replication efficient and rapid, within each set of separated DNA strands, DNA synthesis begins at multiple spots simultaneously on the strands. This allows many areas of the DNA to be replicated at the same time. When replication is complete, the individual newly synthesized pieces are then linked together as a continuous strand.

Many enzymes are involved in DNA synthesis, and these enzymes have different activities important to correct DNA replication. Some of the functions of these enzymes include:

- Relaxing and unwinding the DNA helix
- Breaking the hydrogen bonds of dsDNA and separating it into two single strands (ss) of DNA (ssDNA)
- Keeping the ssDNA separate
- "Reading" the original DNA strands and determining the base order for the new strands
- Placing the nucleotides in the order specified by the template strand
- Linking the separate pieces of newly synthesized DNA into a continuous strand
- "Spell checking" the new strands of DNA to ensure that each base in the new strand is complementary to its base pair on the original strand

Table 1–2 lists some of the different enzymes and their roles in the DNA replication process.

Figure 1–9. The semiconservative model of DNA replication in which the two new sets of dsDNA each retain one of the original strands.

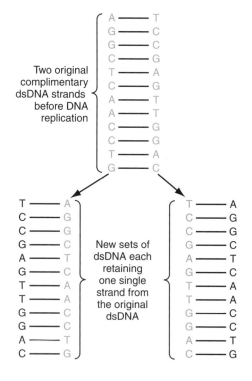

TABLE 1–2

Enzymes Participating in DNA Replication

Enzyme	Action/Purpose
DNA helicase	Unwinds the double helix and initially separates the dsDNA
DNA ligase	Connects or links the individual pieces of newly synthesized DNA during replication, forming a single strand
DNA polymerase (subtypes with different activities)	DNA chain elongation, adding one nucleotide at a time to the new strand while it is being synthesized; editing or proofreading newly synthesized strand, comparing it to the original template strand; exonuclease action, recognizing a misplaced nucleotide, clipping it out, and replacing it with the correct one
DNA topoisomerases	Creates a "nick" in the supercoils of dsDNA, allowing them to loosen so that eventually the two strands can separate; this enzyme also repairs the nick (closes it) so that the DNA can resume its supercoiled helical shape.
Primase	Responsible for initiating DNA synthesis in multiple sites down the single strand being copied
Single-strand binding proteins (SSB proteins)	Helps keep the two single strands separated long enough for initiation of DNA replication

---

Chromosomes

Chromosomes form during the metaphase (M phase) of mitosis in the cell cycle. During M phase of the cell cycle, one complete set of DNA moves into one of the two new cells made during mitosis, and the second complete set moves into the other new cell. As a result, the two new cells have the right amount of DNA with all the genes. The correct movement of the DNA into the two new cells requires that the 46 separate chunks of DNA twist very tightly, forming dense *chromosomes,* which can be seen (when stained) using a standard microscope. Chromosomes, as temporary structures, have the important job of the precise delivery of DNA to the two new cells. This is critical for the new cells to be able to function and, eventually, to be able to reproduce.

After the original DNA has completely replicated, the DNA of each of the 46 chunks forms chromosome structures during mitosis. These structures are needed to make delivery of DNA to each of the two new cells precise so that one new cell does not get more or less than the correct amount of DNA and the correct distribution of the genes.

CHROMOSOME FORMATION

Figure 1–10 shows the formation of one chromosome from its helical DNA after DNA replication has occurred. This means that the visible chromosome now contains twice the DNA and will split in half during mitosis, allowing one new cell to receive the left half of the chromosome and the other new cell to receive the right half. With each chromosome splitting in half during mitosis, each of the two new cells receives the one complete set of the entire human genome at completion of cell division.

Chromosome formation begins with the chunk of DNA (after replication) corresponding to the chromosome supercoiling on itself and becoming a shorter but much denser structure. This is similar to an old-fashioned spiraled telephone cord that is 12 feet long. Over time, the long cord twists around itself until it is much shorter (perhaps only a foot long) and thicker. When DNA supercoils,

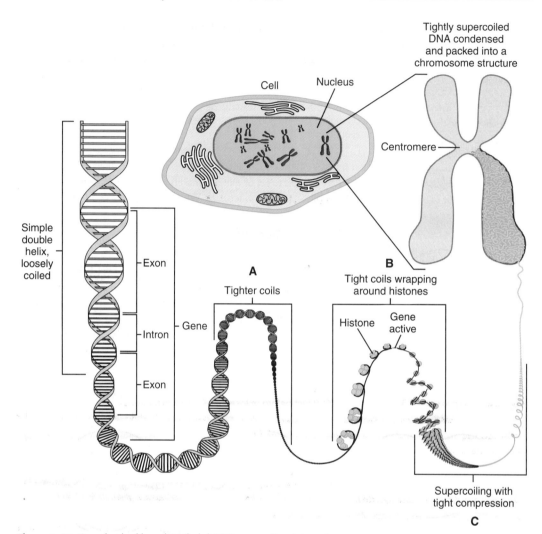

Figure 1–10. One chunk of loosely coiled dsDNA supercoiling into a chromosome.

it is done in multiple organized steps rather than just as a random tangle. As shown in part A of Figure 1–10, the dsDNA starts to coil up more tightly. Then the tighter structure begins to wind around a set of globular protein balls known as **histones**, forming a "bead" on the DNA strand (part B of Fig. 1–10). There are different types of histones, but the important issue to remember about histones is that by having tightly coiled DNA wrap around them, the DNA compacts itself without creating tangles or damaging its basic structure (base pairs are not broken or lost during this process). Individual DNA-wrapped histones continue to wind, which clusters them, forming larger "bead" groups that are packed closely together (part C of Fig. 1–10). These thicker beaded groups continue to coil neatly and form the basic structure of the chromosome. In this way, millions of base pairs now occupy a much smaller space. Chromosomes are so dense that they can be stained and are visible using a standard microscope.

As shown in Figure 1–10, a chromosome is a specific large chunk of double-stranded DNA that has already undergone DNA replication and contains millions of bases and hundreds (and sometimes thousands) of genes. During M phase (metaphase of mitosis), each chromosome forms and moves to the center of the cell that is about to divide. Just before the cell splits into two cells *(cytokinesis)*, each chromosome is pulled apart *(nucleokinesis)* so that half of each chromosome goes into one new cell, and the other half goes into the other new cell. This action is illustrated in Figure 1–11, showing just 2 chromosomes rather than 46.

CHROMOSOME STRUCTURE

Ploidy is the actual number of chromosomes present in a single-cell nucleus at mitosis. Humans have 46 chromosomes divided into 23 pairs. A complete set of *one* of each chromosome is the **haploid chromosome number** (1N) representing 23 individual chromosomes. When the nucleus contains *both* pairs

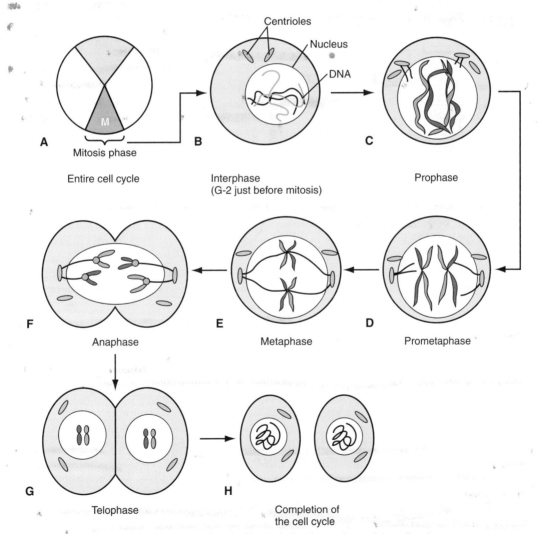

A   Entire cell cycle
    Mitosis phase
    M

B   Interphase
    (G-2 just before mitosis)
    Centrioles
    Nucleus
    DNA

C   Prophase

D   Prometaphase

E   Metaphase

F   Anaphase

G   Telophase

H   Completion of
    the cell cycle

Figure 1–11. Chromosome formation and nucleokinesis during the M phase of the cell cycle.

of all chromosomes, the number present is the **diploid chromosome number** (2N). When additional whole sets of extra chromosomes are present, the condition is termed **polyploidy** (such as 69 chromosomes [triploidy or 3N] and 92 chromosomes [tetraploidy 4N]. Normal human somatic cells (body cells that are not reproductive cells) with a nucleus have the diploid number of chromosomes, 23 pairs. Mature human germ line cells (reproductive cells: ova [eggs] and spermatocytes [sperm]) each have the haploid number of chromosomes, 23, half of each pair. Germ line cells have the haploid number so that fertilization (union of an ova and spermatocyte) results only in the normal diploid number. When a cell's nucleus contains the normal diploid number of chromosomes for the species, the cell is termed **euploid.** When a cell contains more or fewer chromosomes than the normal diploid number for the species, it is termed **aneuploid.**

Figure 1–2 shows a chromosome after DNA replication right before cell division, and Figure 1–3 shows a Giemsa-banded chromosome after the chromosome has been pulled apart. At the tips of this chromosome are the *telomeres* (telomeric DNA), which act as a chromosome cap that holds the DNA strands together similarly to the way a small plastic tube keeps the ends of a shoestring from raveling. (The structure and function of telomeres are discussed in Chapter 3.) As shown in Figures 1–2 and 1–3, the pinched-in area of the chromosome connecting the two sides is the **centromere.** The centromere also connects the chromosome segments above it and below it. Each longitudinal left and right half of the chromosome is a **chromatid.** The two chromatids of a chromosome are termed *sister chromatids.* The segments of chromosome extending above the centromere are known as the *short arms,* or the **p arms** (*p* is for "petite"). The segments of chromosome below the centromere are the *long arms,* or the **q arms** (because *q* is the next letter of the alphabet after *p*). The locus of a gene on a chromosome is pinpointed using these names (see Fig. 1–3). A discussion of what terms are used to identify a gene locus is presented in Chapter 4.

CHROMOSOMAL ANALYSIS

A limited amount of genetic information can be determined by examining a person's chromosomes, a process known as *chromosomal analysis.* This information is limited because each chromosome is composed of a large chunk of DNA. Thus, only large changes with tens of thousands of base pairs of DNA can be seen at the chromosome level as rearrangements, deletions, or additions. As shown in the nucleus of Figure 1–1, just before cell division, individual chromosomes are scattered. Photographs of these metaphase chromosomes can be taken through the microscope to examine and analyze them closely.

The first step in chromosomal analysis is to count the chromosomes in one cell that is in metaphase of mitosis (M phase) to determine how many chromosomes are present (the normal cell should have 46 chromosomes consisting of 23 pairs). After the chromosome number per cell has been established, further analysis requires organizing the chromosomes into a karyotype. A **karyotype** is an organized arrangement of all the chromosomes within one cell during the metaphase section of mitosis. A technician first organizes the chromosomes into pairs and then arranges them by number according to size and centromere position (Fig. 1–12). The largest chromosome pair is number 1, and this pair has the centromere nearly in the middle of the chromosomes so that the p arms and q arms are close to the same length. When the centromere is close to the center of the chromosome, it is termed a *metacentric chromosome.* The next largest chromosome pair is the number 2 chromosomes. Their centromeres are not in the center, so the p arms are clearly shorter than the q arms. This type of centromere location is termed *submetacentric.* The chromosome pairs continue to be arranged by size, from the number 1s to the number 22s. When chromosome pairs are nearly the same size, the one with the more metacentric centromere has a lower number than the pair (or pairs) of the same size with a submetacentric centromere.

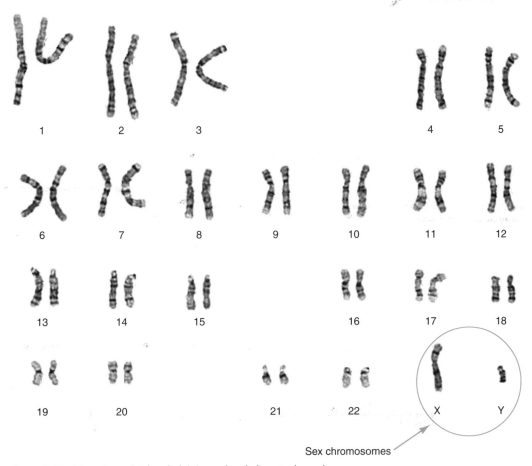

Figure 1–12. A karyotype of G-banded (Giemsa-banded) metaphase chromosomes.

Some chromosomes have the centromere at the top of the q arms, and there is little or no p arm material. These chromosomes are termed *acrocentric*. In Figure 1–12, pairs 13, 14, and 15 and pairs 21 and 22 are acrocentric chromosomes. The sex chromosomes are positioned last in a karyotype even though the X is a medium-sized chromosome. Of the 23 pairs of chromosomes, **autosomes** are the 22 pairs of human chromosomes (numbered 1 through 22) that do not code for the sexual differentiation of a person. These chromosomes contain the genes for all the structures and regulatory proteins needed for normal somatic function. The **sex chromosomes** (circled on the karyotype in Fig. 1–12) are the pair that contains the genes for sexual differentiation. Most commonly, males have an X and a Y as the sex chromosomes, and females have two X chromosomes.

The chromosomes in Figure 1–12 have been processed to enhance the accuracy of identifying each chromosome. One way to increase the accuracy of chromosomal analysis is by treating the chromosomes with special enzymes and stains so that each pair of chromosomes has a unique and consistent striped pattern. The most common way to enhance chromosome appearance is through the G-banding

(Giemsa banding) process. Notice how different the banding patterns are for pairs 4 and 5, which are the same size and shape, and for the acrocentric, same-sized pairs of 13, 14, and 15. With this G-banding–enhanced karyotype, it is possible for a genetics technician to accurately distinguish a pair of number 13 chromosomes from a pair of number 14 chromosomes. What can be learned about the person from whom the karyotype in Figure 1–12 was made? The person is human, male, and euploid (diploid, 2N), having chromosomes that are normal for number and appear normal in structure. What this karyotype cannot tell us is whether any genes are mutated or nonfunctional.

Single-Gene Traits

As described earlier, a gene is a specific segment of DNA that contains the code (recipe) for a particular protein. Thus, a gene is the smallest functional unit of the DNA. Although genes vary in size, even a large individual gene containing a million bases is a very small segment of DNA.

Most of what is known currently about specific genes is related to those genes in which one gene controls the expression of a specific structure, protein, or function. These conditions are known as single-gene traits (monogenic traits). For example, a single gene determines whether a person can synthesize normal beta chains of hemoglobin or has some degree of sickle cell disease. Another single gene determines whether a person has a widow's peak hairline or a straight hairline. Expression of blood type also is a single-gene trait. Table 1–3 lists some single-gene traits and common health problems related to changes in single genes.

In examining one woman's single-gene trait for blood type, the blood type gene is located on chromosome 9 (locus is 9q34). This woman has two copies for this single gene, with one copy on the number 9 chromosome inherited from her father and the other copy on the number 9 chromosome inherited from her mother. These two copies of the single gene for blood type are known as *gene alleles*.

TABLE 1–3

Examples of Common Single-Gene Traits and Disorders

Normal Traits	Disorders
A, B, O blood groups	Achondroplasia
Blood-clotting factors (individual)	Cystic fibrosis
Color vision (red/green)	Hemophilia (classic)
Dimples (facial)	Hereditary hemochromatosis
Earlobe position	Huntington disease
Hair texture	Hurler syndrome
Male pattern baldness	Marfan syndrome
Rh blood groups	Muscular dystrophy
Taste discrimination	Phenylketonuria
Tongue rolling	Sickle cell disease
Widow's peak	Sickle cell trait
	Syndactyly
	Tay-Sachs disease

An **allele** is an alternative form or variation of a gene at a specific location. For each single gene at a specific chromosome location, two alleles together control how that gene is expressed. In the world population, there are three possible gene alleles for blood type: A, B, and O. However, each person has only two of the three specific gene alleles for blood type (unless the person has trisomy 9 with three number 9 chromosomes, an abnormal condition). Some single-gene traits have even more than three possible alleles; however, regardless of how many possible different alleles are present in the entire human population, each person has only two, because he or she has only two chromosomes per pair with one allele on each chromosome. A person's blood type is determined by which blood type gene alleles were inherited from his or her parents.

DOMINANT AND RECESSIVE SINGLE-GENE TRAITS

When a person inherits a blood type A allele from one parent and a type B allele from the other parent, he or she has the A and B alleles and expresses blood type AB. Another factor that determines which blood type is expressed with different alleles is whether the allele is dominant or recessive. The A and B blood type alleles are dominant. A dominant gene allele is always expressed when it is present. This is why the woman who as an A blood type gene allele and a B blood type gene allele expresses both alleles as type AB blood. A person who has two blood type A gene alleles has type A blood, and a person who has two blood type B gene alleles has type B blood. A **dominant trait** is expressed even when the two gene alleles for that trait are different. When two alleles are different and each is dominant, they are both expressed; the expression is termed **codominant** because they are expressed equally.

The alleles for type O blood are recessive and are expressed only when both O alleles are present. For a person who has one blood type B gene allele and one blood type O gene allele, the expressed blood type is B, not OB. A **recessive trait** is a single-gene trait that is expressed only when both gene alleles are the same. When a recessive gene allele is paired with a dominant allele, the recessive allele is *silent* (not expressed), and only the dominant allele is expressed.

GENOTYPE AND PHENOTYPE

The exact gene allele composition a person has for a specific single-gene trait is the person's **genotype** for that trait. The **phenotype** of a trait is the person's observed expression of any given single-gene trait. Thus, a person with the genotype of AO for blood type and a person with the genotype of AA for blood type both express the phenotype of type A blood, even though their genotypes are different. When a person has two identical gene alleles for a single-gene trait, the alleles are termed **homozygous.** When homozygous gene alleles are present for a single-gene trait, the genotype and phenotype for that trait are the same. When a person has two different gene alleles for a single-gene trait, the alleles are termed **heterozygous.** For heterozygous alleles, the actual genotype may be different from the phenotype.

Normally, recessive single-gene traits are expressed only when the person is homozygous for the two gene alleles. Thus, for recessive traits, phenotype and genotype are always the same. Dominant single-gene traits are expressed whether the person is homozygous or heterozygous for the gene alleles. Thus, for dominant traits, phenotype and genotype *can* be the same but do not have to be. More information about dominant, recessive, and codominant expression of single-gene traits and health problems is presented in the discussion for patterns of inheritance in Chapter 4.

GENE GEMS

- Genetics and genomics are similar concepts, but genomics has a broader scope.
- All human nucleated somatic cells contain two sets of the human genome.
- Germ cells are the cells for sexual reproduction (spermatocytes and ova) and contain only one set of the human genome.
- Larger chromosomes contain thousands of genes, and smaller chromosomes may have fewer than 100 genes.
- More than 99% of human DNA is in the nucleus, and a small amount is in the mitochondria.
- Thymine and cytosine are pyrimidines; adenine and guanine are purines.
- Adenine and thymine are complementary to each other and always pair together; cytosine and guanine are complementary and always pair together.
- When the base sequence of one strand of dsDNA is known, the opposite strand's sequence can be predicted accurately.
- When mitosis is normal and the parent cell divides correctly, each new cell has the correct amount of DNA and genes, identical to each other and to the parent cell.
- The complete genome within any one cell is present as 46 separate sets of dsDNA, not as one very long double strand of DNA.
- The semiconservative model of DNA replication results in two complete sets of dsDNA, with each set containing one DNA strand from the parent cell and one newly synthesized strand.
- The initiation of DNA synthesis begins at multiple spots simultaneously on the parent strands of dsDNA.
- The most important feature of mitosis is the delivery of the correct amount of DNA to each of the two newly created cells.
- Chromosomes can be seen only with a standard light microscope during metaphase of mitosis.
- In a karyotype, one cell's metaphase chromosome pairs are organized by size from largest to smallest and by position of the centromere.
- Chromosomal analysis is enhanced by techniques that "band" chromosome pairs with a unique striped pattern.
- For each single gene at a specific chromosome location, two alleles together control how that gene is expressed.
- Some single-gene traits have even more than three possible alleles; however, regardless of how many possible different alleles are present in the entire human population, each person only has two, because he or she has only two chromosomes per pair with one allele on each chromosome.
- When homozygous gene alleles are present for a single-gene trait, the genotype and phenotype for that trait are the same.
- For recessive traits, the genotype and the phenotype are the same.
- For dominant traits, the genotype and the phenotype can be the same but do not have to be.

Self-Assessment Questions

1. What is the normal number of autosomal chromosomes for humans?
   a. 42
   b. 44
   c. 46
   d. 48

2. Which substance is present in a nucleotide but not in a nucleoside?
   a. Uracil
   b. Nitrogen
   c. Phosphorus
   d. Pentose (ribose) sugar

3. What would be the sequence of DNA that is complementary to a DNA strand with the base sequence of ACCTGAACGTCGCTA?
   a. TGGACTTGCAGCGAT
   b. ACCTGAACGTCGCTA
   c. ATCGCTGCAAGTCCA
   d. TAGCGACGTTCAGGA

4. Why is hydrogen bonding of human DNA into double strands more advantageous than covalent bonding?
   a. Hydrogen bonds are incompatible with proteins.
   b. Hydrogen bonds increase the fidelity of transcription and translation.
   c. Covalent bonds are more at risk for mutations than hydrogen bonds.
   d. Covalent bonds are tighter and more permanent than hydrogen bonds.

5. Which genetic process would be disrupted in one cell if it could not form chromosomes?
   a. DNA replication
   b. Gene-directed protein synthesis
   c. Delivery of genetic information to new cells
   d. Conversion of a nucleoside into a nucleotide

6. A person's karyotype shows 44 autosomes and one X chromosome. What is the best interpretation of this karyotype?
   a. The karyotype is aneuploid, and the individual has only one allele for each of the genes on the X chromosome.
   b. The karyotype is aneuploid, and the individual is experiencing the pathologic condition of haploidy.
   c. The karyotype is euploid, making the individual a genotypic female and a phenotypic male.
   d. The karyotype is euploid, making the individual a genotypic male and a phenotypic female.

Continued

7. Which statement regarding genotype and phenotype is true?
   a. For autosomal recessive traits, the phenotype is the same as the genotype.
   b. The only trait in which phenotype *always* follows genotype is physiologic gender.
   c. When a phenotype is fully penetrant, the trait is expressed in the heterozygous person.
   d. Genotype changes as a person ages, while phenotype is not affected by the aging process.

8. What are the expected blood types of children from a mother who is AO for blood type and a father who is OO for blood type?
   a. All children will have type A blood.
   b. All children will have type O blood.
   c. 50% will have type A blood; 50% will have type O blood.
   d. 25% will have type A blood; 75% will have type O blood.

References

National Cancer Institute. Dictionary of Cancer Terms. Retrieved March 2011 from www.cancer.gov/dictionary?cdrid=446543.

National Human Genome Research Institute. A Brief Guide to Genomics. Retrieved March 2011 from www.genome.gov/18016863.

National Human Genome Research Institute. Educators. Retrieved from www.genome.gov/Educators/.

Self-Assessment Answers

1. b 2. c 3. a 4. d 5. c 6. a 7. a 8. c

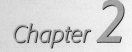

Chapter 2

Protein Synthesis

Learning Outcomes

1. Use the genetic terminology associated with protein synthesis.
2. Compare the locations, processes, and purposes of transcription, translation, and post-translational modification of proteins.
3. Explain the differences, functions, and interactions of DNA triplets, RNA codons, and tRNA anticodons.
4. Analyze the factors that influence when and how transcription of a gene occurs.
5. Explain the structure and function of introns and exons.
6. Describe the relationships among the primary, secondary, tertiary, and quaternary protein structures.
7. Compare the implications of different types of mutations on protein synthesis and protein function.
8. Explain how and why not every mutational event has a deleterious result.

KEY TERMS

Anticodon

Codon

DNA antisense strand

DNA coding region

DNA noncoding region

DNA sense strand

DNA triplet

Exons

Frameshift mutations

Gene expression

Germline mutation

Introns

MicroRNA

Mutagen

Mutation

Point mutation

Post-transcriptional modification

Post-translational modification

Protein synthesis

Ribonucleic acid (RNA)

Ribosome

Single nucleotide polymorphism (SNP)

Somatic mutation

Transcription

Transfer RNA (tRNA)

Translation

Uracil

Introduction

Genes provide the codes for the making of the specific proteins used by a cell, tissue, organ, or even the whole body. As discussed in Chapter 1, the hormone insulin is a protein produced by the beta cells of the pancreas that works to maintain blood glucose levels within the normal range. When the blood glucose level rises above normal, the pancreatic beta cells rapidly synthesize insulin, which then binds to in-sulin receptors on cell membranes, making the cells permeable to glucose. This action allows glucose in the blood and other extracellular fluids to move across cell membranes into cells, reducing blood glucose levels. For the person who does not have diabetes, enough insulin is synthesized each time blood glucose levels begin to rise to return glucose levels back to the normal range. An important concept to consider is that the protein insulin is not stored in large quantities. Thus, every time insulin is needed for blood glucose con-trol, the protein must be newly synthesized. Many proteins are synthesized only "on demand" rather than made and stored in any significant amount. **Protein synthesis** is the selective activation of a gene, resulting in its transcription and translation into the production of the appropriate protein. For this reason, proteins are called *gene products*. Figure 2–1 shows the sequential processes involved in protein synthesis.

When a gene product is synthesized, the gene is turned on, or *expressed*. **Gene expression** is the activation of a gene leading to the transcription, translation, and synthesis of a specific protein. All of the hormones, enzymes, growth factors, and other protein-based chemicals needed for normal human physiologic function are protein gene products that are produced when the correct genes are activated and expressed. A few examples of common gene products include insulin, hemoglobin, erythropoietin, angiotensin, thyroid hormones, antibodies, collagen, fibrinogen, and various intracellular proteins.

The basic structure of a protein is its amino acid sequence. There are 20 different amino acids, often called the *building blocks of life*. Every active protein has a specific amount of the amino acids and a unique sequence in which they are connected. The exact sequence is critical for protein function. It is possible for two separate proteins to have the same total number of amino acids and perhaps even the same numbers of individual amino acids. However, the sequencing order of the amino acids is what makes one protein different in structure and function from another protein. If one amino acid is out of order or completely deleted from the sequence, the protein will be affected and may not perform its function well. For example, the beta chain of hemoglobin (also known as *beta globin*) is a protein that is part of the group of four proteins that form each hemoglobin molecule. Beta globulin contains 146 amino acids connected in a specific order. A change in the sixth amino acid in the sequence reduces

Figure 2–1. The sequential processes involved in protein synthesis.

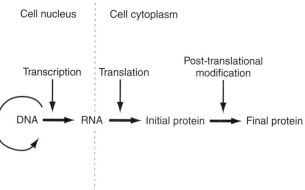

Cell nucleus   Cell cytoplasm

Transcription   Translation   Post-translational modification

DNA → RNA → Initial protein → Final protein

how well hemoglobin retains its shape and carries oxygen. This change is responsible for sickle cell disease. Sickle cell hemoglobin bends improperly causing red blood cells (RBCs) to assume a sickle shape. RBCs with this type of hemoglobin have a life span of only about 20 days instead of the 120 days of an RBC that contains normal hemoglobin. Thus, the order of the amino acids is critical for the final function of any protein, and even one amino acid change can alter the protein's function. Figure 2–2 shows an example of a short protein made up of only eight amino acids.

So, how does a gene direct the correct placement of amino acids to result in a normal and active protein? Each amino acid has at least one specific code within the DNA (Table 2–1). These codes are each

Figure 2–2. The sequence of amino acids in a very short protein.

PRIMARY PROTEIN STRUCTURE

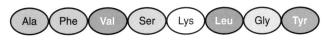

Ala   Phe   Val   Ser   Lys   Leu   Gly   Tyr

TABLE 2–1

The DNA Triplets and RNA Codons for the 20 Amino Acids

Amino Acid	Abbreviations	DNA Triplets	RNA Codons
Alanine	ala (A)	CGA, CGG, CGT, CGC	GCU, GCC, GCA, GCG
Arginine	arg (R)	TCT, TCC, GCA, GCG, GCT, GCC	AGA, AGG, CGU, CGC, CGA, CGG
Asparagine	asn (N)	TTA, TTG	AAU, AAC
Aspartic acid	asp (D)	CTA, CTG	GAU, GAC
Cysteine	cys (C)	ACA, ACG	UGU, UGC
Glutamic acid	glu (E)	CTT, CTC	GAA, GAG
Glutamine	gln (Q)	GTT, GTC	CAA, CAG
Glycine	gly (G)	CCA, CCG, CCT, CCC	GGU, GGC, GGA, GGG
Histidine	his (H)	GTA, GTG	CUA, CAC
Isoleucine	ile (I)	TAA, TAG, TAT	AUU, AUC, AUA
Leucine	leu (L)	GAA, GAG, GAT, GAC, AAT, AAC	CUU, CUC, CUA, CUG, UUA, UUG
Lysine	lys (L)	TTT, TTC	AAA, AAG
Methionine	met (M)	TAC	AUG
Phenylalanine	phe (F)	AAA, AAG	UUU, UUC
Proline	pro (P)	GGA, GGG, GGT, GGC	CCU, CCC, CCA, CCG
Serine	ser (S)	AGA, AGG, AGT, AGC, TCA, TCG	UCU, UCC, UCA, UCG, AGU, AGC
Threonine	thr (T)	TGA, TGG, TGT, TGC	ACU, ACC, ACA, ACG
Tryptophan	trp (W)	ACC	UGG
Tyrosine	tyr (Y)	ATA, ATG	UAU, UAC
Valine	val (V)	CAA, CAG, CAT, CAC	GUU, GUC, GUA, GUG
Start			AUG
Stop			UAA, UAG, UGA

three nucleotide bases long and are called **DNA triplets**. As described in Chapter 1, a gene is a specific segment of DNA that contains the directions (recipe) for making a specific protein (see Figs. 1–2 and 1–10). It contains all the DNA triplets of amino acid codes in exactly the right order for that protein. For example, the final active form of beta globin has 146 amino acids. Thus, the minimum number of bases needed in the gene for beta globin is 438 (three bases per amino acid multiplied by 146 amino acids).

The gene for beta globin (the *HBB* gene) is located on the short arm (p arm) of chromosome 11. The synthesis of beta globin occurs only in immature RBCs, although the *HBB* gene is present in the nucleus of every cell. This means that the *HBB* gene is part of the cellular proteome for RBCs. Synthesis of beta globin, just like for any protein, involves the processes of transcription, translation, and protein modification.

Transcription

Overview

Transcription is the process of making a strand of RNA that is complementary to the DNA sequence that contains the gene for the protein needed. This phase of protein synthesis takes place completely within the nucleus. In examining DNA, there are DNA coding regions separated by noncoding regions. **DNA coding regions** contain many genes, and the sequences of these genes are largely the same from one person to another. **DNA noncoding regions** are sections of DNA that contain multiple repeat sequences that are not parts of genes and that do not code for specific proteins. These noncoding regions make up about 95% of nuclear DNA and have been referred to as *redundant DNA* and *desert DNA*. These regions vary from one person to another and are used to identify the DNA from a specific individual. The noncoding regions of DNA do influence protein synthesis, but not all of its functions are yet known.

Some of the steps used in protein synthesis involve similar enzymes and processes as those used in DNA synthesis during DNA replication; however, there are some differences. One of the biggest differences is the extent of the process. During DNA replication, both of the double strands of *all* the DNA within one cell are entirely copied, resulting in the total synthesis of two new complete strands of each chunk of nuclear DNA. During protein synthesis, only the segment of DNA that contains the actual gene for the protein needed is involved in the process, not the entire genome. This means that only a segment of *one* DNA strand is read and transcribed into RNA.

Process

Using the cookbook analogy with the cookbook containing all the genes for the entire genome, consider each chromosome to be a separate chapter of recipes in a very large book located in a library. To make a specific dish or meal, the cook must look up the correct recipe (gene). For example, if the cook wants to make chocolate chip cookies, he or she opens the chapter that contains cookie recipes, rather than vegetable recipes. The cook then determines on which page (gene locus on the chromosome) the chocolate cookie recipe is located. After finding the correct recipe, the cook writes down (transcribes) this recipe and takes it to the kitchen, where the ingredients and processes for translating the recipe into actual cookies are located.

In protein synthesis, only the area of DNA that contains the actual "recipe" for the protein is read (transcribed) and a complementary strand of RNA synthesized. **RNA** is **ribonucleic acid**, a single strand of nitrogenous bases constructed during transcription from a segment of DNA containing the gene for a specific protein. There are several types of RNA, and the ultimate purpose of all types is to ensure that the information held in the genes reaches cell areas where formation of the actual proteins needed for normal human function can occur. In this sense, RNA is a molecular interpreter of the DNA information stored in the genes.

Newly transcribed RNA functions as the initial template for protein synthesis. RNA is very similar to DNA with a few differences. First, functional RNA is single-stranded (ss) rather than double-stranded (ds). The sugar component of RNA is ribose rather than deoxyribose, which just means that it contains one more oxygen molecule than does the sugar in DNA. Another difference is that RNA does not contain the pyrimidine base thymine. The base **uracil** is used in place of thymine. It is a pyrimidine base with a structure that is almost identical to thymine. The only difference is that uracil does not contain the methyl group (CH_3) that thymine has. However, this difference is important because molecules in the nucleus that contain a methyl group remain trapped inside the nucleus. Because the remaining phases of protein synthesis occur outside the nucleus, the newly transcribed RNA must be able to exit the nucleus.

Sense Versus Antisense

To synthesize beta globin, chromosome 11 is the correct chapter. In one gene-coding region of chromosome 11, many genes are located, including the gene for beta globin *(HBB)*. When more beta globin is needed, the gene-coding region on chromosome 11 containing the beta globin gene area loosens (Fig. 2–3). Some of the same enzymes involved in DNA synthesis assist in the loosening and unwinding of the DNA coding region that contains the beta globin gene. Once this DNA is loosened and unwound, the two strands are slightly separated into a sense strand and an antisense strand (Fig. 2–4). The **DNA sense strand**, also known as *sense DNA*, contains the actual gene-coding sequence for the protein to be synthesized, in this case beta globin. The **DNA antisense strand**, also known as *antisense DNA*, contains the complementary base sequence to this gene, not the gene itself. After the strands are slightly separated, an enzyme known as *RNA polymerase II* reads and then transcribes the gene sequence on the sense strand of DNA resulting in the formation of a complementary strand of RNA. The DNA information is transcribed using the bases adenine, guanine, cytosine, and uracil into a single RNA strand that is now complementary to the gene (see Fig. 2–4). Because this RNA is used as a recipe to

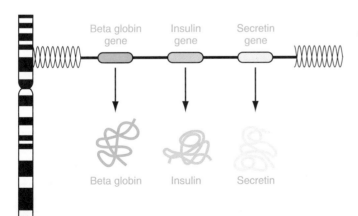

Figure 2–3. Gene-coding region with the genes for beta globin, insulin, and secretin.

Beta globin gene   Insulin gene   Secretin gene

Beta globin   Insulin   Secretin

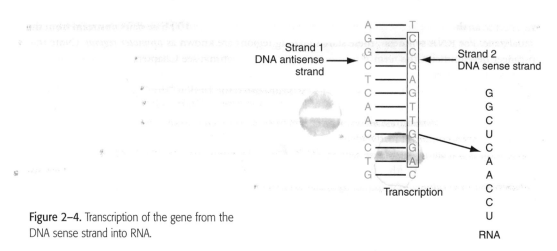

Figure 2–4. Transcription of the gene from the DNA sense strand into RNA.

direct the building of the actual protein coded for by the gene, it is known as *messenger RNA*, or *mRNA*. The DNA triplets in the gene have now been read and converted into RNA codons by the process of transcription (Fig. 2–5).

Starting and Stopping

So how does the enzyme know where to begin synthesizing RNA from the gene? Within the DNA around the gene for beta globin (and all other genes) are codes that direct the starting and stopping of RNA synthesis. The start signal is located in front of or "upstream" from the gene triplets that code for

Figure 2–5. A demonstration of the codons present in a specific segment of RNA.

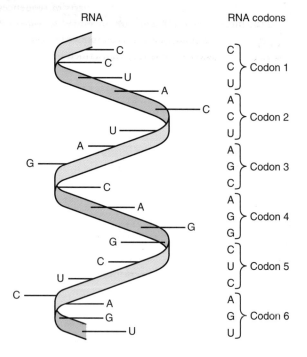

the specific amino acids in the protein. Start signals can be more than 100 base pairs upstream from the actual gene. For RNA synthesis, these start-signaling regions are known as *promoter regions*. (Note that in cancer development, the term *promoter* has a different meaning; see Chapter 12.) One of the most common of the known promoter sequences contains many thymine and adenine bases and is known as *TATA boxes*. In the DNA after the gene (downstream) are transcription "stop" signals. These result in the inhibition of further transcription of DNA triplets into RNA codons and in the addition of a *poly-A tail* to the newly transcribed RNA. Development of a poly-A tail is known as *polyadenylation*. This segment of RNA contains mostly adenine and is not translated into part of the protein.

A **codon** is a specific RNA base sequence containing the complementary code to each amino acid's DNA triplet. For example, the DNA triplet for the amino acid methionine is TAC—thymine, adenine, and cytosine (see Table 2–1). Remember that RNA contains uracil instead of thymine. Thus, everywhere an adenine is positioned in the gene's DNA, a uracil is positioned in the complementary strand of RNA. This makes the RNA codon for methionine AUG—adenine, uracil, and guanine.

So what is the purpose of the DNA antisense strand, and is it always the same strand? The answer to these questions is a little complicated. The DNA antisense strand of a specific gene has no purpose for that gene. However, the DNA antisense strand of one gene is usually the sense strand of a different gene. So when looking at double-stranded DNA in a gene-coding region, one gene in the region, the gene for protein A, is on strand 1 and therefore is the DNA sense strand for protein A. The DNA antisense strand (strand 2) for protein A is the DNA sense strand for protein B. Thus, the answer to the second part of the question is no. Each strand is the DNA sense strand for some proteins and the DNA antisense strands for other proteins. It all depends on the gene.

Results

An interesting fact is that the sequence for a single gene in the DNA is not continuous. Instead, the sequence for one gene is separated by parts of sequences for other genes. So, our genes are in pieces, and the pieces of several genes are integrated together within a gene-coding region. (Incidentally, having genes in pieces made early attempts at sequencing and locating genes more difficult.) This issue means that when a gene is first transcribed into RNA, the initial RNA contains extra sequences that belong to other genes. In a sense, this is like having the recipe for chocolate chip cookies containing all the usual ingredients for chocolate chip cookies (flour, sugar, eggs, butter, salt, baking soda, water, vanilla, chocolate chips) and also containing the ingredients for peanut butter cookies and molasses cookies. The sectional parts of the gene that actually belong in the gene are known as **exons** (for expressed sequences). The additional sequences that are part of other genes and not part of the gene being expressed are known as **introns** (for intervening sequences). For example, the beta globin gene area contains three exons and multiple introns. When the initial mRNA is transcribed, it contains both the needed exons and the extra introns. If the introns remain and are translated, the resulting protein would not be functional.

Post-Transcriptional Modification

Once the gene has been initially transcribed into mRNA, the RNA must be further processed to its mature form through **post-transcriptional modification**. This is a process that eliminates the introns before the mRNA can be translated and used to direct the precise synthesis of the protein coded for by the gene (Fig. 2–6). Removing the introns and connecting the exons is known as *RNA splicing*. After the initial mRNA transcript has been processed and the introns eliminated, the mature mRNA is moved out from the cell nucleus into the cytoplasm where actual translation into a protein occurs.

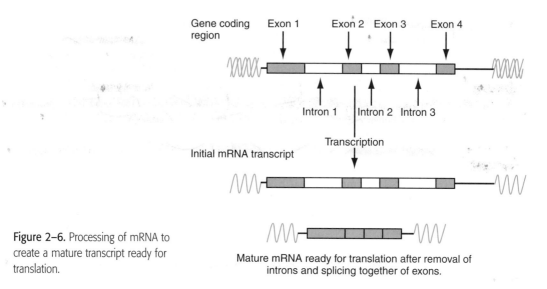

Figure 2–6. Processing of mRNA to create a mature transcript ready for translation.

Mature mRNA ready for translation after removal of introns and splicing together of exons.

Translation

Overview

Translation is the process of using a mature mRNA molecule as the directions for placing amino acids in the correct sequence to synthesize a protein. This energy-requiring activity involves the interaction of amino acids and mRNA along with two other types of RNA: transfer RNA (tRNA) and ribosomal RNA (rRNA). Translation occurs in the cytoplasm. Consider the cytoplasm to be the kitchen of the process where all the ingredients and the appliances for cooking are available for translating the transcribed recipe into an actual product (like chocolate chip cookies).

Transfer RNA molecules are specialized carrier molecules that can move an amino acid into position to be incorporated correctly into a growing peptide chain during protein synthesis. There are 20 separate types of tRNAs in a cell's endoplasmic reticulum, each produced by transcription from a different tRNA gene. Each type of tRNA can carry and transfer only one specific amino acid. For example, there are alanine tRNAs that attach to and transfer only the amino acid alanine, whereas valine tRNAs attach to and transfer only the amino acid valine. The tRNAs have an upside-down, three-leaf-clover appearance with two important areas for protein synthesis—the amino acid attachment site and the anticodon (Fig. 2–7).

The amino acid attachment site is the location that a specific amino acid can attach to and be carried by any one tRNA. Which amino acid attaches depends on the tRNA's anticodon. An **anticodon** is the tRNA complementary code for an amino acid codon. For example, the amino acid methionine has the RNA codon of AUG. The corresponding anticodon on the tRNA that can attach and carry methionine is UAC. Because the anticodon is complementary to the methionine RNA codon, this tRNA can bind with and carry only methionine. It does not recognize or attach any other amino acid. This means that every amino acid has its own specific tRNAs. (Remember, some amino acids have more than one codon and anticodon.)

A **ribosome** is a cytoplasmic adapter molecule containing a complex of proteins and some RNA that essentially decodes the mRNA and ensures the placement of the proper individual amino acid into the

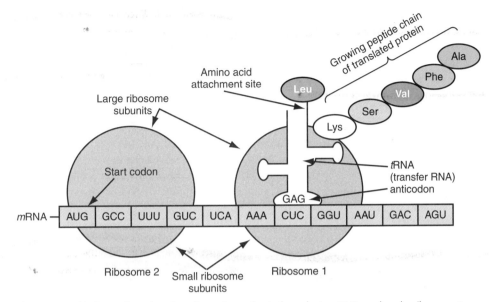

Figure 2–7. Initiation and continuation of protein synthesis through six mRNAs codons by ribosome 1.

growing peptide chain during protein synthesis. Ribosomes have two subunits, both containing small amounts of RNA. These two separate subunits join together around the mRNA strand to perform actual translation and protein synthesis. Ribosomes are nonspecific and will translate any mature mRNA molecule present in the cytoplasm into protein for as long as the mRNA exists.

Process

In a healthy cell about to perform protein synthesis, all the needed "ingredients" must be present along with adequate amounts of the body's usual high-energy chemical adenosine triphosphate (ATP). An especially important ingredient is the amino acids. Without adequate amounts of each individual amino acid, protein synthesis does not occur. Cellular amino acids do not stay in the cytoplasm long as individual amino acids for several reasons. One reason is that they are small molecules that can move out of a cell and down a concentration gradient. Another reason is that as individual molecules, amino acids contribute to the osmolarity of a cell and would make the cytoplasm hyperosmolar compared with the interstitial fluid and the plasma. The hyperosmolarity could then disrupt cell fluid homeostasis. Thus, the intracellular amino acids available for protein synthesis are joined together in no particular order as *storage proteins* within the cytoplasm. When mRNA reaches the cytoplasm, the storage proteins are signaled to break themselves down into groups of individual amino acids. So, when translation is ready to begin, think of these groups as separate buckets of individual amino acids.

Starting

When the mature mRNA reaches the cytoplasm, storage proteins are broken down into individual amino acids, tRNAs attach the amino acids to themselves, and ribosome subunits are activated. One large and one small ribosomal subunit form a complex that fits together around the five prime ends of the mRNA where the translational start signal (AUG) is located (see Fig. 2–7). The start signal tells the ribosome complex to move from the five prime ends toward the three prime ends of the mRNA, decoding and uncovering each codon one at a time. When the first mRNA codon is uncovered, all the different tRNAs enter the open site and try to unload their specific amino acid. For example, in Figure 2–7, the first codon in the mRNA after the start signal codes for alanine (GCC), which means that the first amino acid in this particular protein should be alanine. Although all the tRNAs enter and try to unload their specific amino acid as the first one in the protein, only the tRNA carrying alanine can transfer it into the ribosome. This tRNA has the anticodon that is complementary to the alanine mRNA codon, CGG. The tRNA with the anticodon of CGG temporarily connects to the alanine codon (GCC) and removes its alanine, leaving it in the ribosome complex. This tRNA then leaves the ribosome complex and is recycled by picking up a new alanine molecule from the alanine bucket. At this time, the ribosome complex moves down the mRNA to the next codon (in Figure 2–7, the next codon is for phenylalanine, UUU) and uncovers it. Again, all the tRNAs come in, but only the one with the anticodon AAA (complementary to UUU codon) temporarily connects with the codon and transfers the amino acid phenylalanine into the ribosome complex. The ribosome complex then links the phenylalanine with a peptide bond to the first amino acid, alanine. Now we have a short two-amino-acid peptide, with the sequence alanine and phenylalanine. After linking the second amino acid to the first, the ribosome continues to move down the mRNA, uncovering the codons and linking the appropriate amino acids together in the coded sequence, forming an ever-elongating peptide chain (see Fig. 2–7).

Stopping

The ribosomal complex continues to build the protein, one amino acid at a time in the correct order, until a stop signal is reached. The stop signal causes the ribosomal complex to separate from the mRNA into the two original subunits, releasing the completely translated protein. Protein synthesis is an efficient process, which means that one mRNA molecule can be translated more than once. In this way, if 100,000 molecules of the protein insulin are needed, it is not necessary to form 100,000 insulin mRNAs. Instead, perhaps 100 insulin mRNAs are produced and each one is translated 1000 times. Not only can each mRNA molecule be translated more than once, but also multiple ribosomal complexes attach and begin translation as soon as the first ribosomal complex moves down the mRNA away from the start signal.

Results

Synthesis of a specific protein continues as long as mRNAs coding for that protein are present, along with adequate amounts of all other ingredients and energy. For this reason, mRNA transcription is rapid and so is mRNA breakdown. For example, if a person's blood glucose level suddenly shoots up to 200 mg/dL, the beta cells of the pancreas respond to the need to lower this level by very rapidly transcribing the insulin gene into insulin mRNA. (After all, the pancreas does not know just how many candy bars the person ate to get the blood glucose level that high, and it does not know if the person has stopped eating candy bars.) All of these mature insulin mRNA molecules are rapidly moved into the cytoplasm for translation into insulin.

Once in the cytoplasm, mRNA molecules have a very short life span, only seconds, before they are degraded by enzymes known as *ribonucleases* (RNases for short). This rapid degradation of mRNA is important in preventing such an overproduction of insulin that the person's blood glucose level becomes dangerously low. The idea is to make just enough active insulin to reduce the blood glucose level back into the normal range without making the person become hypoglycemic, a tricky feat requiring continuous feedback of blood glucose levels to the pancreatic beta cells. As the newly produced insulin does its job and blood glucose levels decrease, transcription of new insulin mRNAs slows at the same time that degradation of the initially transcribed bunch of mRNAs occurs. As a result, insulin synthesis decreases so that hypoglycemia does not occur. When the person's blood glucose level reaches the normal range, further transcription of insulin mRNAs stops and existing ones are degraded so that no further insulin is produced at this time.

Another way that gene expression is regulated after transcription of a specific gene is through microRNA activity. **MicroRNA** is a small, noncoding piece of RNA that regulates gene expression at the RNA level. These 20 to 25 base segments of RNA can inhibit translation by binding to parts of specific (targeted) mRNA molecules, making them partially double-stranded, which cannot be translated. It also increases the rate at which mRNA is degraded. As a result, even when gene transcription overproduces specific mRNA, the presence of microRNA can prevent overproduction of the final protein. This type of regulation is very important in controlling the cell cycle, differentiating stem cells into a specific mature cell type, controlling viral replication, and modulating critical metabolic pathways. Chapter 4 discusses some of the ways that mutations that affect microRNA function interfere with health.

All protein synthesis appears to work in a similar manner. Although some proteins are stored to a greater extent than insulin—for example, thyroid hormones are stored in large amounts—each protein is produced when an appropriate signal indicates that more of that specific protein is needed.

Post-Translational Modification

Primary, Secondary, Tertiary, and Quaternary Protein Structures

Getting the right amino acids in the right order through translation is the protein's *primary structure*. However, most proteins are not in their final forms for active function when they are first synthesized and thus require **post-translational modification**. This is the further processing of the newly translated primary protein structure into its secondary and tertiary structures (and sometimes even a quaternary structure) needed to make it fully functional. Although further processing leads to these formations, correct secondary, tertiary, and quaternary protein forms all depend on accurate primary structure.

Secondary protein structure is a twisting of the linear primary structure as a result of the interaction of amino acids located near each other. Thus the sequence of amino acids does not change, but now the structure has more three-dimensional depth as parts of individual amino acids project out differently from the main structure. *Tertiary structure* is the folding of the linear structure and occurs as a result of remote amino acids interacting with each other. These interactions allow parts of the linear structure to draw closer together in some areas and have greater distances in other areas. Folding often creates a "pocket" within the protein that becomes an "active site," able to interact with other structures or substances. Folding in some proteins is enhanced when "bridges" are formed that connect distant amino acids. The most common bridges are formed by linking two sulfide molecules (known as *disulfide bridges*). Some proteins are active after proper folding into the tertiary structure; others require associations with additional protein molecules to be active. For example, one tertiary beta globin molecule cannot carry oxygen. It must associate properly with another beta globin molecule, two alpha globin molecules, and a heme molecule to form the oxygen-carrying compound hemoglobin. Thus, a protein's *quaternary structure* is its needed association with one or more specific other proteins.

Additional Modification

Other types of post-translational modification may be needed for protein activity. Some amino acids may need to be removed to activate a protein. For example, the protein insulin is first translated into a "preprohormone" that contains more than the 51 amino acids that compose active insulin. The *pre* part of the preprohormone is a signaling peptide that is removed in the endoplasmic reticulum shortly after insulin is translated, converting it to a prohormone that contains 84 amino acids. (The 33 amino acid *pro* part of the prohormone is later removed in the liver right before active insulin is present in the blood and binds to its membrane receptor.)

Another type of post-translational modification involves adding other substances to the protein to make it functional. These other substances may include various types of sugar molecules, lipid molecules, or additional peptides. Once again, the proper order of amino acids in the primary structure is important for these other substances to be correctly attached in order to result in the most functional form of a protein.

In addition, many proteins need to leave the cell in which they were synthesized to produce a functional effect. For example, if insulin remained in pancreatic beta cells, it would not be able to change membrane permeability to glucose and reduce blood glucose levels. One common way of processing proteins synthesized in one cell for use in other body areas involves packaging the new protein within a secretory vesicle in the Golgi apparatus of the cell. This processing surrounds the new protein with plasma membrane components that allow the vesicle to fuse with the cell's plasma membrane. After the vesicle membrane fuses with the cell's plasma membrane, the vesicle opens on the outer aspect of the cell, and the newly synthesized and processed protein is released into the circulatory system. Once in the blood, the protein can travel to other body areas for final function.

Mutations

Overview

A **mutation** is an alteration in the base sequence of DNA or RNA. Although mutations can occur anywhere in the DNA or RNA, they are most noticed when they occur in a gene-coding region. When a mutation becomes a permanent part of one cell's DNA, it can be passed on to other generations of cells (it is inherited or passed from one *cell* generation to another). Some mutations occur daily within one person and do not produce problems, especially if only a few cells or tissues are affected. Mutations that occur after birth in general body cells *(somatic cells)* are known as **somatic mutations.** Because these mutations are present only in a person's somatic cells, somatic mutations cannot be passed on to offspring. One problem of somatic mutations is an increased risk for cancer in cells with such mutations.

Germline mutations occur in germ cells (sex cells, sperm or ova) and can be passed on to one's children at conception. When a child inherits a germline mutation, each of that child's cells contains the mutated DNA, including the child's sex cells. This means that the mutation can be passed to many generations as long as the mutation does not interfere with the person's fertility.

Generally, more is known about gene mutations that result in serious health problems; however, some gene mutations do have beneficial results. An example of a helpful mutation is the one that prevents a person from producing a specific receptor on the white blood cells known as *helper/inducer T lymphocytes* (CD4-positive cells). Without this receptor, the white blood cell is not invaded and destroyed by the human immunodeficiency virus (HIV). Thus, people with this mutation who have been infected with HIV do not develop the progressive immunosuppression associated with HIV disease and AIDS. So, mutations that result in gene variations may cause one person to have a higher risk for developing a disease, whereas a different mutation in the same gene may cause another person to have a lower risk for developing the same disease. Discussions of specific mutations affecting health are presented in the clinical chapters of this textbook.

Point Mutations

Point mutations include substitutions of one base for another and can occur in DNA or RNA. This type of change does not result in an extra base or a lost base, just a substitution. Thus the DNA triplets remain intact, although one may be incorrect. This change may or may not alter amino acid position or protein synthesis, depending on where it occurs. When a single point mutation occurs in a DNA coding region or in mature RNA, the result can change one amino acid in the protein's primary structure with a resulting change in protein function, but it also may have little or no effect. When a point mutation has little or no effect on a protein's function, it is known as a *benign mutation* or a *normal variation*.

Think of the sentences below as an analogy to a point mutation. The top sentence represents the correct reading sequence for a specific gene:

THE RED BUG BIT THE DOG

THE RED BUG BIT THE HOG

A point mutation, as seen in the bottom sentence, has substituted the *d* in dog with an *h*. The coded message is similar but not exactly the same.

Can a point mutation alter protein function or protein synthesis? No, some, and yes. First, point mutations occur much more often in noncoding regions of DNA rather than in coding regions, because noncoding regions make up about 95% of total nuclear DNA. This makes the noncoding regions bigger targets for mutational events. Point mutations and other types of mutations in these noncoding regions are actually responsible for making one person's DNA different from and identifiable from another person's DNA. Even identical twins (monozygotic twins) do not have absolutely identical DNA by the time they are born, although they probably did when the embryo first split into two embryos. By the time identical twins are born, they usually have at least 100 base pairs different from each other in the noncoding regions. As they live their lives, each twin continues to accumulate more and different mutations, so as they age, these identical twins become less identical in their DNA.

Silent Point Mutations

Even when a point mutation is part of a gene-coding region, it may have no effect, a mild effect, or a major effect on synthesis of the protein coded by that gene. Sometimes a point mutation does not alter the final amino acid sequence of the protein because the substitution occurs in the third base in the triplet, and the resulting RNA codon still codes for the same amino acid. This type of point mutation is known as a *silent point mutation* (Fig. 2–8).

Missense Point Mutations

A point mutation that does change the amino acid sequence is a *missense point mutation* and does affect protein function, usually reducing it to some extent (see Fig. 2–8). Some missense point mutations reduce protein function only slightly, and others cause a more profound change in protein function. For example, in normal adult beta globin, the sixth amino acid in the sequence is glutamine. This is the correct sequence for hemoglobin A (HbA), and the beta globin folds are proper, allowing hemoglobin to maintain its shape and bind well with oxygen. In people who have sickle cell disease, a single base substitution in the DNA changes the sixth amino acid to valine instead of glutamine, creating hemoglobin S (HbS). While this form of beta globin (when combined with two alpha globin molecules and a heme molecule) can still carry oxygen, its folds are different, which make it function less well than HbA. In addition, under conditions of low-tissue-oxygen levels, the folds become more abnormal, causing the blood cell to form a "sickle" shape. The protein produced as a result of this missense point mutation has significantly reduced function.

Normal sequence			
DNA code ACA	GAC	CCC	CAC
Amino acid Cys	Leu	Gly	Val

A silent mutation with a single base change in the DNA but no change in amino acid sequence.			
DNA code ACA	GAC	CCG	CAC
Amino acid Cys	Leu	Gly	Val

A missense mutation with a single base change that causes a different amino acid to be placed within the protein.			
DNA code ACC	GAC	CCC	CAC
Amino acid Trp	Leu	Gly	Val

A nonsense mutation with a single base change that results in a "stop signal" that halts protein synthesis.			
DNA code ACT	GAC	CCC	CAC
Amino acid Stop	Leu	Gly	Val

Figure 2–8. Comparison of the effects of a silent point mutation, a missense point mutation, and a nonsense point mutation on protein synthesis.

Nonsense Point Mutations

A point mutation that results in an inappropriate placement of a stop signal is known as a *nonsense point mutation*, which has a negative effect on protein function. This type of mutation, also shown in Figure 2–8, prevents the completion of a protein. The protein may not be synthesized at all if the stop signal is present early in the reading sequence. If it is present later in the sequence, protein synthesis stops prematurely and results in a short, or *truncated*, protein that usually has little, if any, function.

Single Nucleotide Polymorphisms

The correct sequences for every gene are not yet known. Among the ones that have been sequenced most, people have the same DNA sequence for most genes. However, some of the known gene sequences have small variations from the most common sequences in some groups of people. (The most known common sequence of a gene in a population is known as the *wild type* sequence rather than the normal sequence.) Usually, these variations are the result of missense point mutations and may affect protein function to varying degrees. These differences or variations are known as **single nucleotide polymorphisms**, or SNPs ("snips"). An example of a group of genes with considerable personal variation that results in protein function changes is the cytochrome P450 enzyme system.

The cytochrome P450 system of enzymes is coded for by a 10-gene family that may have subsets of as many as 100 genes. The genes in this family have names that all begin with CYP. These genes are large, and there are many variations in the exact sequence of these genes, making some more active and others less active than "normal." Function of the proteins produced by these genes is very important in drug metabolism. Chapter 15 provides a more in-depth discussion about the issues related to SNPs in these genes.

Frameshift Mutations

Frameshift mutations are disruptions of the DNA reading frame as a result of having one base or number of bases that are not multiples of three added or deleted. (A frameshift mutation involving only one base is a specific type of point mutation.) When this type of mutation occurs in gene-coding regions, it always disrupts the reading frame from the start of the mutation to the end of the gene. The result is complete alteration of amino acid position and prevention of synthesis of a functional protein. A normal protein cannot be made from a gene with a frameshift mutation.

Think of the sentences below as an analogy to a frameshift mutation. The top sentence represents the correct reading sequence for a specific gene:

THE RED BUG BIT THE DOG
THR EDB UGB ITT HED OG
THE RED GBU GBI TTH EDO G

A base deletion mutation, as seen in the middle sentence, has removed the *E* in the first *THE*, shifting the rest of the bases to the left (for the three base codes) and disrupting the reading frame. A base addition mutation, as seen in the bottom sentence, has added a *G* to *BUG*, shifting the three-base reading codes to the right from that point and disrupting the reading frame. The coded message from either a deletion or an addition is essentially garbage and no functional protein can be generated.

Sometimes a mutation involves the deletion or insertion of a number of bases, and the number is one that is a multiple of three. When these deletions or insertions occur in a gene coding region, the actual reading frame is not disrupted, but either some amino acids will not be present in the final protein synthesized or other unneeded amino acids will be present somewhere within the final protein. So even though the reading frame is not shifted, the final protein synthesized is not normal and may not be functional.

One example of this type of mutation is the founder mutations in the *BRCA1* gene. This very large gene codes for a protein that controls cell growth and protects against cancer development, especially breast and ovarian cancer. Mutations that eliminate function in this gene are several large areas of base deletions causing the loss of many amino acids although much of the rest of the amino acid sequence in the synthesized protein remains intact. When a person inherits the mutated form of this gene in one gene allele and produces a nonfunctional protein, her or his risk for cancer greatly increases because the protection provided by the protein is not in place. More information about this specific gene mutation is presented in Chapter 12.

Mutational Events

Mutations can occur at any genetic level and in any genetic process. Thus, mutations can involve individual nucleotides; DNA segments; genes; RNA; chromosomes; the genome; or, in any step of the various processes involved in DNA replication, cell division and protein synthesis. While some causes of mutations appear random, the location of uncorrected mutations appears less random. This means that some areas and some processes are more susceptible to development of mutations. Individuals vary in their susceptibility to mutation development and mutation retention. In addition, both internal and external environmental conditions influence mutation susceptibility and consequence. Some known causes of mutations include:

- Spontaneous DNA replication error
- Poor DNA repair function
- Exposure to environmental mutagens (biological, chemical, physical, viral)

Mutation Mechanisms and Repair

These are many causes and mechanisms of mutations. The most well-studied mechanism is spontaneous DNA replication error. Recall from Chapter 1 that with every cell division, the entire genome within the cell must replicate. The average human produces about a trillion new cells daily through mitosis, providing lots of opportunity for spontaneous mutational events. Although DNA synthesis is a process with *high fidelity*, meaning that errors are relatively few because replication of the new strand is faithfully complementary to the template strand, errors do occur. If an incorrect base were placed in the new DNA strand at a rate of 1 out of every 1000 bases (and who among us can do the same thing over and over again 1000 times correctly each time), the overall result would be 1,000,000,000,000,000,000 mutations daily (1 trillion cells times 1 billion base pairs divided by 1000). This rate is not really compatible with health. With "antimutation" mechanisms in place, however, one mutation for every million base pairs is estimated to be the final daily average spontaneous mutation rate during cell division. This basal rate varies with personal and environmental conditions.

As DNA synthesis during mitosis progresses, a variety of DNA repair processes help discover and correct errors. In a sense, a backup "editing" or "spell-checking" function occurs, with enzymes actually comparing the sequence of the template DNA strand to the newly synthesized strand. Recall that the newly synthesized strand should be complementary to the template strand. Thus, the sequence A-G-T-C in the template strand should be T-C-A-G in the new strand. What happens if instead of a G, a T is placed in the new strand (T-C-A-T)? The DNA repair system of enzymes should recognize that the T is incorrect, clip it out, and insert a G as the correct base in the sequence. Mutation fixed! Still, the process is not perfect, allowing for about one in every million base errors to remain and to be passed down to the next cell generation. When these mutations occur in the vast areas of DNA noncoding regions, they have little effect on overall body function but do account for increasing DNA variations from one person to another as people age.

Even the effectiveness of the DNA repair mechanisms is an inherited trait. Most people have "average" repair function that can correct or manage well the day-to-day spontaneous replication error mutations and even the mild-to-moderate mutations that occur as a result of exposure to environmental mutagens. A **mutagen** is any substance or event that can inflict temporary or permanent changes in the normal DNA sequence. Other people have inherited repair mechanisms with greater-than-average function that serve to protect them from allowing excessive mutational events to result in permanent DNA mutations. Still others have inherited poor repair mechanisms that do not recognize DNA mutations or that make further mistakes during the repair process. For example, instead of correcting the error of placing a T instead of G in the new strand complementary to A-G-T-C (T-C-A-T), it replaces the incorrect T with an incorrect C.

Even the most outstanding repair mechanisms can be overwhelmed if environmental exposure to mutagens is excessive. Consider the person who has a huge mutagen exposure by smoking four packs of cigarettes daily, drinking a liter of whiskey daily, mining asbestos for a living, and lying out in the sun without protection for hours daily. Then consider that this same individual has a house that was built in an area where radon gas is very high. Not only will there be a greater rate of spontaneous errors that become permanent, but also other direct damage to the DNA can occur, such as the creation of extra bonds or cross-links between double-stranded DNA so that it cannot separate for synthesis. This damage results in large areas of DNA deletions in some of the new cells made daily. Health problems are likely, especially different types of cancer and birth defects in any offspring produced by this individual.

Mutation Locations

At one time, mutations were thought to occur only in DNA and be totally random. It is now clear that mutations can occur in many places, not just in the DNA, and that the process is less random. "Hot spots" for mutations exist. These are largely areas where extra events or processes are needed for normal function. Recall, for example, that DNA replication is not a continuous process during cell division. Rather, synthesis of new DNA strands complementary to the original strands in a cell occurs in many sites along the length of the template. After these individual new DNA pieces have been synthesized, they must be spliced together. These splice sites are areas that are more susceptible to the occurrence and retention of mutations. This is also true during mRNA maturation. The splice site areas where introns are removed and the exons are spliced together also provide hot spots for mutations. Also consider that misreading can cause an intron to remain when it should have been removed or, conversely, can cause an exon to be removed when it should have remained. Start and stop codes can be misplaced or deleted. Transfer RNAs (tRNAs) can be synthesized incorrectly and not bind with the appropriate amino acid. Any of these mutational events can disrupt protein synthesis; however, unless the disruption is widespread within a person, a problem may never develop.

Summary

Protein synthesis is an essential process for all life-forms. It is complex and requires precision in all steps for proper outcomes. Changes in protein synthesis are a common factor in many health problems. These changes can occur as a result of somatic cell mutations, which are a problem only to the person who developed the mutation. Protein synthesis changes also can occur as a result of germline mutations and thus may be inherited. Specific health problems associated with changes in protein synthesis form the foundation of the clinically focused chapters of this text.

GENE GEMS

- All of the hormones, enzymes, growth factors, and other protein-based chemicals needed for normal human physiologic function are protein gene products that are produced when the correct genes are activated and expressed.
- The sequencing order of the amino acids is what makes one protein different in structure and function from another protein.
- Only about 5% of nuclear DNA contains gene-coding regions, and these are largely the same from one person to another.
- DNA noncoding regions are different from one person to another, even between identical twins.
- DNA sequences are read from the 5 prime (5') to the 3 prime (3') direction.
- The transcription phase of protein synthesis takes place completely within the nucleus.
- The DNA sense strand contains the actual triplets coding for a specific protein, and the complementary strand to this is the DNA antisense strand.
- The DNA antisense strand for one protein is the sense strand for a different protein.
- DNA sequences of one gene are in pieces within a coding region and are separated by areas of DNA that are not part of that gene.
- RNA is single-stranded (ss) and serves as the interpreter of information stored within the genes of DNA.

Continued

- RNA contains the base uracil in place of thymine.
- When messenger RNA is first constructed, it contains segments of the gene to be expressed (exons) and segments of other genes (introns) that are not to be expressed at this time.
- Introns must be removed from messenger RNA before protein synthesis can occur properly.
- The translation phase of protein synthesis takes place in the cytoplasm, often in an organelle known as the *endoplasmic reticulum*.
- Translation requires sufficient amounts of amino acids, ribosomes, mRNA, and tRNAs.
- Each tRNA is specific for only one amino acid and can be used more than once.
- Each mRNA is translated multiple times for as long as it is present.
- Molecules known as microRNA can regulate the translation of mRNA by either binding to it so that translation does not occur or by increasing the rate at which mRNA molecules are degraded.
- Initial translation that produces a peptide with all the amino acids in the correct order is a protein's primary structure.
- Further modification of a protein's primary structure is needed for function.
- Although DNA synthesis is a process with high fidelity, errors do occur.
- Mutations can involve individual nucleotides, DNA segments, genes, RNA, chromosomes, and genomes, and can occur in any step in DNA replication, cell division, and protein synthesis.
- Not all mutations have deleterious results.
- A new somatic cell mutation cannot be inherited by one's children.
- Germline mutations occur in sex cells and can be inherited by one's children.
- A silent point mutation does not change protein function, a missense point mutation usually reduces protein function, and a nonsense mutation often eliminates protein function.
- A normal protein cannot be made from a gene with a frameshift mutation.
- Many cellular repair mechanisms exist to correct mutations or prevent them from becoming permanent.

Self-Assessment Questions

1. What is the best meaning for the term *gene expression*?
   a. The location of a specific gene allele on a specific autosomal chromosome
   b. The specific trait or protein coded for by a single gene is actually present.
   c. The ability of a single gene to code for more than one trait or characteristic
   d. The loss of a trait or characteristic from one family generation to the next generation

2. Which process occurs outside of the nucleus?
   a. DNA transcription
   b. RNA transcription
   c. Splicing out of introns
   d. Translation of mRNA

3. What would be the sequence of RNA complementary to single-stranded DNA with the base sequence of ACCTGAACGTCGCTA?
   a. TGGACTTGCAGCGAT
   b. ACCTGAACGTCGCTA
   c. UGGACUUGCAGCGAU
   d. ACCUGAACGUCGCUA

4. Which events, structures, or processes are likely to trigger transcription of the beta globin gene?
   a. Anemia and TATA boxes upstream from the beta globin gene
   b. Anemia and polyadenylation downstream from the beta globin gene
   c. Polycythemia and TATA boxes upstream from the beta globin gene
   d. Polycythemia and polyadenylation downstream from the beta globin gene

5. Indicate the sequence of the mature mRNA transcribed from the sense strand of DNA having the following sequence, with the underlined letters indicating exons and letters not underlined indicating introns.

   <u>ATCGG</u>TAC<u>C</u>GCG<u>CAC</u>A<u>TTC</u>GCT<u>ATGCCAAAA</u>

6. Which factor has the greatest influence on protein tertiary structure?
   a. The presence of a poly-A tail
   b. The specific amino acids that are in close proximity to each other
   c. Bond formation between amino acids that are distant from each other
   d. The number and position of additional proteins needed to form the complex structure

7. What is the expected result of a "missense" point mutation?
   a. Total disruption of the gene reading frame and no production of protein
   b. Replacement of one amino acid with another in the final gene product
   c. Replacing an amino acid codon with a "stop" codon, resulting in a truncated protein product
   d. No change in amino acid sequence and no change in the composition of the protein product

8. Jack and Jill go up a hill that has high levels of gamma radiation emission. Jack suffers 10 point mutational events in a noncoding region, and Jill suffers only one frameshift mutation in the insulin gene–coding region of her pancreatic beta cells. What are the possible and probable outcomes of these events for both people?
   a. Jack will have major deficiencies in the production of ten proteins; Jill will have reduced insulin activity.
   b. Jack will have less functional proteins and an increased risk for cancer; Jill will have type 2 diabetes mellitus.
   c. Jack will have few, if any, effects on protein synthesis but will have more personal DNA markers; Jill will not produce any functional insulin and will have type 1 diabetes mellitus.
   d. Jack will not have any change in protein synthesis or function; Jill will have an increased risk for developing type 1 diabetes mellitus and can pass this risk on to her children.

Self-Assessment Answers

1. b 2. d 3. c 4. a 5. UAGCCGGUGAAGUACGGUUUU 6. c 7. b 8. c

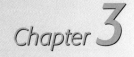

Chapter 3

Genetic Influences on Cell Division, Cell Differentiation, and Gametogenesis

Learning Outcomes

1. Use the genetic terminology associated with cell division, cell differentiation, and gametogenesis.
2. Compare the characteristics and growth regulation of normal cells and early embryonic cells.
3. Analyze the influences of membrane receptors, signal transduction pathways, and transcription factors in the regulation of cell division.
4. Explain the role of apoptosis in normal cell function.
5. Describe the influence of gene expression in cell differentiation.
6. Compare the processes, timing, and outcomes of mitosis and meiosis.
7. Compare the processes and consequences of meiosis I and meiosis II in spermatogenesis and oogenesis.

KEY TERMS

Anaplastic

Apoptosis

Cell adhesion molecules (CAMs)

Contact inhibition of mitosis

Cyclins

Cytokinesis

Differentiation

Fertilization

Gametes

Gametogenesis

Hyperplasia

Hypertrophy

Meiosis

Meiotic Cell Division

Nucleokinesis

Oncogenes

Oogenesis

Phosphorylation

Pluripotent cell

Signal transduction

Spermatogenesis

Suppressor genes

Transcription factors

Tyrosine kinases (TKs)

Zygote

Introduction

Human health is dependent on the efficient and correct function of normal cells in every tissue and organ. In addition to ensuring proper cell function, an important aspect of health is the tight regulation of when cells divide, when they die, and how or if they are replaced. The process of cell division is complex and common, occurring millions of times every minute throughout one's life span. Genetic regulation ensures that the process occurs at the right time and at the right rate. Interference with genetic regulation of cell division can result in developmental abnormalities of anatomy and function and is a major factor in cancer development.

Normal Cell Biology

Overview

Some human organs continue to grow and increase in size after development is complete because of **hyperplasia**, mitotic cell growth in which the tissue or organ increases in size by increasing the number of cells within it (Fig. 3–1). (Recall from Chapter 1 that mitosis is a duplication cell division that results in two new cells that are identical both to each other and to the parent cell that began the mitosis cell duplication division.) Examples of tissues and organs that continue to grow or replace themselves by mitosis and hyperplasia throughout the life span include the skin, liver, bone marrow, and the linings of the intestinal tract and blood vessels. Some human cells no longer grow by mitosis after tissue or organ maturation in fetal life or infancy. Examples of tissues and organs that do not grow by mitosis after maturation include cardiac muscle cells, skeletal muscle cells, and neurons. Instead, these tissues increase from infant size to adult size by **hypertrophy**, the expansion of the size of each individual cell rather than by generating new cells to increase the number of cells (see Fig. 3–1). A disadvantage of organs that have attained their final size by hypertrophy is that when these nondividing cells die, they are replaced by scar tissue cells rather than by the same type of cells that were lost. For example, if a person had a myocardial infarction and 30% of the ventricular myocardial cells died from ischemia, the dead cells slough. Rather than leave the ventricle with a hole, these dead myocardial cells are replaced with collagen and fibrous connective tissue that forms a scar or *patch* in the area. The scar tissue cells are not cardiac muscle tissue and do not contract or contribute to cardiac output—they merely keep the chamber from leaking. Whenever normal cells are replaced with scar tissue, some tissue or organ function is reduced. The degree of function lost is proportionate to the amount of scar tissue present.

Figure 3–1. Tissue growth by hyperplasia and hypertrophy.

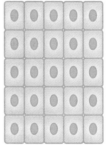
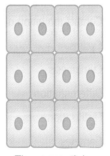

Original tissue   Tissue growth by   Tissue growth by
                          hyperplasia   hypertrophy

Many tissues and organs continue to replace cells by mitotic cell division throughout one's life span, although the rate of cell division decreases with age. Often, these tissues and organs are located where constant damage or wear occurs and continued cell division is needed for replacement. A major advantage of tissues and organs retaining mitotic ability is the replacement of dead, aged, or damaged cells with new cells, thus ensuring optimal tissue or organ function, although more energy is used in the replacement process. In those tissues and organs that retain mitotic ability, the growth of new cells is well controlled so that the optimum amount of maximal functioning cells is present. For example, unlike the heart, the liver is composed of cells that retain mitotic ability. In a healthy person who is 90 years old, all of his or her liver cells are much younger than 90 years. Each liver cell performs its physiologic function, ages, and eventually dies. Cell aging in tissues capable of mitosis is determined by *quantal mitosis*, or the number of preprogrammed cell divisions it can undergo. As a person's liver cells age, wear out, are damaged, or become less functional in some way, they undergo a process of programmed cell death or cellular suicide, known as **apoptosis.** These poorly functional cells are removed from the liver, making room for new liver cells to generate by mitosis so that the liver continues to be populated throughout life by optimally functional cells. If apoptosis did not occur, the liver would contain too few functional cells to perform its work efficiently and effectively. For optimum function, mitosis must be balanced with apoptosis. Normal cell function requires strict genetic regulation over both of these processes.

Characteristics of Normal Cells

Appearance

Every normal cell has a distinctive or differentiated appearance, including size and shape. The structural appearance of normal cells reflects their function. The nucleus within a normal cell takes up very little space compared with the size of the rest of the cell, resulting in a small nuclear-to-cytoplasmic cell ratio.

Function

All normal cells perform at least one specific job, called a *differentiated function,* that helps whole-body function. For example, skin cells synthesize keratin, testicular cells secrete testosterone, skeletal muscle cells contract, neurons generate action potentials, and adrenal cortex cells secrete cortisol. Some cells, such as liver cells, have more than one differentiated function.

Adherence

Normal cells have several different cell surface proteins that allow normal cells of the same type to adhere tightly together. These proteins are known as **cell adhesion molecules, or CAMs.** Some of the most well-known CAMs include fibronectin, the cadherins, and a variety of integrins. They each work in slightly different ways. Having normal cells within one tissue or organ that remain bound tightly together prevents cell migration. Thus, normal cells do not leave their parent organ or tissue. On the other hand, erythrocytes and leukocytes, although they are normal, do not adhere tightly together and are able to move about the body as part of their function. These cells do not produce fibronectin or other CAMs.

Ploidy

Normal human somatic cells have a nucleus and are diploid, containing 23 pairs of human chromosomes (or 46 individual chromosomes), a condition known as *euploidy.* The only normal mature human cells that are not diploid are erythrocytes, which have extruded the nucleus and do not contain any chromosomes, and mature sex cells (oocytes or eggs and spermatocytes or sperm), which are haploid, containing only half of each pair of chromosomes (23 total chromosomes).

Cell Growth

Normal cells that have retained mitotic ability are inhibited from mitosis when their membranes are completely in contact with the membranes of other cells, a condition known as **contact inhibition of mitosis.** One of the signals for when mitosis is needed is the presence of cell surface membranes that are untouched by the membrane of another cell. Once a normal cell is completely surrounded by other cells and its membrane is contacted directly on all surface areas with the membranes of other cells, it no longer undergoes mitosis. Another term for this characteristic is *density-dependent inhibition of cell growth.* The purpose of this feature is to prevent inappropriate tissue overgrowth. Think about what would happen if you skinned your knee and the remaining normal cells were not contact inhibited. They could continue to divide after wound closure and form excess (and unsightly) skin flaps or folds on your knee (keloid formation is a type of abnormal cell growth).

Cells that retain mitotic ability have choices to make. They can divide, perform differentiated functions, or undergo apoptosis, depending on age, body conditions, and body needs that are communicated as signals to the cell.

Normal cells have well-regulated mitosis in response to the need for cell division. Mitosis in all cells that retain mitotic ability occurs in a well-recognized pattern described by the cell cycle. The length of the cell cycle varies by tissue and by the person's age, but the process and its regulation are the same. The phases and normal regulation of the cell cycle is described in detail in the next section, "Controlled Mitosis."

Even cells that retain mitotic ability are restricted from entering the cell cycle unless new cells are essential for growth and development or when cells that are damaged or dead must be replaced. These restrictions are part of the genetic regulation for cell growth. Specific gene products are needed to promote cell division, and other gene products inhibit cell division. Normal cells are able to respond appropriately to the presence of these products. Normal cell populations are regulated by a balance between products produced by **oncogenes,** which promote entering and completing the cell cycle, and products produced by **suppressor genes,** which restrict or inhibit entering and moving through the cell cycle. Thus, oncogene products are *promitotic* and induce cells to divide. Suppressor gene products inhibit all aspects of mitosis and also trigger apoptosis.

Consider the control of cell division to be the same as that which controls the movement of a car. The controller is the person driving the car (the suppressor gene). In order to move, the car's accelerator (oncogene) is activated, and enough fuel reaches the engine for the car to go. When the car needs to stop, the driver stops pressing the gas pedal (inhibits it) and steps on the brake so that the brake disks or drums slow and stop the wheels. The driver is responsible for preventing the car from moving when movement is not needed, for determining when movement is needed, for allowing the car to move when movement is needed, and for maintaining the right speed for driving conditions. A car set into motion without a driver or brakes is a disaster (cancer).

Controlled Mitosis

As discussed earlier and in Chapter 1, cells not actively reproducing (undergoing mitosis) are outside of the cell cycle in G_0, the reproductive resting state, and continue to perform all their usual differentiated functions. Cells that retain mitotic ability must exit the G_0 state in order to enter the cell cycle.

Among all normal cells capable of mitosis, the step of leaving G_0 and entering the first phase of the cell cycle, G_1, is severely restricted. This restriction includes the presence or absence of external and internal signals, many of which are gene products. Once a cell enters the cell cycle, it responds only to internal signals. Cells in the cycle must either progress through the cycle or be arrested at some point in the cycle. Cells that are arrested are nonfunctional and usually die.

As you recall from Chapter 1, mitosis allows one cell to divide into two new cells that are identical to each other and to the original cell that started the mitotic cell division (see Fig. 1–7 and Fig. 3–2). The steps of entering and completing the cell cycle are tightly controlled by suppressor gene products. These genes are activated at checkpoints and determine how much oncogene expression is needed to allow sufficient cell division to occur for events such as normal wound healing but not lead to excessive cell division.

Some of the checks, known as *restriction point controls,* that are placed on a cell before it can enter the cell cycle include:

- The cell has retained its mitotic ability.
- A need exists for cell division in the specific tissue where the cell resides. Are more cells needed in this tissue as a result of previous cell damage or loss? Are more cells needed in this tissue because the tissue needs to increase in size (as in normal development)?
- Adequate nutritional stores are present (especially protein, glucose, and oxygen) to support existing and new cells.
- The cell has a sufficient energy supply or is capable of producing enough energy to participate in cell division and synthesize additional membranes, proteins, and organelles.

The presence of external events that inform the cell of a need for cell division are sent to the cell's nucleus through a process known as **signal transduction.** This communication system chain allows information about events, conditions, and substances external to the cell to reach the nucleus and then influence whether the cell divides, undergoes apoptosis, or performs its differentiated functions. There are many signal transduction pathways within cells that have retained mitotic ability. These pathways usually have multiple feedback loops and often interconnect with each other. Some pathways are promitotic, and others transfer signals to suppress cell division. Known factors that are external promitotic signals

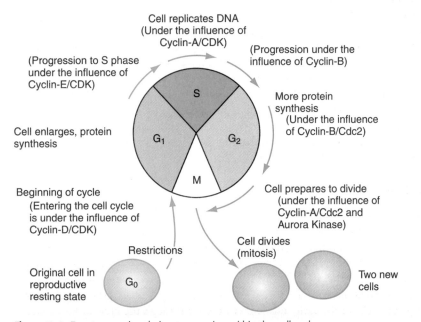

Figure 3–2. Events occurring during progression within the cell cycle.

include growth factors (such as epidermal growth factor [EGF] and vascular endothelial growth factor [VEGF]); CAMs; steroid hormones; and cell-to-cell contact through direct touching, chemical transmission, and electrical interactions. Most of these pathways involve the activation of membrane receptors. Most cells have multiple receptor types and complicated interconnecting signal transduction pathways. Not all pathways have been completely characterized, and different cell types express and activate different pathways. Thus, general control of cell division is very complex.

Figure 3–3 presents a single promitotic signal transduction pathway in a cell segment that, when activated as a result of external conditions, leads to oncogene activation and the promotion of cell division. Any of several conditions can initiate activation of this pathway, including growth factors that bind to receptors, the interaction of drugs with the cell plasma membrane, the presence of adhesion proteins, changes in ion movement (especially sodium and calcium), ligand binding, and other cell-to-cell interactions. When the pathway is activated, one of the first responses is the activation of enzymes that increase the intracellular concentration of a variety of **tyrosine kinase (TK)** enzymes. The end result of the activation of any promitotic signal transduction pathway is the increased production of transcription factors. **Transcription factors** are a variety of promitotic substances that enter a cell nucleus and signal to the cell that a specific gene transcription or mitosis is needed. Some of these

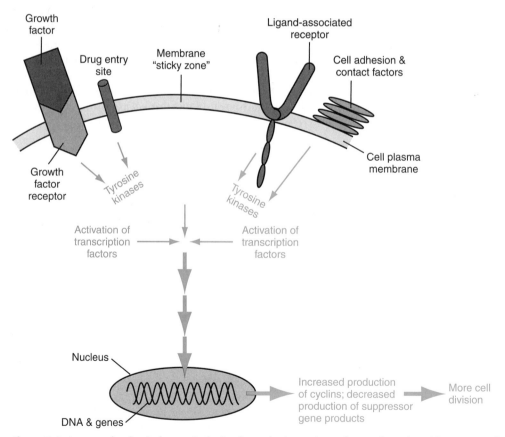

Figure 3–3. An example of a single promitotic signal transduction pathway that can be activated by any one of several external factors or conditions.

substances are proteins and others are electrolytes. (These transcription factors are reminding the driver of all the errands he or she needs to run and are helping the driver prioritize them.)

The remaining discussion about cell cycle control may appear complicated because of the many different gene products that interact to control the process. For most nurses and other health-care professionals, memorizing the activity of these different gene products is less important than understanding the following concepts:

- Suppressor gene products control the expression of oncogene products.
- Oncogene products are always promitotic.
- Control is exerted at every phase of the cell cycle.
- Activation of most of the promitotic gene products requires the addition of a phosphate group to their structures.
- These promitotic products can be deactivated by removing a phosphate group from their structures.

To help you understand the "big picture" of normal genetic control over cell division, please read the following sections, which describe the activities that occur during the phases of the cell cycle.

G_1 Phase

When external promitotic signals reach the cell's nucleus and the checkpoint information indicates that the resources are adequate, the cell exits G_0 and enters G_1, the first phase of the cell cycle. Progression to the next phase is determined by the presence of cyclins. **Cyclins** are a group of promitotic proteins produced by specific oncogenes that, upon activation, propel the cell forward through all phases of the reproduction cycle. (Think of the cyclins as the gas released into the engine by the accelerator that allows a car to move.) Normally, the oncogene expression of cyclins is carefully regulated by suppressor gene products. Cyclin activation requires the attachment of a phosphorous molecule to the cyclin structure, a process known as **phosphorylation**. Phosphorylation is performed by a variety of TKs. TKs activate many transcription factors at different steps in the signal transduction pathway, and they activate cyclins in the cell cycle. There is a wide variety of TKs, most of which are products of oncogenes. Some are unique to the cell type; others are produced only in cancer cells that express a specific oncogene mutation.

Cyclins are activated by cyclin-dependent kinases, or CDKs. The CDKs combine with cyclins to form complexes that start the cellular reproductive processes. In normal cells, cyclins and CDKs are carefully regulated by suppressor genes (the driver) so that cell division occurs only when it is needed and to the degree it is needed. (The driver keeps the car at the correct speed when it needs to move.)

The type of cyclins present in a cell during mitosis varies by the phase of the cycle. Differences in cyclin types determine whether the cell progresses through the phases of the cell cycle and whether the cycle is completed so that two new cells are generated. More than 20 different families of cyclins have been identified (A through T). The A, B, and D cyclin families are the most well characterized. The most common signal for leaving G_0 and entering G_1 is the formation of the complex cyclin-D/CDK, which is formed by combining cyclin-D with its specific CDK. Additional complexes of other cyclins and their specific CDKs form to allow progression through each phase of the cell cycle. All of the cyclins and CDKs are made in the cell in response to specific oncogene activation. Figure 3–2 shows the activity of various cyclin complexes in the cell cycle.

Late in G_1, additional cyclin-CDK complexes form to move the cell into S phase. These complexes promote DNA transcription and protein synthesis. The resulting response is a greater expression of promitotic cyclins by oncogenes and a reduced expression of suppressor gene products that inhibit cell division. Progression into S phase requires that regulator proteins be phosphorylated to work with transcription factors. All of these processes are under genetic control. A major regulator of the cell cycle for many types of normal cells is the *Tp53* suppressor gene product. It is known as the "guardian of the genome," and its activation restricts the progression of cells from G_1 into S phase. Anything that damages the *Tp53* gene results in less restriction for progression of the reproductive cell cycle.

S Phase

DNA replication is the major activity of S phase. The result is two complete sets of DNA. The cyclin-E/CDK2 complex drives DNA replication by activating the enzymes needed to produce nucleotides. Another complex, the cyclin-A/CDK complex, then permits the synthesis of all substances needed for DNA replication. After DNA is replicated, cyclin-B activates other kinases for completion of S phase and progression into the G_2 phase.

G_2 Phase

This phase of the cell cycle is characterized by intense protein synthesis for proteins that are important in M phase and for those that provide routine cell maintenance. The cyclin-B/Cdc2 complex drives these actions and then moves into the nucleus to trigger gene expression for the production of other complexes and proteins of cell structures needed for M phase (e.g., centrioles and spindle fibers).

M Phase

M phase is the part of the cell cycle in which true mitosis, which results in two new daughter cells, occurs. It is during this phase that DNA is organized into chromosomes. As discussed in Chapter 1, the subphases of M phase are prophase, prometaphase, metaphase, anaphase, and telophase (see Fig. 1–11). Microtubular spindle fibers form from the centrioles as a result of the interaction of cyclins and an activating enzyme called *aurora kinase*. As each chromosome forms, it moves to the center of the cell and attaches each chromatid to one end of a spindle fiber under the influence of aurora kinase and the protein survivin. At this point, **nucleokinesis** occurs in which each chromosome is pulled apart at the centriole so that the two sets of chromosomes are separated within the single large cell. This process is immediately followed by **cytokinesis**, which is the separating of this cell into two new cells that each have a complete set of chromosomes.

Apoptosis

As discussed earlier, some cells also have to die for the optimum function of a tissue and the human body, a process known as *apoptosis* or *programmed cell death*. Cells are programmed to undergo this cellular "suicide" after a specified number of rounds of cell division. When cells are damaged, apoptosis is triggered at earlier cell ages. (Sometimes even a new car is totaled, damaged beyond the point that repair is possible and just has to be junked.)

A major signal for normal apoptosis is the shortening of the telomeric DNA at the tips of the cell's chromosomes, which occurs with each round of cell division (see Fig. 1–3). When the cell is healthy, telomeric DNA is maintained by the enzyme telomerase that was produced in the cell during fetal life. The cell has achieved its preprogrammed number of cell divisions when telomerase is depleted and the telomeric DNA is completely gone. Loss of the telomeres leads to chromosomal unraveling and fragment formation. This response triggers a variety of genetic and intracellular signals for self-destruction.

A major protein for apoptosis is the product of the *Tp53* tumor suppressor gene. This gene is expressed when cells reach their preprogrammed age or are damaged. The response to this protein is either apoptosis or the arrest of these cells at the G_1 or G_2 phases of the cell cycle. Other substances synthesized and released in response to the *Tp53* gene product include cytochrome c and the p21 protein, both of which are important in apoptosis.

The sequence of events in which apoptotic signals are received by normal cells starts with endonuclease enzymes degrading the DNA and the mitochondria in the cell releasing cytochrome c. This substance activates apoptotic protease activation factor (Apaf-1), which then activates the enzyme caspase 9. Activation of caspase 9 starts a cascade reaction to activate the whole family of caspases, resulting in the degradation of the cell's internal structures and fracturing the cell membrane. The cell breaks into smaller fragments (apoptotic bodies) that are eliminated as debris by white blood cells. Again, the genetically controlled processes of apoptosis balanced with the strict controls of cell growth ensure that organs remain optimally functional.

When cell division is not needed, external signals (such as growth factor inhibitors and the surrounding of a cell plasma membrane with other cells) are sent that inhibit the promitotic cell division signal transduction pathways (Fig. 3–4). This inhibition leads to low levels of TKs and reduced levels of promitotic transcription factors. Suppressor gene activity is increased, resulting in the production of more suppressor gene products that inhibit the synthesis of cyclins and CDKs by oncogenes.

Internal cell conditions, such as poor cell nutrition and reduced energy stores, can trigger the activation of suppressor genes to disrupt the promitotic signal transduction pathways, even when external conditions indicate a need for cell division (Fig. 3–5). Thus, healthy and active suppressor genes guard against cell division when it is not in the body's best interest.

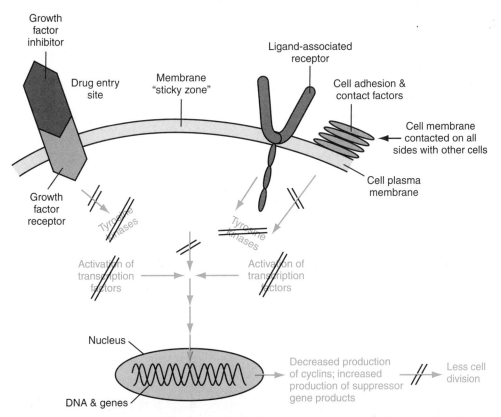

Figure 3–4. External signals that inhibit the sample signal transduction pathway, resulting in greatly reduced cell division.

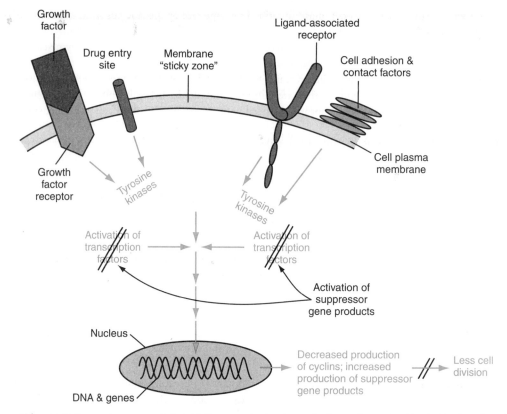

Figure 3–5. Suppressor gene activity inhibiting sample signal transduction pathway, resulting in greatly reduced cell division.

As you can see, apoptosis is regulated by different gene products, particularly suppressor gene products. There are many suppressor genes, and although all are present in every cell type, specific suppressor genes may be more active in selected types of tissues. For example, the *BRCA1* suppressor gene appears most active in suppressing excessive cell division in breast, ovary, and genitourinary tract tissues.

Early Embryonic Cell Biology

Early embryonic cells are normal cells; however, in the first 8 days after conception, they more closely resemble cancer cells in their growth patterns. Some of what has been learned about the genetic origins of cancer has come from studying early embryonic cells.

Characteristics of Early Embryonic Cells

Appearance

Early embryonic cells are anaplastic in appearance. **Anaplastic** means without a specific shape *(morphology)* or differentiation. At this stage of development, the embryo is a ball of cells that look like each other rather than like the mature cells they will eventually become. They are all small and rounded with a large nuclear-to-cytoplasmic ratio. The large size of the nucleus indicates continuing DNA replication.

Function

Early embryonic cells do not perform any specific differentiated functions because they have not yet differentiated into any mature cell type. At this point in development (up to day 8 in humans), they have unlimited potential for differentiation, a feature known as *pluripotency*. A **pluripotent cell** can, under the right conditions, become any cell type in the human body. These are the original "stem" cells. (**Differentiation** is the process by which a cell leaves the pluripotent stage and acquires the maturational features and functions of a specific cell type.)

Adherence

Cell adhesion molecules are not produced by early embryonic cells. These cells adhere very loosely to each other. As a result, early embryonic cells migrate within the early embryo.

Ploidy

When early embryonic cells are generated from normal germ cells (the sex cells of one mature ovum and one mature spermatozoa), they are diploid. This is the only characteristic that early embryonic cells share with normal differentiated human cells.

Cell Growth

Early embryonic cells do not display contact inhibition of cell growth, even when all sides of these cells are in continuous contact with the surfaces of other cells. These cells perform rapid and continuous cell division with a minimal amount of time spent in G_0. They reenter the cell cycle nearly as soon as they leave it and do not respond to signals for apoptosis. These cells have long telomeres that do not shorten with each cell division, and they have a relatively large amount of the enzyme telomerase. (Later in fetal life, apoptosis is needed for normal development; however, it is not a characteristic of early embryonic cells.) The only job for an embryo during the first week after conception is to increase the number of cells within it.

Commitment and Differentiation

Obviously, early embryonic cells have to change in some way so that humans are not born as large balls of undifferentiated cells. The change that occurs is known as *commitment* and involves adjusting the activity of the promitotic oncogenes and the genes that regulate differentiation. At about day 8 after conception, early embryonic cells each commit to a differentiation pathway and are no longer pluripotent. At this stage, cells have not yet taken on any differentiated features, but they begin to position themselves within the embryo in areas that will eventually become specific organs or tissues. Suppressor gene activity increases so that greater control and limits are placed on oncogenes, usually slowing cell division somewhat. In addition, whatever genes are important for structure and function within specific organs are selectively expressed. Thus, the genes for pancreatic structure and function are expressed within the cells destined to become pancreatic cells and are not expressed in cells destined to become cardiac muscle cells. This selective gene expression directs the normal growth and differentiation into specific body tissues and organs.

Note that commitment comes with strict regulation over cell division. The genes that control cell division in the embryo and during fetal life are the same as the ones that control cell division for normal differentiated cells that retain their mitotic ability. The difference is one of timing and the degree of expression.

Early Embryo Stage

Just after conception and for the next 14 days, an unborn baby is known as an *early embryo*. The cells in this early embryo have not yet started to differentiate into specific organs or tissues. Because the placenta has not yet completely formed, very few drugs affect an unborn baby at this stage unless the mother is harmed. However, toxins and infectious organisms can damage the early embryo at this stage and can cause a spontaneous abortion (miscarriage). More commonly, though, genetic issues that disrupt commitment and differentiation are responsible for miscarriage at this stage.

Embryonic Stage

From the third week of pregnancy to the eighth week of pregnancy (days 15 through 60), the unborn baby is called an *embryo*. This pregnancy stage is when most of the important organs are beginning to differentiate and form and is when some, such as the heart, begin to function. It is the most sensitive time when birth defects are more likely to occur if a pregnant woman takes a drug or is exposed to toxins and infectious agents. Such exposures can interrupt organ development. Unfortunately, some women in this stage are not yet aware they are pregnant. The most dangerous time of pregnancy for external or internal conditions to induce birth defects is the embryonic stage from the third week to the eighth week of pregnancy.

   Failure of a pregnancy to progress from the embryonic stage to the fetal stage is a very common feature of many genetic problems, especially the inheritance of more or less than the correct amount of genetic material. In fact, a high number of spontaneous abortions may be the first clue that one member of a couple has a genetic or chromosomal abnormality that affects his or her germ cells.

Fetal Stage

From the ninth week of pregnancy until birth, the unborn baby is called a *fetus*. In this stage, the organs have most of their structures organized as a result of selected expression of structural genes. These structures, for the most part, just continue to grow and get larger. However, tight regulation by suppressor gene products over oncogene expression is still needed to ensure that organ development continues to proceed at the right rate and does not overgrow. Although these organs are less likely to be damaged during middle and late pregnancy, it is still possible for drugs and toxins to disrupt gene activity and development. Many birth defects are attributable to such environmental exposures rather than to genetic issues. However, variation in gene sequencing and expression can alter (increase or decrease) the susceptibility to embryonic or fetal damage from environmental exposures.

   The interplay of all genes is a keystone for development. The timing of expression and suppression is critical for development to proceed normally. As strange as it may sound, even *apoptosis* (programmed cell death) is an absolute requirement for normal development but must occur within a narrow time frame. For example, when the face and head structures begin to form, the right half and the left half first develop separately. Thus, early in development, we all have a cleft palate (in fact, we have a cleft face). The two halves of the palate first grow vertically in the head rather than horizontally. In order for the palate to develop correctly as a single, closed structure, the two halves must rotate upward into a horizontal position. Then the cells on the very middle edges of the two halves become "sticky" as a result of limited apoptosis in this region. The stickiness of the two halves allows tissue fusion to occur. Timing here is critical. The edges are sticky for only about 24 hours. So, if the two halves of the palate rotate a day later than usual, they will not fuse. This results in the palate remaining as a cleft rather than as a fused single palate. The timing of gene expression determines which day the palate halves rotate and when apoptosis occurs to make the edges sticky.

Another example of the need for apoptosis in normal development is the growth of separate fingers and toes. When these digits first form, the hands and feet are actually paddles. The areas between the digits are solid tissue. This tissue must undergo apoptosis for the digits to separate and function individually. If apoptosis occurs too early, the digits will be underdeveloped. If it occurs too late, one or more digits may be fused.

Think about all of prenatal development as a very complex dance with thousands of participants each simultaneously performing separate steps and maneuvers that interact. The choreography and timing of all actions must be precise for the outcome to appear as a unified performance. Think how unfortunate it would be for one performer to leap out from a balcony and no other performers were present at the right time to catch him or her. Various genes control the expression and the timing of all events related to development. Although external conditions can influence how well development proceeds, genetic influences determine whether it proceeds.

Gametogenesis

Overview

Gametogenesis is the conversion of diploid germ cells into haploid gametes that are capable of uniting at conception to start a new person. It represents a specific type of cell differentiation and maturation. Converting precursor diploid germ cells into haploid gametes requires the process of meiosis. **Meiosis or meiotic cell division** is a special type of cell division in which the chromosome number per cell is reduced to half. This type of cell division occurs only in germ cells. The process of meiosis for gamete formation involves only one episode of DNA synthesis and two separate rounds of meiotic cell divisions. This process takes time and occurs at different rates for the ova compared with the sperm. The final outcome in terms of gamete numbers also differs between the ova and sperm. For sperm, one precursor diploid germ cell undergoing meiosis results in the eventual formation of four haploid mature sperm, each capable of fertilization. For ova, one precursor diploid germ cell that completes meiosis results in the formation of only one haploid mature ovum capable of being fertilized along with up to three haploid small cells, known as *polar bodies*, that contain almost no cytoplasm. Table 3–1 summarizes the key differences in meiosis between spermatogenesis and oogenesis.

The term haploid during the process of gametogenesis refers to both chromosome number and DNA content. This distinction is important in understanding how we can have haploid numbers after both meiosis I and meiosis II. The two cells resulting from meiosis I are haploid for chromosome number (23), but because each chromosome at that point has two chromatids that have not separated, the DNA content is still diploid. At meiosis II, the chromatids of each of the 23 chromosomes separate. Thus, the two cells undergoing meiosis II do not replicate either chromosomes or DNA, and each produces two cells that are haploid for both chromosome number and DNA content.

Spermatogenesis

Immature male germ cells, known as *spermatogonia*, are produced in the seminiferous tubules of the testes late in fetal development. These cells are nonfunctional (dormant) throughout late pregnancy and childhood. The conversion of the diploid spermatogonia into mature sperm, **spermatogenesis**, does not

TABLE 3–1

Comparison of Spermatogenesis and Oogenesis

Spermatogenesis	Oogenesis
Converts diploid precursor germ cells into mature haploid sperm	Converts diploid precursor germ cells into mature haploid ova
Requires the process of meiosis	Requires the process of meiosis
Begins at puberty and continues throughout the life span	Begins in fetal life and stops when menstruation stops
Is a continuous process	Is a cyclical process
Completion of meiosis I and meiosis II takes days to weeks	Completion of meiosis I and meiosis II takes years and is not complete until after fertilization.
Prophase I is hours to days long	Prophase I is years long
One diploid precursor cell can ultimately result in the formation of four haploid sperm capable of fertilizing a mature ovum	One diploid precursor cell can result in the formation of one haploid ovum capable of being fertilized by a mature sperm and up to three haploid polar bodies

begin until the individual enters puberty. At that time, the spermatogonia exit dormancy under the influence of a variety of hormones and start to develop further. They also become mitotically active, greatly increasing their numbers. At any one time after puberty, the seminiferous tubules contain hundreds of millions of spermatogonia in various stages of development. The final developmental stage before the process of meiosis is the *primary spermatocyte*, which is still diploid.

Meiosis I

The primary spermatocyte, which has 46 chromosomes (23 pairs), enters meiosis I, which is the type of cell division that reduces the chromosome number and has multiple stages or steps. Some of these stages are similar to those in mitosis, whereas others are unique to meiosis. (See Chapter 1 to review the stages of mitotic cell division.) Figure 3–6 shows the stages of the process of meiosis. (Stages that are also part of meiosis II are labeled with a Roman numeral I when the stage occurs during meiosis I and with a Roman numeral II when the stage occurs during meiosis II.) The primary spermatocyte enters the cell cycle and progresses through the phases of G_1 and S in the same way as for mitosis, including DNA replication during S phase. However, G_2 phase does not really exist for meiosis. Shortly after S phase, M phase for meiosis begins and has additional steps compared with M phase of mitosis.

PROPHASE I

On entering M phase, the spermatocyte has double the DNA and chromosome content from DNA replication during S phase, just like in mitosis. Because each chromosome has sister chromatids, tetraploidy (4N) now exists, just like in mitosis. During prophase I, the DNA of the replicated chromosomes continuously condenses. Remember that the metaphase of mitosis is a relatively rapid process. However, in meiosis, it is much longer. For spermatocytes, the prophase of mitosis is days long (for oocytes, prophase is years long).

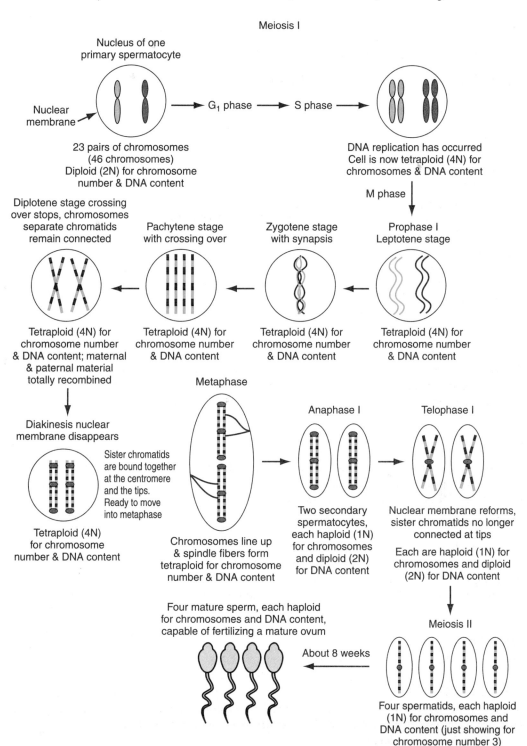

Figure 3–6. Overview of spermatogenesis from the primary spermatocyte through sperm maturation using one pair of number 3 chromosomes to show the steps. (Blue = paternally derived chromosome 3; gray = maternally derived chromosome 3.)

LEPTOTENE STAGE. The leptotene stage of prophase I is similar to the early prophase of mitosis. At this time, the four chromatids of each chromosome pair are long, thin threads. These threads become looser and slightly unwind.

ZYGOTENE STAGE. Chromosome movement occurs during the zygotene stage. The chromosome pairs, with a total of four chromatids each, line up next to and even on top of each other. For example, the pair of chromosome number 3 gets very close to each other, lining up the entire length of the four chromatids along their axis, a process called *synapsis*.

PACHYTENE STAGE. Because the four chromatids of each chromosome pair are lined up lengthwise and touch, the exchanges of chromosome material occur through breaks and rearrangements. The exchanges are called *crossing over*, and they occur not just between chromatids from one parent but also among the four chromatids for both the maternal and paternal chromosomes of the pair. This results in a huge but usually even "shuffling" of genetic material, so at the end of the pachytene stage, the two chromosomes (with two chromatids each) are now combinations of maternal and paternal genes, rather than one purely maternal-derived chromosome and one purely paternal-derived chromosome. Think about what that means for any one person and how that person receives bits and pieces of genetic material in combination from many, many parental ancestors (Fig. 3–7).

DIPLOTENE STAGE. At the diplotene stage in spermatogenesis, the recombined chromosome pairs now separate, but the chromatids for each chromosome remain connected. Crossing over halts and the two-armed (bivalent) chromosomes coil and condense in preparation for segregation.

DIAKINESIS

At this point, the 46 chromosomes are coiled into very compact structures. The two chromatids of each chromosome are firmly attached at the center and at the terminal areas. The nuclear membrane disperses and these chromosomes move into the cytoplasm.

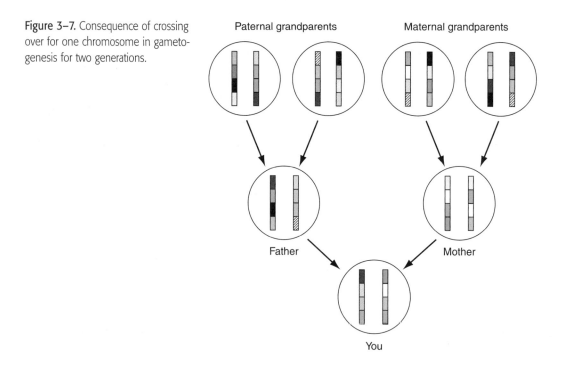

Figure 3–7. Consequence of crossing over for one chromosome in gametogenesis for two generations.

Paternal grandparents   Maternal grandparents

Father   Mother

You

METAPHASE I

The homologous chromosome pairs move to the center of the spindle area of the cell, much like what occurs in mitosis. Spindle fibers form and attach to each chromosome.

ANAPHASE I

Complete separation of the chromosome pairs (not the chromatids) occurs at this time, resulting in two secondary spermatocytes that are now haploid for chromosome number (23 individual chromosomes) and diploid for DNA content. Those recombined chromosomes that are each a mixture of maternal and paternal genes sort randomly into the two secondary spermatocytes.

TELOPHASE I

The telophase I stage of meiosis I is similar to the interphase stage for mitosis. The coiled single chromosomes (with two chromatids) in each secondary spermatocyte relax somewhat. These two secondary spermatocytes are structurally alike in terms of chromosome number, cytoplasm, and intracellular organelles. Their genetic material is very different in terms of which gene alleles came from which parent. Under normal circumstances, these two secondary spermatocytes will each enter meiosis II without further DNA synthesis or replication.

Meiosis II

For both ova and sperm, meiosis II is a relatively rapid process. This division is sometimes called an *equational* division because the number of chromosomes remains the same (23). In many ways, meiosis II resembles mitosis. Within each of the two secondary spermatocytes, the individual chromosomes line up in the center, spindle fibers attach to the kinetochores, and the chromatids are pulled apart. Each chromatid segregates independently, so each secondary spermatocyte produces two spermatids that are haploid both for chromosome number and DNA content.

Sperm Maturation

Although the spermatids generated at the end of meiosis II are genetically correct, they are not yet mature **gametes** capable of fertilizing an ovum. (**Fertilization** is the union of one mature haploid sperm with one mature haploid ovum to form a diploid zygote.) Over a period of about 2 months, these spermatids continue to develop and change. Changes include losing most of the cytoplasm, condensing the nucleus, developing a functional tail (flagellum), and acquiring the acrosomal material and cap. These mature sperm are stored in a tubular environment just outside of the testes called the *epididymis* before exiting the male reproductive system.

After puberty, men produce mature sperm throughout their life spans. The rate of sperm production decreases with age but does not stop. Even though the sex chromosomes in a male are not completely homologous, they do line up as a pair during meiosis I and meiosis II. The final result of normal, complete spermatogenesis from one spermatogonium is the generation of four haploid spermatocytes, with two having 22 autosomes and one X, and two having 22 autosomes and one Y.

Oogenesis

Oogenesis is the process of forming oocytes from precursor germ cells. Although oogenesis, just like spermatogenesis, requires converting diploid cells into haploid cells through the process of meiosis, the timing and overall results differ significantly.

Immature female diploid germ cells, known as *oogonia,* undergo quite a lot of cell division in both embryonic and fetal life. At 9 weeks after conception, the early ovary contains at least half a million oogonia. By the fifth month, several million diploid oogonia are present in each of the two ovaries.

Many of these diploid cells undergo degeneration without further maturation. Those that progress to mature ova begin this journey by entering meiosis I during the fetal period.

Meiosis I

For the early part of meiosis I, oogonia undergo the same processes at the same rate as spermatogonia. They first start by entering the cell cycle and proceeding through S phase with DNA replication. Like spermatogonia, they bypass G_2 and enter prophase of metaphase I. The leptotene, zygotene, and pachytene stages continue, and the events that occur in these stages are very similar to those that occur during prophase I for spermatogenesis.

The events in the diplotene stage for oogenesis differ from those occurring during spermatogenesis. The four chromatids per chromosome pair lengthen rather than contract, and the nucleus becomes quite large. The chromatids become very loose, taking on a brushlike appearance. The threads of DNA unwind at many points, and much more crossing over among homologous chromatids occurs. Not only is more DNA in close contact for crossing over, but also this stage lasts for years, at least until puberty. Thus, prophase I of meiosis I is arrested for a prolonged period of time during oogenesis. By birth, most female infants have about a million primary oocytes trapped in meiosis I in both ovaries, and no further proliferation of these cells occurs. The majority of primary oocytes regresses and degenerates so that by the time a girl begins puberty, only about 40,000 oocytes remain.

During the diplotene stage, other non-nuclear but essential growth of the oocytes occurs, especially of the proteins, fats, developmental information, and organelles of the cytoplasm. (This content is critical for proper development after fertilization occurs.) So, the extended diplotene stage is not truly dormant, although the process of meiosis is on hold.

After puberty, groups of primary oocytes continue meiosis I as a result of hormonal influences. In these cells, diakinesis occurs with events similar to those in spermatogenesis. In anaphase I, however, the results are different. Complete separation of the chromosome pairs (not the chromatids) occurs at this time, resulting in one secondary oocyte and the first polar body (Fig. 3–8). Both of these new cells are now haploid for chromosome number (23 individual chromosomes) and diploid for DNA content. Those recombined chromosomes that are each a mixture of maternal and paternal genes sort randomly into the two new cell structures. However, they are not equal in terms of cytoplasm and size. The secondary oocyte essentially has all of the extremely important cytoplasm, and the first polar body has minimal cytoplasm. Another difference at this point is that the polar body usually does not separate completely from the secondary oocyte. It remains connected by the plasma membrane.

Completion of meiosis I of the primary oocyte into a secondary oocyte and a polar body does not happen until just before ovulation. This means that if a girl begins menstruating at 10 years of age and has her first ovulatory cycle that year, the ova released at ovulation that year have been trapped in prophase of meiosis I for more than 10 years. If she continues to menstruate and is ovulatory until age 50, the last ovum has been trapped in prophase of meiosis I for that entire time! During that long time, there is plenty of opportunity for chromosome breaks and rearrangements. Therefore, in women, oogenesis is a limited process that occurs cyclically only during the menstrual years. By the time a woman stops menstruating, she may have fewer than 1000 primary oocytes left in both ovaries. On average, a woman forms only about 400 secondary oocytes in her lifetime.

Meiosis II

In theory, meiosis II occurs in both the secondary oocyte and the first polar body. It has been speculated that the first polar body might not always undergo meiosis II (it certainly is not needed).

Meiosis II of the secondary oocyte occurs only if fertilization takes place. The result of meiosis II of the secondary oocyte is a maintenance of chromosome number (23) and a reduction of DNA so that

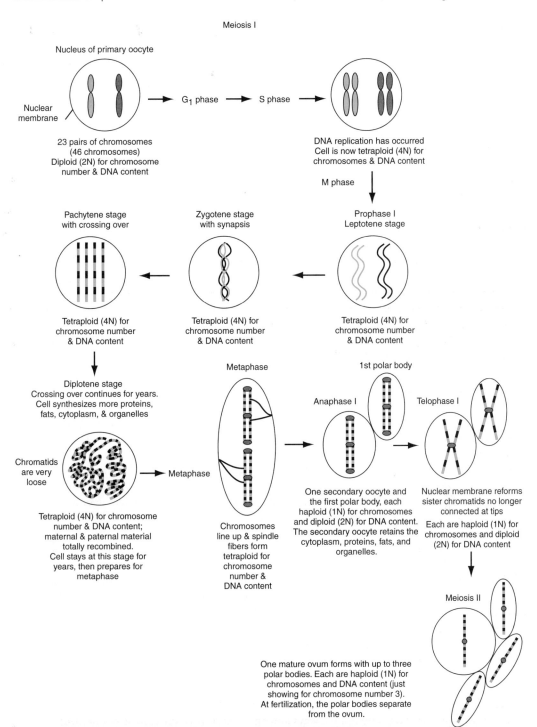

Figure 3–8. Overview of oogenesis from the primary oocyte through maturation of one mature ovum using one pair of number 3 chromosomes to show the steps. (Blue = paternally derived chromosome 3; gray = maternally derived chromosome 3.)

the ovum is haploid for both the chromosome number and the DNA content. Another polar body is formed and also is haploid for chromosome number and DNA content. If the first polar body also undergoes meiosis II, the final outcome of meiosis of one oogonium is the formation of one mature haploid ovum that is fertilized and three haploid polar bodies that are not capable of supporting fertilization (see Fig. 3–8).

Fertilization

Each month, usually one ovum matures and gets larger under the influence of several hormones. This mature ovum has a plasma membrane that is surrounded by a thicker membrane *(zona pellucida)* and a layer of follicle cells within a "shell" that also contains a gelatinous fluid. At ovulation, this entire mature ovum and its shell are released from the ovary. The shell separates from the ovum, although some follicular cells remain, surrounding the ovum like a halo known as the *corona radiata*. At fertilization, the sperm must penetrate this halo of cells, liquids, and the zona pellucida before penetrating the ovum's plasma membrane. The acrosomal area of the sperm head contains enzymes that allow the corona radiata to be penetrated (and the acrosome falls off the sperm). When the sperm binds with and then penetrates the plasma membrane of the ovum, several different processes occur. The ovum's plasma membrane changes its electrical charge, preventing any other sperm from entering. The sperm's tail and midsection drop off and do not enter the ovum. The sperm's haploid nucleus fuses with the haploid nucleus of the ovum. The result of this action is a **zygote** (a single diploid cell formed as a result of fertilization that is capable of developing into a multicelled embryo). At the same time, the polar bodies separate completely from the oocyte.

Summary

Strict genetic control over cell division is required throughout a person's lifetime, from conception to death, to ensure optimal physiologic function. Loss of genetic control not only forms the basis for many anatomic and physiologic problems, but also it is the source of all types of abnormal cell growth, such as cancer.

GENE GEMS

- Whenever normal cells are replaced with scar tissue, some tissue or organ function is reduced.
- The maintenance of healthy tissues and organs is dependent upon the proper balance of cell division with apoptosis.
- Suppressor gene products limit cell division by controlling the expression of oncogenes so that mitosis occurs only when it is needed and to the extent it is needed.
- Oncogenes are normal genes, and their products are promitotic. The controlled expression of oncogenes is needed for normal cell division.
- Oncogenes are heavily expressed during early embryonic development.
- Apoptosis of differentiated cells ensures that a greater number of optimally functional cells populate a tissue or organ that retains its mitotic ability.
- Commitment is an event critical to the development of an embryo that has the potential to differentiate into a fetus.
- Tight genetic regulation of cell growth is essential for health throughout the life span, not just for prenatal development.

- The mature ovum is the largest single cell in the human body, and the mature sperm is the smallest single cell in the human body.
- The process of meiosis for gamete formation involves only one episode of DNA synthesis and two separate rounds of meiotic cell divisions.
- The end result of meiosis I is two pregametes that each are haploid for chromosome number (23) and diploid for DNA content.
- Meiosis II does not involve any additional replication of DNA or chromosomes.
- The end result of meiosis II is the formation of four cells, totally haploid for chromosome number and DNA content.
- The entire process of meiosis for spermatogenesis occurs after puberty, takes days, and continues throughout the life span.
- The entire process of meiosis for oogenesis begins in fetal life, is not completed until fertilization occurs, and stops when menstruation stops.

Self-Assessment Questions

1. How are gametes different from zygotes?
   a. Zygotes are usually haploid, whereas gametes are usually diploid.
   b. Zygotes are the cells that result from fertilization, and gametes are the mature sex cells of both genders.
   c. Zygotes are fertilized ova with a 46, XX karyotype, and gametes are fertilized ova with a 46, XY karyotype.
   d. Zygotes are fertilized ova with 46, XY karyotypes, and gametes are fertilized ova with 46, XX karyotypes.

2. Which cell feature is common to normal human differentiated cells and to early embryonic human cells?
   a. Growth by hypertrophy
   b. Contact inhibition
   c. Tight adhesion
   d. Euploidy

3. How do transcription factors influence cell division?
   a. They directly transmit external signals to the cell's nucleus.
   b. When transcription factors are present, gene expression for cell division is enhanced.
   c. Loss or inactivation of transcription factors disrupts or disables the suppressor gene regulation of cell division.
   d. Transcription factors are enzymes that activate promitotic substances by adding a phosphate group to the chemical structure.

4. How does apoptosis contribute to healthy organ and whole-body function?
   a. Maintains telomeric DNA
   b. Allows cells to differentiate rather than to undergo mitosis
   c. Removes old or damaged cells from an organ population
   d. Activates oncogenes when cells are damaged or necrotic

Continued

5. Which mechanism allows cell differentiation?
   a. Increased expression of oncogenes
   b. Decreased expression of suppressor genes
   c. Selected expression of individual structural genes
   d. Enhanced expression of promitotic transcription factors

6. Which process is unique to spermatogenesis?
   a. Synapsis during the zygotene stage
   b. Equal distribution of cytoplasm during meiosis I
   c. Elongation of chromatids during the diplotene stage
   d. Degeneration of germ cells between fetal life and the onset of puberty

7. Why is crossing over a more amplified process in oogenesis than in spermatogenesis?
   a. The final outcome of oogenesis is the formation of one mature ovum, whereas the final outcome of spermatogenesis is the formation of four mature sperm.
   b. Prophase I in spermatogenesis is hours to days in length and is years in length for oogenesis.
   c. Women undergo the process of meiosis for less of their lifetimes than men do.
   d. The completion of meiosis II in oogenesis occurs after fertilization.

Self-Assessment Answers

1. b 2. d 3. b 4. c 5. c 6. b 7. b

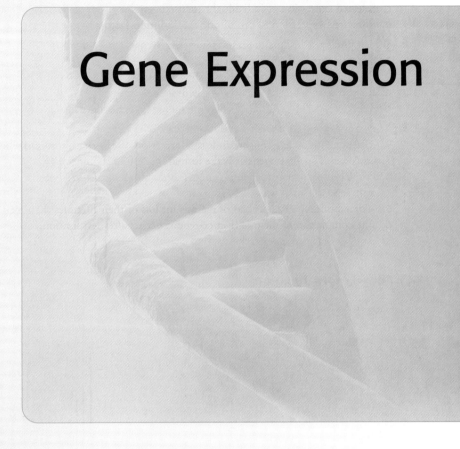

Gene Expression

Chapter 4

Patterns of Inheritance

Learning Outcomes

1. Use the genetic terminology associated with patterns of inheritance.
2. Identify the characteristics of autosomal dominant, autosomal recessive, sex-linked recessive, and sex-linked dominant patterns of inheritance for monogenic traits.
3. Explain how penetrance and expressivity change the expected expression of some autosomal dominant traits and disorders.
4. Explain why X-linked recessive disorders are expressed at a higher rate in males than in females.
5. Use a Punnett square to predict the probability for transmitting a monogenic trait to offspring.
6. Explain how complex diseases differ from diseases that are transmitted following Mendelian patterns.
7. Describe the impact of modifier genes on expression of a genetic trait.
8. Explain how the liability model is used to describe genetic risk in complex disease.
9. Describe how the epigenome is related to the genome.

KEY TERMS

Carrier	Hemizygosity	Polygenic traits
Codominant expression	Kindred	Recurrence risk
Complex traits	Liability model	Regression to the mean
Epigenome	Mendelian inheritance	Risk alleles
Expressivity	Modifier genes	Threshold
F generations	Monogenic trait	Transmission
Genetic resistance	Penetrance	Twin concordance
Genetic susceptibility	P_1 generation	

Introduction

As discussed in Chapter 1, traits are inherited directly from one's parents and indirectly from more remote ancestors. **Mendelian inheritance** refers to the rather strict rules for inheritance of monogenic traits as first recognized by Gregor Mendel in the 19th century. A **monogenic trait** or *single gene trait* is one in which the expression is determined by the input of the two alleles of a single gene. The same rules or patterns do not apply for traits or structures that involve the input of more than one gene, known as **polygenic traits**. In addition, other types of inheritance exist, and other factors influence the expression of monogenetic gene traits and polygenetic gene traits. Family history information in the form of a pedigree is essential to recognizing patterns of mendelian inheritance. Although information for constructing and interpreting pedigrees is presented in Chapter 6, pedigrees that exemplify specific patterns also are used in this chapter.

Mendelian Inheritance

Overview

Mendel first worked out patterns of inheritance for what we now know as single gene traits using plant models in the 19th century. These patterns were then applied using animal models rather than humans. Plants were used in this early work because it was possible to observe the inheritance of certain characteristics over many generations in a single year. Obviously, waiting to observe inheritance from one generation to the next in the human situation would take many years and would make drawing conclusions more difficult. Some of Mendel's conclusions regarding the patterns of inheritance for single gene traits were quite remarkable and accurate considering he never saw a chromosome or DNA.

Dominant and Recessive Expression

Mendel's work explained the concepts of dominant traits and recessive traits. His observations over 10 years of different types of garden peas led Mendel to determine that specific varieties of peas had unique traits. For example, one variety of peas always produced wrinkled seeds when fertilized with pollen from the same pea type, while another variety of peas always produced smooth seeds when fertilized with pollen from its same pea type.

Modeling out this information yielded the patterns shown in Table 4–1 wherein **P_1 generation** indicates the initial parental generation of a family or group (in this case peas) being observed for a specific trait or traits; for example, if you were examining your family history, starting with your great-grandparents, they would be the P_1 generation. The **F generations** are the succeeding generations of offspring or progeny produced from the parental generation. Each succeeding generation is designated by a numeric subscript (F_1, F_2, F_3, etc.), so that F_1 is the first-generation offspring or progeny after the parental generation, F_2 is the second-generation offspring or progeny, F_3 is the third-generation offspring or progeny, and so forth, for succeeding generations. So, if your great-grandparents are the P_1 generation, your grandparents are the F_1, your parents are the F_2, you and your siblings are the F_3, and your children are the F_4 generations. In Mendel's famous pea experiment, after the parental generation, each generation of progeny was fertilized with pollen from the same generation.

When Mendel experimented with cross-pollination (cross-breeding) of the two pea varieties, the expected response was that the F_1 generation would have 50% smooth seeds and 50% wrinkled peas. However, the inheritance of seed texture came out differently than expected. Table 4–2 shows Mendel's

TABLE 4–1

Mendel's Observations of Seed Texture Inheritance With Self-Pollination

Generation	Seed Texture	Seed Texture
P_1 (parental generation)	Smooth seeds pollinated with smooth seeds	Wrinkled seeds pollinated with wrinkled seeds
F_1 (first generation after parental generation)	All smooth seeds produced Self-pollination of F_1 seeds:	All wrinkled seeds produced Self-pollination of F_1 seeds:
F_2 (second generation)	All smooth seeds produced Self-pollination of F_2 seeds:	All wrinkled seeds produced Self-pollination of F_2 seeds:
F_3 (third generation)	All smooth seeds produced Self-pollination of F_3 seeds:	All wrinkled seeds produced Self-pollination of F_3 seeds:
F_4 (fourth generation)	All smooth seeds produced	All wrinkled seeds produced

TABLE 4–2

Mendel's Observations of Seed Texture Inheritance With Cross-Pollination

Generation	Seed Textures
P_1 (parental generation)	Smooth seeds cross-pollinated with wrinkled seeds
F_1 (first generation after parental generation)	All smooth seeds produced Self-pollination of F_1 smooth seeds:
F_2 (second generation)	Smooth and wrinkled seeds produced in a ratio of three smooth seeds to one wrinkled seed

results of using a smooth seed pea variety fertilized with the pollen of a wrinkled seed pea variety. Note that the F_1 generation showed only smooth seeds, although wrinkled seed peas were half of the parental generation used in the fertilization process. It is not until the second F generation that wrinkled seed peas finally appear, and even then, they are not present as 50%.

From this and other experiments, Mendel correctly concluded that two elements control the inheritance of a trait (one from each parent)—in this case, seed texture—and that the elements were not always equal in strength. We now know that these two hereditary elements are the two alleles of a single gene. As described in Chapter 1, variation in allele "strength" is responsible for the variable expression of a single gene trait when the pair of alleles are mixed (heterogeneous). When both parent pea seeds have the same hereditary element or *genotypes* (homogeneous), all the offspring in succeeding generations have the same appearance or *phenotype* expression. For homogeneous pairs, the phenotypes and the genotypes were identical. When the parent seeds are heterogeneous for seed texture alleles, the first-generation offspring express only the stronger or *dominant* allele even though both alleles are present in all offspring. In this situation, the appearance or phenotype is different from the genotype (the appearance of the peas in the F_1 generation is smooth even though the seed texture alleles consisted of one gene allele for smooth texture and one gene allele for wrinkled texture).

The mixed seed textures in the F_2 self-fertilized generation led Mendel to determine that the hereditary element (*gene allele*) for smooth texture was *dominant*, and the hereditary element for wrinkled texture was *recessive*. He predicted that dominant traits could be expressed in the phenotype when the genotype for that trait was either homogeneous or heterogeneous, but recessive traits could only be expressed in the phenotype when the genotype for that trait was homogeneous.

Codominant Expression

Mendel also defined the issue of *incomplete dominance* or *codominant* inheritance using cross-pollination of the colorful four-o'clock flower. In cross-pollinating red flowers with white flowers in the parental generation, Mendel predicted that only the dominant color trait would be expressed in the F_1 generation, with both colors being expressed in the F_2 generation (in a 3:1 ratio). Because red was a stronger, bolder color, Mendel expected that the first-generation flowers from this cross-pollination would all be red. Instead, as shown in Table 4–3, the flowers in the first-generation progeny were all pink, indicating that the gene allele for red and the gene allele for white (flower color being a single gene trait) were expressed equally, known as **codominant expression.** Flowers in the second generation of this cross-pollination were red, pink, and white in a 1:2:1 ratio. Thus, in codominant inheritance, the phenotype accurately expresses the genotype. Red flowers must have two red gene alleles *(homogeneous),* pink flowers must have one red gene allele and one white gene allele *(heterogeneous),* and white flowers must have two white gene alleles *(homogeneous).*

Transmission of Monogenic Inheritance Patterns

Expression of any monogenic trait depends on inheritance of dominant or recessive alleles and also depends on whether the gene is located on an autosome or on a sex chromosome. Specific inheritance patterns of a monogenic trait can be assessed without knowing a person's genotype based on family history. **Transmission** is the term used to describe how a trait is inherited or passed from one human generation to the next. Transmission patterns are determined by examining the way a trait is expressed through several generations of a family. A common method of examining emerging transmission patterns is by pedigree analysis of a kindred. A **kindred** (sometimes termed a *kinship*) is the extended family relationships over several generations.

As described in Chapter 6, a *pedigree* is a pictorial or graphic illustration of family members' places within a kindred and their history for a specific trait or health problem over several generations. The

TABLE 4–3	
Mendel's Observations of Flower Color With Cross-Pollination Showing Codominant Expression	
Generation	**Flower Colors**
P_1 (parental generation)	White flowers cross-pollinated with red flowers
F_1 (first generation after parental generation)	All pink flowers produced Self-pollination of F_1 pink flowers:
F_2 (second generation)	White, red, and pink flowers produced in a ratio of one white to two pink to one red

pattern of inheritance for a single gene trait can be identified by examining the expression of the trait as it is transmitted over several family generations. At least three family generations must be explored to draw supportable conclusions about trait transmission. (Remember that Mendel examined hundreds of plant generations to develop the rules regarding specific patterns of inheritance.)

Autosomal-Dominant

Autosomal-dominant (AD) single gene traits have the controlling gene alleles located on an autosomal chromosome. The trait is expressed regardless of whether the person is homozygous or heterozygous for the dominant allele. Criteria for AD patterns of inheritance include the following:

- The trait is found in approximate equal distribution between male and female family members.
- The trait has no carrier status (the person with even one dominant allele expresses the trait).
- The trait appears in every generation with clear transmission from parent to child.
- The risk for an affected person who is heterozygous for the dominant allele to pass the trait to his or her child is 50% with each pregnancy.
- The risk for an affected person who is homozygous for the dominant allele to pass the trait to his or her child is 100% with each pregnancy.
- Unaffected people do not have the allele and have essentially zero risk for transmitting the trait to their children.

Figure 4–1 shows a typical pedigree with transmission of an AD trait. Table 4–4 lists common physical characteristics and disorders that have AD transmission. A key feature of AD traits is that they are expressed whether both alleles are dominant or only one allele is dominant. Thus, when a dominant allele is paired with a recessive allele, only the dominant allele is expressed.

TABLE 4–4

Three Most Common Mendelian Patterns of Inheritance for Monogenic Traits and Disorders

Pattern of Inheritance

Autosomal Dominant	• Traits
	• Blood type A
	• Blood type B
	• Free earlobes (not attached to head)
	• Taste sensitivity to phenylthiocarbamide (PTC)
	• Widow's peak
	• Disorders
	• Achondroplasia
	• Diabetes mellitus type 2*
	• Ehlers-Danlos syndrome
	• Familial adenomatous polyposis
	• Familial melanoma
	• Familial hypercholesterolemia
	• Hereditary nonpolyposis colon cancer (HNCC)
	• Huntington disease
	• Long QT syndrome and sudden cardiac death**
	• Malignant hyperthermia (MH)

Continued

TABLE 4–4

Three Most Common Mendelian Patterns of Inheritance for Monogenic Traits and Disorders—cont'd

Pattern of Inheritance

	• Marfan syndrome
	• Myotonic dystrophy
	• Neurofibromatosis (types 1 and 2)
	• Polycystic kidney disease** (types 1 and 2)
	• Polydactyly
	• Porphyria
	• Retinitis pigmentosa**
	• Syndactyly
	• von Willebrand disease
Autosomal-Recessive	• Traits
	• Earlobes attached to head
	• Middle finger shorter than second or fourth finger
	• Lack of taste sensitivity to phenylthiocarbamide (PTC)
	• Disorders
	• Albinism
	• Alpha-1 antitrypsin deficiency
	• Ataxia telangiectasia
	• Beta thalassemia
	• Bloom syndrome
	• Cystic fibrosis
	• Gaucher disease
	• Hereditary hemochromatosis
	• Hurler syndrome
	• Lesch-Nyhan syndrome
	• Phenylketonuria
	• Sickle cell disease
	• Tay-Sachs disease
	• Xeroderma pigmentosum
Sex-linked Recessive	• Disorders
	• Duchenne muscular dystrophy
	• Fragile X syndrome
	• Glucose-6-phosphate dehydrogenase deficiency
	• Hemophilia
	• Hunter syndrome
	• Red-green color blindness
	• Severe combined immune deficiency (SCID)**

*Some disorders have both a genetic and a nongenetic form.
**Some disorders have more than one genetic form and can be autosomal recessive.

One important distinction must be made between normal traits with an AD transmission and disorders with an AD transmission. A person can be homozygous for the dominant alleles of a normal trait with an AD transmission pattern, such as taste sensitivity or widow's peak. However, many health problems that have an AD transmission pattern do not show homozygous genotypes. For these disorders, the homozygous AD genotype appears lethal, with loss at the embryonic or fetal pregnancy stages or

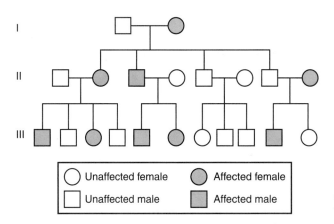

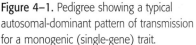

Figure 4–1. Pedigree showing a typical autosomal-dominant pattern of transmission for a monogenic (single-gene) trait.

within the first 12 months after birth. Examples include Huntington disease (HD) and achondroplasia. Living people with these disorders are heterozygous for the mutated dominant allele. This distinction slightly changes the predictability of the disorder.

Some health problems inherited as AD single gene traits are not apparent at birth but develop as the person ages. Two examples are Huntington disease and some forms of hearing loss among older adults. Even when a single gene trait is present at birth, variation in expression is possible. Two factors that affect the expression of some AD single gene traits are penetrance and expressivity.

PENETRANCE

Penetrance is how often a gene is expressed within a population when it is present. Penetrance is calculated by examining a population of people known to have the gene mutation and assessing the percentage of people in that population who actually express the condition coded by the gene. Some AD genes have greater penetrance than others. For an AD genetic disorder that has high penetrance, among 100 individuals who have one allele, nearly 100% will express the disorder. For example, the gene for HD, which is a degenerative neurologic disorder, has an AD pattern of transmission with a high degree of penetrance. Therefore, the risk for a person who has one HD allele to develop this disease approaches 100%, although gender differences and other factors influence the age of disease expression and the rate of neurologic deterioration.

Some dominant gene alleles have "reduced" penetrance. This means that a person who has the gene mutation has a risk of less than 100% for expressing the gene. One example of an AD gene allele is *polydactyly*, a condition in which a person has one or more extra digits on the hands or feet. This gene has a penetrance rate of about 80%, which means that of 100 individuals who actually have the gene, only about 80% have one or more extra digits. However, even those individuals who have the gene mutation but do not express it can transmit the gene to their children, who may express the trait and have extra digits. So, having a gene mutation does not absolutely predict that the person will express the health problem, but the risk is higher than for an individual who does not have the gene mutation.

EXPRESSIVITY

Expressivity is a personal issue (rather than a population issue) in which the degree of gene expression varies by the person who has a dominant gene for a health problem. The gene is *always* expressed, but some people have more severe problems than do other people. For example, the gene mutation for one form of neurofibromatosis (NF1) is dominant. Some people with this gene mutation express it as only a few light brown skin tone areas known as *café au lait spots*. Other people, even within the same family who have the same gene mutation, develop hundreds of tumors (*neurofibromas*) that protrude through the skin. A person with low expression of this problem can transmit the gene to his or her child who then may have high expression of the disorder. The reverse also is true. A person with high expression can transmit the gene to his or her child who then may have low expression of the disorder.

Autosomal-Recessive

Autosomal-recessive (AR) traits have the controlling gene alleles on an autosomal chromosome. These traits are expressed *only* when both alleles are present. Table 4–4 lists some AR traits and disorders. Figure 4–2 shows a typical pedigree with transmission of an AR disorder. The trait is expressed only when the person is homozygous for the recessive alleles. Criteria for AR patterns of inheritance include the following:

- The trait is found in approximate equal distribution between male and female family members.
- The trait often appears first in siblings rather than in the parents of affected children.
- The trait may not appear in all generations of any one branch of a family.
- The risk for children of two affected parents to also be affected is close to 100%.
- About 25% of the members of a family with an AR trait will express the trait or disorder.
- AR traits do have a carrier status in which those individuals who have only one affected allele may not express any level of the trait.
- Unaffected carriers of AR traits *can* transmit the trait to their children if their partner is either a carrier or is affected.
- An AR allele may be present in a family for many generations without overt expression.

An example of an AR trait is type O blood in which both alleles must be type O (homozygous) for the person to express type O blood. If only one allele is a type O allele and the other allele is either type A or type B, the dominant allele will be expressed and the O allele, although present, is not expressed and cannot be detected by standard blood type analysis. The phenotype and genotype are the same for expressed AR traits and disorders.

CARRIER STATUS

A person who has one mutated allele for a recessive genetic disorder is a **carrier**. A carrier, even though he or she may have one mutated allele, does not usually have any manifestations of the disorder but can pass this mutated allele on to his or her children. For some AR disorders, a carrier may have very mild manifestations. One example is *sickle cell trait*. A person with two sickle cell gene alleles for the beta chain of hemoglobin (beta globin) expresses all the health problems associated with sickle cell disease. However, a person who has only one sickle cell gene allele and one normal gene allele for beta globin usually has about 50% normal hemoglobin and rarely expresses sickle cell health problems. This carrier

Figure 4–2. Pedigree showing a typical autosomal recessive pattern of transmission for a monogenic (single-gene) trait.

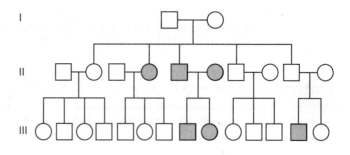

has sickle cell trait and can transmit the mutated allele to his or her children. (Chapter 9 provides a full discussion of sickle cell disease.) Figure 4–3 shows an AR pedigree with affected individuals, unaffected individuals, and carriers identified. Remember that a child of a person who expresses an AR trait will have at least one of the two recessive alleles. This person is termed an *obligate carrier* of that trait even if he or she does not express it.

GENE SURVIVAL

People have wondered how it is that recessive gene alleles in humans have survived for hundreds or even thousands of years when they are not expressed in the heterozygous state. The most reasonable explanation for this gene allele survival is the fact that the recessive allele is not expressed when paired with a dominant allele. In a sense, the lack of expression allows a recessive allele to "hide" for many generations without expression. So, what does this really mean for humans?

Humans are sentient beings who can think, assess their surroundings, and make choices. In many cultures, humans choose with whom to have children, and usually the selection is made from outside one's family. Think about a scenario in which family A has two or more developmentally delayed siblings in every generation, which suggests a genetic cause that has an AD transmission. It is likely that some people would avoid having children with members of family A to prevent such an occurrence in their own offspring. But what about family B, many of whose members carry a recessive allele for severe developmental delay, but because it is not expressed in the heterozygous form, no one is aware of this possibility? Perhaps as many as 10 generations have passed without any child expressing developmental delay. Thus, outsiders (and current family members) would have no reason to believe such a problem is possible. Then, if a carrier from family B has children with a carrier for the same problem from family C, a child is born with the severe developmental delay. If only one child expresses the problem, it could be perceived as a random event, not one associated with a familial disorder. Thus, a true genetic problem can go unrecognized as one that can be transmitted. This "hiding," or lack of frequent expression, has allowed AR mutations to continue to exist. Now that genetic testing is possible and being used, the frequency of AR transmission of genetic problems could change.

Sex-Linked Inheritance

The sex chromosomes (the X and the Y) have some genes that are not present on other chromosomes. The Y chromosome is small and has less than 300 protein-encoding total genes. Most of these genes are important for male sexual development and are transmitted only from father to son. Only a very few gene alleles, located at the tips of the Y chromosome, actually pair with homologous alleles on the X

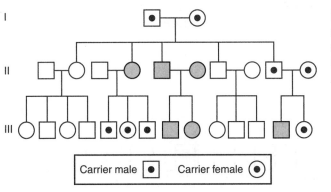

Figure 4–3. Pedigree showing affected, unaffected, and carrier status for an autosomal-recessive monogenic (single-gene) trait.

chromosome. The X chromosome is much larger than the Y chromosome (Fig. 4–4) and has about 1500 single gene alleles, most of which are not present on the Y chromosome or on any autosome. Some of these genes are specific for female sexual development, but there are also several hundred gene alleles on the X chromosome that code for nonsexual functions for both males and females.

Normally, men have one X and one Y chromosome. Mature sperm cells are haploid and contain only one chromosome of each pair, including the sex chromosomes. Thus, each sperm contains *either* one X chromosome or one Y chromosome, not both. Normally, a woman's ova also contain only one chromosome of each pair, but each has only an X chromosome for the sex chromosome and never a Y chromosome. When a sperm fertilizes an ovum (egg), the resulting cell should contain 46 chromosomes (23 pairs), including one pair of sex chromosomes. If the sperm that fertilized this ovum had a Y chromosome, the new cell would be male, with an X from the mother and a Y from the father. If the sperm that fertilized the ovum had an X chromosome, the new cell would be female, with an X from the mother and another X from the father.

Y-LINKED TRANSMISSION

Genes on the Y chromosome are termed *Y-linked*. All males inherit their Y chromosomes from their fathers (because Mom doesn't have one). Thus, the unique genes on the Y chromosome are all paternal in origin and are expressed only in males. Most of these unique genes are important for male anatomic and sexual development and fertility. This includes penis size and relative fertility in terms of amount of different types of testosterone produced and rate of *spermatogenesis* (development of mature, fertile sperm). Timing of the onset of puberty in males also appears related to Y-linked inheritance.

Figure 4–4. Comparison of the X and Y chromosomes for size and loci.

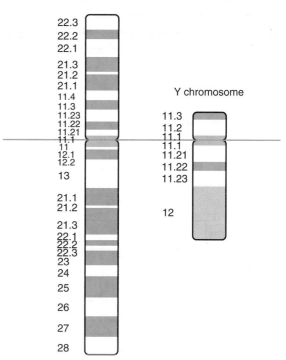

X-LINKED TRANSMISSION

The number of X chromosomes in males and females is not the same, with females having twice the number of X chromosomes than males, making the number of X-linked chromosome gene alleles unequal between males and females. Because males have only one X chromosome, they have only one allele for every gene on the X chromosome and thus have only half of the X gene alleles that a female has. Because these alleles have no corresponding allele in the Y chromosome, any X-linked allele in a male is expressed as if it were a dominant allele, a condition known as **hemizygosity.** As a result, *X-linked recessive genes have dominant expression in males and recessive expression in females.* This difference in expression occurs because males do not have a second X chromosome to balance the presence of a recessive gene allele on the first X chromosome.

X-LINKED RECESSIVE. X-linked recessive traits and disorders are relatively common and sometimes called *sex-linked recessive* because there really are no Y-linked recessive issues. Expression of X-linked recessive monogenic traits occurs differently for males than females. For such a disorder to be expressed in females, the gene allele must be present on *both* of the X chromosomes (the female must be homozygous for the trait). In males, expression of an X-linked recessive allele occurs when the allele is present on only one X chromosome. Table 4–4 lists traits and disorders associated with X-linked recessive transmission. Figure 4–5 shows a typical pedigree for an X-linked recessive trait or disorder, including carrier status. Features of a sex-linked recessive pattern of inheritance include the following:

- The incidence of the trait is much higher among males in a family than among females (and may be exclusive to males).
- The trait cannot be transmitted from father to son.
- Transmission occurs from an affected father to all daughters (who will be obligate carriers) and from a carrier mother to both sons and daughters.
- Female carriers have a 50% risk of transmitting the gene to their children with each pregnancy.
- If no sons are born to carrier mothers, the trait may not be expressed overtly for many generations.
- If no daughters are born to affected fathers who have children with noncarrier mothers, the trait is not transmitted further.
- Depending on the disorder, females who are homozygous may not survive pregnancy or will have more severe disease.

X-LINKED DOMINANT. X-linked dominant disorders are rare. Two examples include hypophosphatemic rickets (males and females) and Rett syndrome (females only). Females do express the disorder in the heterozygous state and have a 50% chance of transmitting the trait with each pregnancy to children of either gender. Males who are hemizygous for the allele are more profoundly affected than heterozygous females. For some disorders, the severity is so strong for males that the disorder is lethal and they die in utero or shortly after birth. The most outstanding feature of X-linked dominant disorders is that an affected father transmits the disorder to all of his daughters (who then express the disorder) and to none of his sons. An affected woman generally has unaffected daughters, affected daughters, unaffected sons, and affected sons in equal proportions. The most notable feature that distinguishes this transmission from that of autosomal recessive is the complete lack of father-to-son transmission.

X CHROMOSOME INACTIVATION. A special genetic feature is present in the somatic cells of females related to the issue of unequal gene alleles for the approximate 1500 genes on the X chromosome. Most of the genes on the X chromosome code for somatic cell functions important to both males and females, and relatively few genes code for female sexual differentiation. To prevent XX females from having an excessive "dose" of the X chromosome genes coding for somatic cell function, one of the X chromosomes in

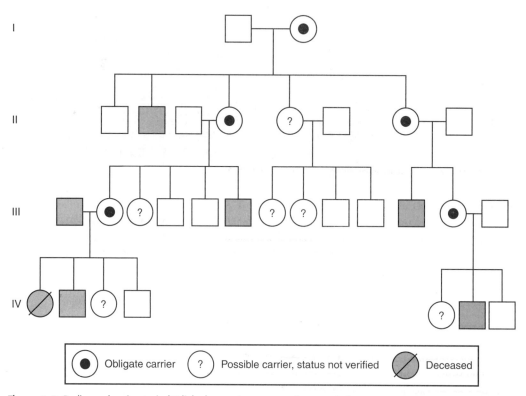

Figure 4–5. Pedigree showing typical X-linked recessive monogenic transmission.

every somatic cell is randomly inactivated. This random inactivation means that in some cells the paternally derived X chromosome is inactivated and exists as a Barr body, and only the maternal genes are expressed in those cells. In other cells, the maternally derived X chromosome is inactivated and exists as a Barr body, and only the paternal genes are expressed in those cells (Fig. 4-6).

An interesting result of this random X inactivation is that, for any particular organ, the majority of cells may express more of one parent's X chromosome, which can affect the function of the organ. For example, the gene for the muscle protein dystrophin is on the X chromosome. When this gene is mutated, the person may express Duchenne muscular dystrophy, a sex-linked recessive disorder of progressive muscle weakness. A grandmother who is a carrier for this disorder transmits the X with the mutation to her daughter. The daughter also inherits a normal X chromosome from her father. This daughter is now a carrier and transmits the affected X chromosome to her son. Because the dystrophin gene is on the X chromosome, her son expresses the disorder even though his carrier mother, who has two X chromosomes, does not. However, if this mother has the majority of her cardiac muscle cells with her paternally derived X chromosome inactive, these cells will express the mutated maternally derived dystrophin gene and her heart function is reduced below normal.

So, how does it happen that this woman's heart has more paternally derived X chromosomes inactivated and expresses more maternally derived X chromosome function if the process is random? Given the large number of cells in the heart, why isn't the maternal-to-paternal percentage of X inactivation just about equal (50-50)? The answer to these questions lies in the timing of embryonic X inactivation and the fact that the inactivation is "fixed," meaning that it is an irreversible event. In Figure 4-6,

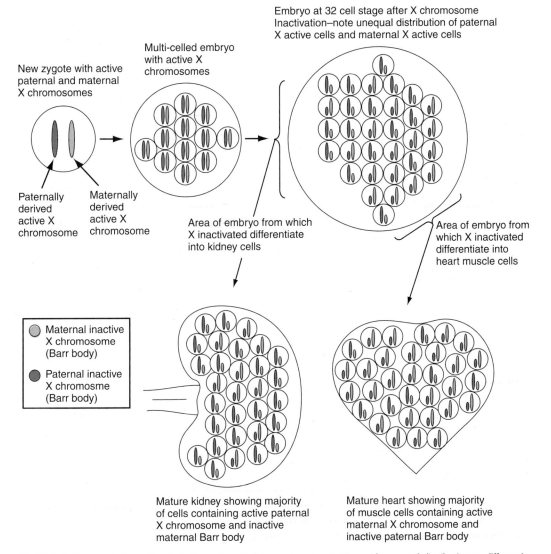

Figure 4–6. Demonstration of embryonic random X chromosome inactivation with unequal distribution to differentiated tissues.

notice that when the fertilized egg first forms a zygote, both parental X chromosomes are active. As the zygote becomes an early embryo and the cells divide to increase in number, both X chromosomes are still active. Within the first week of embryonic life and before commitment occurs, these cells will randomly inactivate one X chromosome in every cell. At this time the maternal-to-paternal percentage of X inactivation within this early embryo is nearly equal. However, as cells each commit to become a specific type of tissue or organ, the early organ contains only a few cells, and usually this small number of cells is not equal in maternal-to-paternal percentage for X inactivation. In Figure 4–6, you can see that in the embryo after X inactivation has occurred, there is an equal number of maternal Xs and paternal Xs inactivated, but they are not evenly distributed throughout the embryo. So, if 10 of these cells are committed to becoming heart muscle and only 2 of the 10 (20%) express the active paternal X chromosome, then 8 of the 10 (80%) are expressing the active maternal X chromosome. As these future heart cells continue to divide and form the heart, these percentages (20% paternal X chromosome active and 80% maternal X chromosome active) remain in the same unequal distribution, and this person's adult heart will have mostly maternal X chromosome influence. In the case of the woman who is a carrier for Duchenne muscular dystrophy, 80% of her heart muscle cells do not make functional dystrophin, and she will have very serious heart function problems. If she had a greater percentage of heart muscle cells actively expressing her father's X chromosome, her heart muscle function would be better.

Punnett Square Analysis and Probability

These mendelian rules for patterns of inheritance apply to only those traits or characteristics that are regulated by a single gene with at least two possible alleles. The relationship between genotype and phenotypic expression as well as predictability can be explained with the use of the Punnett square. This model involves plotting the known maternal genotype of a specific monogenic trait against the known paternal genotype for the same specific trait. The example provided at the top of Figure 4–7 uses blood

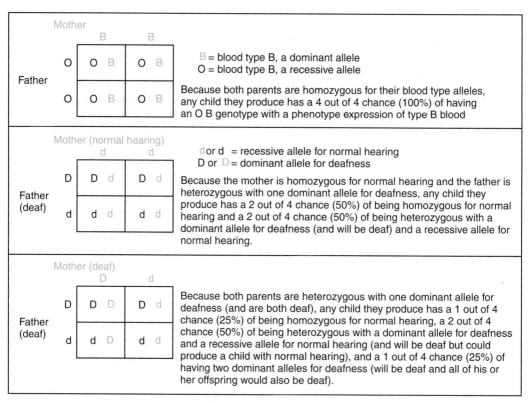

Figure 4–7. Examples of Punnett square analysis of probability for offspring genotypes and expressed phenotypes when parental genotypes are known.

type. The allele for type O blood is recessive and the alleles for either type A or type B are dominant. The mother is phenotypically and genotypically type B (BB) while the father is phenotypically and genotypically type O (OO). The expected genotype for all first-generation offspring is BO with the expressed phenotype for all first-generation offspring expected to be type B blood. The probability of this genotype and phenotype among the children born to this couple is four out of four (100%) with each pregnancy.

The middle section of Figure 4–7 shows Punnett square prediction for hearing in which *D* is an autosomal dominant allele for deafness and *d* is a recessive allele for normal hearing. In this case, the probability is that two out of four pregnancies (50%) will have the Dd genotype and express deafness and two out of four pregnancies (50%) will result in the dd genotype and have normal hearing. The bottom section of Figure 4–7 shows the Punnett square prediction for hearing when both parents are heterozygous for a dominant D (deafness) allele and a recessive d (hearing) allele. The results indicate that with each pregnancy, the allelic risks are one out of four (25%) with a DD genotype and deaf phenotype, two out of four (50%) for a Dd genotype and deaf phenotype, and one out of four (25%) with a dd genotype and hearing phenotype.

One problem that exists with Punnett square analysis for probability is that the model is less reliable when using smaller numbers. If we were using Punnett squares to predict the probable incidence of a single gene trait for two mouse parents that would eventually have 100 offspring, the model would be close to correct. However, human couples do not have 100 children. Think about tossing a coin 100 times and counting the number of times "heads" versus "tails" appears. With just the two possibilities (heads or tails), the probability with each toss is 50% heads and 50% tails. Tossing the coin 100 times will have a reality close to 50 heads and 50 tails. However, if you tossed the coin only four times, you are less likely to have 50-50 heads and tails. So, when the couple in the middle of Figure 4–7 has only three pregnancies, they have a 50% chance with each pregnancy that any one child will be deaf, but with such a small number of children, the probability and the actuality may not be the same. Thus, all three children could be deaf, all three children could have normal hearing, two children could be deaf with one child having normal hearing, or one child could be deaf with two children having normal hearing.

A *probability* is only a chance based on statistics—it is not an absolute—and many people misinterpret these probabilities. For example, a couple with one child who has a genetic health problem is told that the risk is 50%. Their interpretation is that the next child will not have the problem because the first child already does (50% of the two children). It is important to remind parents that these probabilities apply to *each pregnancy* and not to the family as a whole.

Another issue with Punnett square analysis is that it does not take into account any other factors that may influence the expression of monogenic traits. Other factors that can modify the expression of a monogenic trait or problem include the presence of modifier genes, the environment, and epigenetic influences.

Chromosomal Inheritance

Normally, we inherit one copy of each chromosome pair from our mothers and one copy from our fathers. Problems can occur when a child inherits more or less than two copies of a chromosome, or part of a chromosome, from his or her parents. Such inheritance represents a disproportionate or unbalanced inheritance of the gene alleles on that chromosome and usually results in abnormalities in anatomical development. A complete discussion of chromosomal inheritance is presented in Chapter 5.

Complex (Multifactorial) Disease

Overview

Complex traits and diseases are sometimes referred to as *multifactorial traits and diseases* because they result from the actions of several genes working together (polygenic) and/or the combined influences of both genes and environment. Most people who will require hospitalization for a genetic or genomic problem have complex diseases, such as some forms of diabetes mellitus, atherosclerosis, obesity, and cancer.

Complex traits are not dominant or recessive. Each gene variant adds to or takes away from the actual expression of the trait (phenotype). Sometimes the contributions of a particular gene variant are large and sometimes they are small. For example, nearly 20 different regions of the genome have been associated with the onset of multiple sclerosis and another 24 regions have been associated with the development of type 2 diabetes.

Many complex traits are considered quantitative. Height is a good example, because it can be measured on a numerical scale. People are taller when they inherit more alleles that add to height, and many of the genes involved in height are on the X chromosome. If your parents are both tall, there are more tall alleles for you to inherit than if your parents are both short, but with the random assortment of genes that occurs during the formation of mature sex cells, you may end up with many or few of the alleles contributing to greater height. Not all children of tall parents will be tall, but they are more likely to be tall than the children of short parents. Environment is also important in the final phenotype of a complex trait. Imagine someone who has a larger-than-average number of tallness alleles but who is severely malnourished during his or her growth years. That person may end up being much shorter than someone who has the same genomic constitution but was able to eat a diet providing plenty of nutrients and calories.

Francis Galton was a British aristocrat who lived around the time of Mendel and was actually Charles Darwin's cousin. Galton studied multifactorial inheritance and noticed the phenomenon of what he called "regression to mediocrity." This idea today is **regression to the mean**. Extremes of a condition or trait tend to become more average over time in successive generations. For example, a very tall father tends to have sons who are shorter than he is (closer to average height), and a very short father tends to have sons who are taller than he is (again, closer to average height). Galton applied his ideas to all quantitative (continuous) heritable traits, including intelligence. He was the founder of the very controversial eugenics movement in 1883 (see Chapter 17).

Modifier Genes

Genes that contribute to the phenotype but are not the primary cause of its expression are considered **modifier genes**. Even in single gene diseases, there can be other genetic influences in addition to the predominant mutation. For example, two children in the same family (with the same primary mutation) may have cystic fibrosis, but one might be much sicker than the other. Assuming they are both receiving the same quality of care, there is probably some difference in modifier genes. Perhaps one has a gene variant that is somewhat protective while the other has a gene variant that makes things worse. Evidence of the actions of modifier genes are seen in disorders such as Gaucher disease, hemochromatosis, beta thalassemia, and polycystic kidney disease, although not all modifier genes involved have been identified.

Liability Model and Threshold

People carry differing numbers of risk alleles for a given complex trait such as hypertension. **Risk alleles** are gene variants that increase a person's risk of developing the phenotype. If you graphed a population's risk, the combination of genetic and nongenetic factors would be normally distributed in the population and a bell-shaped curve could be drawn. The population numbers (from few to many) would be on the y-axis, and the liability risk (from less to more) would be on the x-axis (Fig. 4–8). The top of the bell curve represents the mean of the population, or the liability (risk) of most of the population. If we are talking about risk for hypertension, some people would be at the low end of the curve because they have very few alleles that increase their risk of becoming hypertensive. A few other people will be at the high end of the curve because they have lots of alleles that increase their risk of becoming hypertensive. Most people would fall somewhere near the middle of the curve; the dotted line represents the average number of risk alleles carried by most of the population.

For every trait, there is a theoretical point called the **threshold,** which indicates the point at which the number of risk alleles needed to express the disorder has just been met. In Figure 4–8, all points to the right of the threshold line are designated as "affected." The threshold for expression of a complex trait or health problem varies with each individual, even within one family.

A model of the liability threshold for a complex trait indicates how high the risk is in the general population and at what point risk is high enough so that having the disease or trait is likely. Thus, a **liability model** is an estimate of the risk an individual has of experiencing a complex disease based on the number of risk alleles in his or her kindred. When one looks at risk in a family with a high incidence of disease, there are more risk alleles present than are in the average family from the general population. For example, in a family where many people are tall, it is likely that there are lots of gene variants that will confer tallness, so the mean for the people in that family is much higher than for the population in general. If someone comes from a family with lots of hypertension, chances are good that he or she has more risk alleles for hypertension than the general population. So, you can use the liability model to plot out the risk for someone who has siblings with hypertension. Though the threshold is at the same place in the population (of siblings of an affected person), the mean has shifted to the right so more people from the population now have sufficient risk alleles to express hypertension.

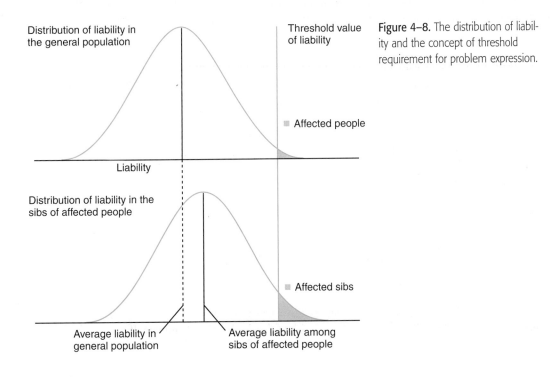

Distribution of liability in the general population

Threshold value of liability

Figure 4–8. The distribution of liability and the concept of threshold requirement for problem expression.

Affected people

Liability

Distribution of liability in the sibs of affected people

Affected sibs

Average liability in general population

Average liability among sibs of affected people

A point to consider regarding why the liability model is used to calculate risk only among kindred rather than for the general population is the issue of the degree of genetic susceptibility to the expression of a disorder versus the degree of genetic protection or resistance to the expression of a specific disorder. Much more is known about susceptibility than about resistance. These issues are discussed later in this chapter.

Twin Concordance

Twin concordance can help determine how much genetics contributes to disease. If twins are *monozygotic* (identical), they share nearly identical genomes. If one twin has a disease that is completely due to genetic variants, then the likelihood of the other twin having the same disease is 100%. If environment plays a role, the likelihood of the second twin having the disease goes down a bit. It goes down as well if environment is important and the monozygotic twins were raised apart, because they did not share the same environment after birth. *Dizygotic* (fraternal) twins share only about 50% of their genomes. Most are raised together and so share much of their environment. If the incidence of a trait being shared by twins is equal for monozygotic and dizygotic twins, it is likely to have a strong environmental component and some genetic contribution. For example, consider a trait like diabetes mellitus type 2 (DMT2). Studies have demonstrated that for this disorder there is a higher twin concordance for monozygotic than dizygotic twins, so the genetic contribution must be stronger than the environmental contribution in DMT2. Chapter 10 has a more in-depth discussion of this issue.

Heritability estimates (the proportion of the variance accounted for by genetic factors) tell us how important genetics is in creating disease risk. Of course, some of these estimates will vary from study to study, depending on the variations in a number of factors, such as the background of genetic traits or variations in the environment being considered; however, you can get a general sense of how heritable something is by looking at a heritability estimate (Table 4–5).

TABLE 4–5

Heritability Estimates of Common Health Problems

Disorder	Heritability Estimate
Schizophrenia	85%
Asthma	80%
Cleft lip/cleft palate	76%
Pyloric stenosis	75%
Coronary artery disease	65%
Hypertension	62%
Congenital hip dysplasia	60%
Anencephaly/spina bifida	60%
Peptic ulcer	37%
Congenital heart disease	35%

Recurrence Risk

Families that already have one child with a genetic disorder are concerned that future children will have the same disorder, which is known as the **recurrence risk.** Providing families with this information is an important service provided by genetic counselors who are educated in both the statistics involved in making accurate estimates and the skills required to counsel worried families. When the disorder follows a clear dominant or recessive pattern, it is a bit easier to provide families with numbers that convey the likelihood that another child will be affected. Remember that if both parents are carriers of a recessive trait, the risk of having an affected child is 25% with each pregnancy. Things are much more complicated when the disorder is complex.

Some factors can help in estimating the recurrence risk for a specific family. For example, the risk is higher if more than one family member is affected. The risk of having a second child with a ventricular septal defect, when a couple already has one affected child, is 3%; however, if this family already has two affected children, the risk of another child being affected goes up to 10%. The risk increases because with two affected children, the parents must be carrying a fairly large number of risk alleles. The family is also at the higher end of the liability curve if their child is severely affected, making it more likely that a sibling will be affected. If the disorder is found more commonly in one sex than the other and the child with the problem is of the less commonly affected sex, the risk to another sibling is also higher. Pyloric stenosis is five times more common among males, so if the child with pyloric stenosis is female, the family probably has a high liability of having other children with this problem. Of course, the more distant the affected relative is, the lower the risk of a child being born with the disorder.

Epigenomics: Gene Expression and the Microenvironment

Overview

Epigenomics is a term that may be new to most people in health care. It adds an interesting layer to our understanding of how genetic information is transmitted and the factors that affect it. The term makes good sense when we break it down into its parts. You already know that the genome is the entire set of DNA in a cell and that contained in the genome is the information needed for constructing every protein needed by the body. You also know that gene expression (resulting in protein production) varies with the physiologic needs of the body and the specific tissue. Genes are turned on or off, depending on the needs of a particular cell.

The word **epigenome** comes from the Greek and means "above" or "on" the genome, just as the term *epicardium* refers to the outer layer of the wall surrounding the heart. The epigenome uses chemicals that affect the structure or that silence parts of the genome, thereby altering gene expression and subsequent protein production. The surprising part is that these modifications can be passed on from generation to generation. As the cell divides, the chemical modifications stay with the parental DNA; these modifications can be altered by interactions with the environment, including things such as parental diet and exposure to environmental toxins. The modifications that science knows most about are DNA methylation, histone modification, and the interaction of microRNAs with the genome.

Methylation

Methylation is the addition of a chemical tag called a *methyl group* to the DNA sequence itself. The presence or absence of methylation can turn gene expression on or off. For example, some genes are expressed only if they are transmitted from the father, and some are expressed only if they are transmitted from the mother. The chemical process of methylation silences the genes from one parent. If a gene with a defect is the only active gene or if there is a deletion and the needed gene is not there, disease will result.

Histone Modification

The DNA double helix winds around histone proteins, which give it structure and stability, allowing the DNA to form chromosomes. Histone (or chromatin) modification involves changes to the proteins around which the DNA double helix winds (see Fig. 1–10). Chemical tags attach to the "tails" of the histones and can alter how tightly the DNA is packaged by adjusting the tension with which it winds. When the DNA is wound tightly around the histones, some sequences of DNA may not be available for transcription, so no protein will be made from that sequence. The gene will appear "turned off." When the DNA is loosened, a gene that was hidden may suddenly be able to interact with the cell's protein-making machinery and appear to be "turned on." In this way, histone modification and DNA methylation can turn gene expression on and off.

MicroRNA

As discussed in Chapter 2, *microRNAs* (miRNA) are small single-stranded pieces of RNA that can bind to messenger RNA, making it double-stranded and preventing protein production. MiRNA can just turn off gene expression. These single-stranded pieces of RNA are only 20-30 bases long, and they do not encode protein. Sometimes they are included as contributing to epigenomic changes. MiRNAs bind to messenger RNA, making it double-stranded; this binding prevents the process of translation. The possibility that miRNA plays a part in the development of cancer is currently being explored.

Epigenomic changes may be caused by a wide variety of environmental factors under prenatal influence, including mother's diet, radiation exposure, foreign chemicals, and even behaviors. Both human and animal studies are supporting these ideas in what is known as the "fetal basis of adult-onset disease" (Jirtle and Skinner, 2007). People with the same genotype (identical or monozygotic twins) often have some phenotype variability. One may have DMT2 while his sibling does not. One may get cancer while her twin remains healthy. All these differences may not be attributable to differences in lifestyle. Both twins may exercise, have a great diet, and deal well with stress, yet one twin still gets sick while the other remains healthy. Epigenomic changes may provide clues about why this happens by altering what scientists call *developmental plasticity* or the ability of the environment to cause different phenotypes from the same genotype (Jirtle and Skinner, 2007).

Identical (monozygotic) twins are most genotypically alike when they are first conceived; the older twins become, the more genotypically and phenotypcially different they become. Epigenomic changes are passed from generation to generation, and they can be the result of environmental influences. Older twins may have been exposed to different environmental influences, such as different diets, living in different geographic locations, or taking different drugs. Epigenomic changes have been implicated in the onset of autoimmune diseases such as systemic lupus erythematosus (Renaudineau, 2010).

Epigenomic changes have also been identified as important contributors to tumor growth in breast cancers and some other cancers. DNA methylation may result in the silencing of tumor-suppressor genes or the activation of oncogenes. Understanding of epigenomics has promising implications for early breast cancer diagnosis and treatment (Dworkin et al., 2009).

A public/private multinational collaboration called the Human Epigenome Project (HEP) is working to identify, record, and interpret DNA methylation patterns throughout the human genome. Because methylation can be altered by environmental influences such as diet, this process is thought to provide the missing link between DNA sequence and the environment. We have known for a long time that environment influences gene expression, but the way this happens has been elusive. Learning about methylation has provided an important step forward in appreciating environmental contributions to our health (Jirtle and Skinner, 2007).

Research studies using agouti mice have taught us a lot about epigenomics and the influence of environmental factors on DNA expression. When mice carry two copies of the dominant agouti alleles, they will be yellow and obese, but the agouti gene *(Avy)* can be methylated (or turned off) to varying degrees. Mice born with variations in methylation vary in color according to the activity of *Avy* activity. Mice with mottled coats will be produced when *Avy* activity varies from cell to cell.

Epigenomic variations occurring while fetal mice grow in their mother's uterus produce offspring with a range of coat colors, despite being genetically identical. In addition to causing variations in coat color, having the agouti gene turned on makes the mice ravenously hungry, resulting in gross obesity. Obese yellow mice have the agouti gene turned on. They are also at a higher risk of cancer and diabetes mellitus type 2. When the *Avy* gene is methylated, it is turned off, and mice have normal appetites and a brown coat color. Scientists have shown that this variation can be manipulated because of the diet's effect on methylation.

Studies with agouti mice have demonstrated some variations in phenotype that can be inherited but are not encoded in the DNA sequence. In 1998, Craig Cooney and his team fed pregnant brown agouti mice different levels of nutrients that supported methylation. These included folic acid, zinc, and the amino acid methionine. The mother mice that were fed higher levels of the supplements produced offspring that were browner in color, leaner, and healthier. This surprising study demonstrated that a mother's diet can affect the offspring's phenotype by altering *Avy* gene expression.

In 2006, Cropley and colleagues completed a study in which pregnant agouti mice were fed a diet rich in methyl donors similar to what Cooney had used. High levels of a methyl-rich diet again produced offspring with browner coats, and this affected not only the offspring of the mice Copley actually fed, but also their grandchildren. It was clear that these changes in methylation were being inherited from one generation to the next. The work by these and other scientists has demonstrated that epigenetic changes are maintained through mitosis and are passed on in the germline during meiosis.

Genomic Variation Influencing Susceptibility and Resistance to Health Problems

Overview

The section of clinical chapters will be discussing how the inheritance of certain gene changes and allele variations increase the risk for developing some health problems. Rarely is the risk as high as 100%, but it can be substantial. Some of these variations have been identified as a result of exploring families who have a higher incidence of single gene-associated disorders, and others have been identified by performing genome-wide association studies (GWAS) to begin to identify groups of changes that together may increase disease risk. In addition to genomic variations that increase risk, scientists believe that some genomic variations exist that actually decrease the risk for disease development. Some of the evidence suggesting this possibility include the observation that longevity seems to "run in some families," just like specific diseases appear to run in others.

Over the years, attention has focused largely on identifying individuals and families at an increased risk for a health problem or birth defect, because often the disorders required significant health-care effort and reduced individual productivity (not to mention quality of life and life span). Attempting to identify a gene for a specific disorder, such as cancer, can be compared to looking for a needle in a haystack. It helps if you start with a haystack that you know contains needles. So, performing genetic studies on family groups who had higher-than-average incidences of a specific disorder was a good start and has led to the identification of many genomic variations that increase the risk for a specific disorder.

Because some families appear to remain free of common disorders and health problems, even when living in geographic areas in which specific problems are common, it is highly likely that some inherited genomic variations actually protect against disease development. Think about the person who has smoked cigarettes since the age of 12 and now continues to smoke four packs daily at the age of 100 with no evidence of lung cancer or chronic obstructive lung disease! Are there such people? Yes, there are; however, they are in the minority and should not be used as role models for living well. Their longevity occurs despite their personal choices and environmental influences, not because of them.

Susceptibility

Variation in allele sequences for single genes does increase the risk for a person to develop a specific disease. As a result, the individual's susceptibility to the disease is greater than that of the general population. For example, having one mutated allele in the *BRCA2* gene increases the risk for a woman who carries that mutation to develop breast cancer from an overall 12% lifetime risk to a lifetime risk of 25% to 50%, and also increases her overall risk for ovarian cancer from less than 1% to 40% to 80%. Because such gene mutations are known to greatly increase risk, they are termed *susceptibility genes.* Thus a **genetic susceptibility** is having one or more gene variations that increase the risk for disease expression. Having a specific mutation that works as a susceptibility gene only increases the risk for disease but does not (often) guarantee it. One exception is mutation of the Huntington disease (HD) gene allele, in which the person who has the mutation has nearly a 100% risk for HD if she or he lives long enough and does not die of something else first. Even when the risk for developing a specific health problem is very high as a result of inheriting one or more susceptibility genes, whether the disease ever occurs appears to be partly determined by the presence of other genetic variations that modify the risk and appear to provide some protective influence.

Many susceptibility genes have been identified that increase disease risk, including those that result in sickle cell disease, colorectal cancer, familial hypercholesterolemia, hereditary hemochromatosis, long QT syndrome, hemophilia, and cystic fibrosis. (The inheritance patterns, pathophysiology, and genetics of these disorders are presented in the clinical chapters.) The susceptibility genes that have been identified are most often those for single-gene disorders that may be inherited in an autosomal dominant, autosomal recessive, or sex-linked recessive manner. It is likely that many more variations exist as multiple gene affects that require interaction to increase susceptibility to disease. Through GWAS, some susceptibility variations have been identified in genes that regulate enzyme activity, inflammation and immune responses, and metabolism.

Resistance

Scientists have termed genes that can protect against the development of a specific disease *resistance genes* or *modifier genes,* which confer **genetic resistance**. Because few genes that may confer disease resistance have been identified currently, they are largely considered "theoretical," but few genetic professionals doubt their existence.

For many decades, health-care professionals and scientists had observed that disease-free longevity was a feature of some families and appeared to be a good predictor of healthy aging. Environmental studies of long-lived individuals do not show consistent lifestyle choices, other than a low animal-fat diet, that contribute to disease-free exceptional longevity. (Remember the *centenarian*—a person who lives to be at least 100 years old—who smoked his way through life.) Although this may represent just good luck, it more likely represents a yet-to-be identified genetic difference that confers protection or resistance to common health problems often associated with aging, such as hypertension, diabetes, and cardiac disease. Of course, the best combinations for healthy aging probably include both a good genetic predisposition to disease-free longevity coupled with a lifestyle that avoids known risky behavior (e.g., sedentary habits, dietary challenges, chemical or radiation exposures, and/or activities associated with a greater possibility of trauma).

For some complex disorders with a strong genetic component, such as diabetes mellitus type 2, disease expression may represent an imbalance among susceptibility genes that promote expression, resistance genes that protect against expression, and personal environmental (lifestyle) choices. For example, a 32-year-old woman has just been diagnosed with gestational diabetes. Although the disorder will resolve within a few weeks after she delivers, this greatly increases her risk (90%) for later developing type 2 diabetes. In examining her family history without performing any genetic studies, her mother and older sister were both diagnosed with type 2 diabetes by age 40. What does this mean for the pregnant woman?

The fact that she has gestational diabetes indicates she has inherited the predisposition for type 2 diabetes and may have few, if any, resistance genes or factors to modify her risk (Fig. 4–9). When the resistance genes and the susceptibility genes are added together, susceptibility wins (Fig. 4–10). Does this mean that her development of type 2 diabetes is inevitable? Not really, because the gene-environment interaction is also in play.

In Figure 4–11, we can see that in considering the risk for developing any disorder, some people have more susceptibility genes with fewer resistance genes, others have more resistance genes than susceptibility genes, and still others have equal input from susceptibility and resistance genes (like offsetting penalties). If people could know their susceptibility versus resistance to a specific disorder, it might be possible to manipulate their environments to support resistance and reduce susceptibility. So, how would this work for the pregnant woman with gestational diabetes?

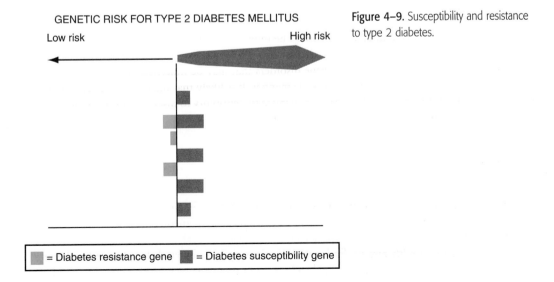

Figure 4–9. Susceptibility and resistance to type 2 diabetes.

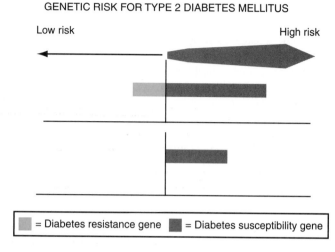

GENETIC RISK FOR TYPE 2 DIABETES MELLITUS

Low risk   High risk

= Diabetes resistance gene   ■ = Diabetes susceptibility gene

Figure 4–10. The interaction of suscepti-bility genes and resistance genes for diabetes mellitus type 2. The top section shows the ratio of one person's suscepti-bility and resistance to type 2 diabetes. The bottom section shows that com-bined, genetic susceptibility to type 2 diabetes greatly overwhelms the person's genetic resistance to the disease.

The two most influential personal environmental factors for the development of type 2 diabetes among people who have a genetic predisposition (susceptibility) to the disorder are a sedentary lifestyle and obesity. If our patient participated in a lifestyle change for either one of these two factors, she might be able to delay the onset of the disorder by as much as 10 years beyond the ages her mother and sister expressed overt diabetes. If she changed both of these factors, she might delay the onset of the disease by 25 or more years, or she might never develop overt type 2 diabetes. Just to illustrate, one of the authors of this text has a friend who really is the 32-year-old described earlier. This friend is now 68 years old and still has a normal fasting blood glucose level and a normal hemoglobin A1c. She started running 5 miles daily after the birth of her 11-pound daughter and has maintained her weight within 5 pounds of ideal for her height (she is 5 foot 9 inches tall and weighs 150 pounds). Will she ever

Figure 4–11. Differences in the risk for disease expression based on the inheritance of specific susceptibility genes and resistance genes.

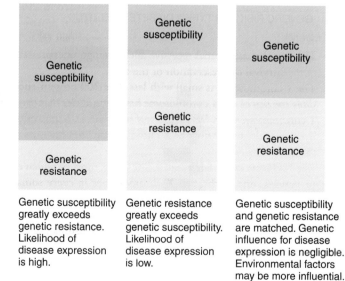

Genetic susceptibility

Genetic resistance

Genetic susceptibility

Genetic resistance

Genetic susceptibility

Genetic resistance

Genetic susceptibility greatly exceeds genetic resistance. Likelihood of disease expression is high.

Genetic resistance greatly exceeds genetic susceptibility. Likelihood of disease expression is low.

Genetic susceptibility and genetic resistance are matched. Genetic influence for disease expression is negligible. Environmental factors may be more influential.

develop type 2 diabetes? Possibly, but she has certainly delayed the onset of the disease and all of its complications by decades. So sometimes you can "beat your genes" by manipulating the disease risk input from the environment.

Summary

Monogenic traits can be explained and shown to follow stable patterns of inheritance with strong patterns of probability prediction. For traits and health problems associated with the input of more than one gene (polygenic input), the probability for expression is more difficult. However, the expression of even monogenic traits can be modified by other genes, the gender of the parent who transmitted the gene, interactions with the environment, and factors that have yet to be identified. Therefore, some of the mendelian rules can be thwarted. In a sense, when we understand how these other factors interact with genetic factors, we may be able to "beat our genes." For example, diabetes mellitus type 2, which is a multifactorial complex disorder, shows a strong autosomal dominant pattern of inheritance, although no specific single gene has been identified as causitive. Environment clearly plays a role because those individuals who have the genetic risk can delay the onset of the disease for two decades (or more) by maintaining a normal weight and participating in a lifelong program of moderate intensity exercise.

GENE GEMS

- Mendelian inheritance applies only to monogenic (single gene) traits and disorders.
- Autosomal dominant traits are expressed whether both alleles are dominant or only one allele is dominant.
- The genotype and phenotype for autosomal dominant traits can be the same but do not have to be the same.
- When a dominant allele is paired with a recessive allele, only the dominant allele is expressed.
- Having a gene for a disorder does not necessarily mean that the disorder will ever develop.
- Many autosomal dominant disorders are lethal in the person who is homozygous for that allele.
- Autosomal recessive traits usually are only expressed in the homozygous state.
- The child of a person who expresses an autosomal recessive trait will have at least one of the two recessive alleles and is an obligate carrier of that trait.
- The fact that autosomal recessive alleles can go unexpressed for many generations contributes to the survival or preservation of the trait.
- The Y chromosome is small with less than 300 protein-encoding gene alleles.
- Only the tips of the Y chromosome have gene alleles that pair with alleles on the X chromosome.
- Y chromosome traits are all paternal in origin and transmitted only from father to son.
- Because males have only one X chromosome, they have only one allele for nearly every gene on the X chromosome.
- The X chromosome has about 1500 genes, most of which code for non–sex-related functions.
- In females, one of the two X chromosomes in every somatic cell is inactivated to prevent a "double dose" of X chromosome alleles.
- X-linked recessive traits and disorders are expressed more frequently among males.
- A man with an X-linked recessive disorder transmits the allele to all daughters and to none of his sons.

Continued

- X-linked dominant disorders are very rare, and males are more profoundly affected than females.
- Punnett square probability is less reliable with smaller numbers of offspring.
- The probability for offspring genotypes and phenotypes is calculated for each pregnancy and not for families as a whole.
- Common disorders that are considered complex multifactorial diseases include some forms of diabetes mellitus, atherosclerosis, obesity, and cancer.
- Complex traits and disorders are neither dominant nor recessive but represent the influence of multiple genes and the environment.
- Complex traits are quantitative expressions that vary within families and within populations.
- Modifier genes are not responsible for an actual genetic feature or product but modify how the trait is expressed.
- Each person has a unique distribution of risk alleles for any complex trait.
- The threshold of expression for a complex health problem or trait varies with each individual, even within a family.
- Heritability estimates help determine how much of the expression of a complex trait is dependent on genetic factors rather than environmental and lifestyle factors.
- When the incidence of trait concordance is higher among monozygotic twins than for dizygotic twins, genetic factors have a stronger influence than environmental factors.
- When the incidence of trait concordance among monozygotic twins is the same as among dizygotic twins, environmental influences are at least equal to or greater than genetic factors.
- Recurrence risks are easier to calculate for monogenic traits or problems than for complex traits.

Self-Assessment Questions

1. What is the difference between the terms *triploidy* and *trisomy?*
   a. Triploidy involves an extra copy of every chromosome, and trisomy involves an extra copy of only one chromosome.
   b. Trisomy involves an extra copy of every chromosome, and triploidy involves an extra copy of only one chromosome.
   c. Triploidies are maternally derived, and trisomies are paternally derived.
   d. Trisomies are fatal more frequently than are triploidies.

2. Which statement is a criterion for an autosomal dominant pattern of inheritance of a specific trait or characteristic that is highly penetrant?
   a. Carriers for the trait may express it but do not necessarily express the trait.
   b. Unaffected family members do not transmit the trait to their children.
   c. Genotypes of individuals expressing the trait must be homozygous.
   d. The trait appears only among male offspring of female carriers.

3. How are *gene penetrance* and *gene expressivity* different?
   a. With penetrance, the gene is either expressed completely or is not expressed at all; with expressivity, the gene is always expressed, but the degree of expression can range from minor to extreme.
   b. Penetrance and expressivity are both related to "gene dosage." With penetrance, only one copy of the gene is expressed, and with expressivity, more than one copy of the gene can be expressed.
   c. Gene penetrance and gene expressivity are different terms for the same concept, which is the excessive expression of recessive alleles.
   d. *Penetrance* refers to the actual gene structure in the DNA, and *expressivity* refers to the chromosome locus of the gene.

4. Why are X-linked recessive disorders expressed in males more frequently than in females?
   a. Hemizygous X alleles in males have homozygous expression.
   b. One X chromosome of a pair is always inactive in all female cells.
   c. Females have more effective DNA repair mechanisms than do males.
   d. Expression of genes from the Y chromosome does not occur among females.

5. If a man with classic hemophilia (X-linked recessive) has children with a woman who is a carrier for the disorder, what is the expected risk pattern?
   a. All sons will be unaffected; all daughters will be carriers.
   b. All sons will be carriers; all daughters will be affected.
   c. All sons have a 50% risk of the disorder; daughters will all either be affected or carriers.
   d. All sons will be carriers; daughters have a 50% chance of being a carrier and a 50% chance of being unaffected.

6. Which statement or condition best demonstrates the concept of "polygenic" inheritance?
   a. A mutation in a single gene results in the expression of problems in a variety of tissues and organs.
   b. The susceptibility to a problem is inherited as a single gene trait, but development of the problem is related to environmental conditions.
   c. A mutated gene is inherited, but the results of expression of that gene are not evident until middle or late adulthood.
   d. Several genes are responsible for the mechanism of hearing and a mutation in any one of them results in hearing impairment.

7. Which situation is an example of modifier gene action?
   a. A mother and father both have type O blood, and their son is born with type B blood.
   b. Two children in the same family both have cystic fibrosis, but one child has more severe symptoms than the other.
   c. Monozygotic twins separated at birth and raised in two different countries are of different heights (3 inches) and different weights (25 pounds).
   d. A woman who has a gene mutation for diabetes mellitus type 2 delays the onset of the disease by exercising and maintaining a normal weight.

Continued

8. Under which condition for a complex disorder is the problem more likely to recur in a family?
   a. The mother's great-grandfather had a milder form of the problem.
   b. The problem is found in only one child in a set of dizygotic twin boys.
   c. The affected child is male, and the disorder usually occurs among females.
   d. The problem has never been seen in the family going back five generations.

9. Which statement regarding the epigenome and its relationship to the genome is correct?
   a. The genome is unchangeable and the epigenome is subject to mutational events.
   b. The epigenome is present only in germline cells, and the genome is present in all cells.
   c. The genome contains the gene coding DNA regions, and the epigenome is composed of other biochemicals that alter gene expression.
   d. The epigenome contains only introns and exons, whereas the genome contains the noncoding DNA regions in addition to the introns and exons.

References

Cropley, J., Suter, C., Beckman, K., and Martin, D. (2006). Germ-line epigenetic modification of the murine A(vy) allele by nutritional supplementation. *Proceedings of the National Academy of Sciences, 103*(46), 17308–17312.

Dworkin, J., Huang, T., and Toland, A. (2009). Epigenetic alterations in the breast: Implications for breast cancer detection, prognosis, and treatment. *Seminars in Cancer Biology, 19*(3), 165–171.

Human Epigenome Project (HEP). Retrieved March 2011 from www.epigenome.org/index.php.

Jirtle, R., and Skinner, M. (2007). Environmental epigenomics and disease susceptibility. *Nature Reviews Genetics, 8*(4), 253–262.

Renaudineau, Y. (2010). The revolution of epigenetics in the field of autoimmunity. *Clinical Reviews in Allergy and Immunology, 39*(1), 1–2.

Self-Assessment Answers

1. a **2.** b **3.** a **4.** a **5.** c **6.** d **7.** b **8.** c **9.** c

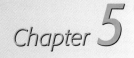

Chapter 5

Chromosomal and Mitochondrial Inheritance and Disorders

Learning Outcomes

1. Use the genetic terminology associated with chromosomal structure, inheritance, and disorders.
2. Apply the basic information about chromosome structure, nomenclature, ploidy, and karyotyping presented in Chapter 1.
3. Compare the developmental, functional, and reproductive consequences for a person who is a balanced translocation carrier with those of a person who has an unbalanced translocation.
4. Identify the common features of people who have the following chromosomal disorders: trisomy 21, trisomy 18, trisomy 13, Klinefelter syndrome, Turner syndrome, and other syndromes with extra sex chromosomes.
5. Explain the consequences of duplicated areas and deleted areas of chromosomal material that contain gene-coding regions.
6. Describe how genomic imprinting can affect the phenotype.
7. Explain how mosaicism of a chromosomal abnormality affects the phenotype.
8. Explain how it is possible for genotypic gender to not match phenotypic gender without artificial intervention.
9. Explain the inheritance pattern for mitochondria and mitochondrial mutations and disorders.

KEY TERMS

Adenosine triphosphate

Balanced translocation

Bipotential gonad

Genomic imprinting

Heteroplasmy

Homoplasmy

Mitochondria

Monosomy

Mosaicism

Nondisjunction

Oxidative phosphorylation

Replication segregation

Reciprocal translocation

Robertsonian translocation

Sex reversal

Translocation

Triploidy

Trisomy

Unbalanced translocation

Uniparental disomy (UPD)

Introduction

As first introduced in Chapter 1, chromosomes are large sections or chunks of DNA that are formed during the metaphase of mitosis in the cell cycle. They are a temporary but consistent state of condensed DNA structure formed for the purpose of cell division, and they are visible during metaphase using a standard light microscope. It is important to remember that although the tightly condensed chromosome structure is temporary, the double-stranded DNA making up each chromosome is a permanent section of the total DNA within one cell's nucleus. Each chromosome contains many genes. Small chromosomes may have as few as 80 to 90 genes, and larger ones have thousands. The most important job of a chromosome is to ensure the precise delivery of the correct amount of DNA to the two new cells generated during mitosis. Please review the "Chromosomes" section of Chapter 1 to become familiar with the basic issues of chromosome structure, nomenclature, ploidy, and karyotyping.

Humans have 46 chromosomes in each somatic cell that has a nucleus. These are arranged in 23 pairs consisting of 22 pairs of autosomes and one pair of sex chromosomes (see Fig. 1–12). One chromosome of each pair was inherited at conception from your father, and the other was inherited from your mother. Thus, in every cell, half of the chromosomes are paternal in origin and half are maternal in origin (see Fig. 1–1). The process of forming mature sex cells that are capable of uniting at conception to start a new person is *gametogenesis*. This process is described in detail in Chapter 3.

Chromosomal Inheritance

Normally, we inherit one copy of each chromosome pair from our mothers and one copy from our fathers. This occurs when each sperm and each ovum have only half of each chromosome pair so that the fertilization of an ovum by a sperm results in one new cell with 23 pairs of chromosomes that can develop into a new person. The cells that become the germ cells (sperm and ova) start out diploid with 23 pairs of chromosomes. During the formation of germ cells through the process of meiosis, the cells become haploid, containing half of each chromosome pair. For ova, most of meiosis occurs in the fetal female ovary, so a girl is born with all of the ova she is ever going to have. For sperm, spermatogenesis (the forming of mature sperm) and meiosis begin at puberty and continue throughout life. For both ova and sperm, the diploid cells become haploid. When conception occurs, the two haploid cells fuse, forming a single diploid cell called a *zygote* that contains the entire human genome.

Although we do inherit half of each chromosome pair from our fathers and half from our mothers, these chromosomes are a mixture of chromosome parts inherited from each of our four grandparents. During the process of making mature gametes, pieces of homologous chromosomes are often exchanged between chromatids, resulting in a "shuffling" effect of our paternal grandparent genes in our father's chromosomes and of our maternal grandparent genes in our mother's chromosomes. This phenomenon is discussed in Chapter 3, in the "Gametogenesis" section.

The most important part of this beginning process in which a zygote is formed is that it inherits exactly the right amount of genetic material from each parent—half from its father and half from its mother. The actual location of the genetic material is less important for normal growth, development, and function. When the location of some genetic material is translocated from one chromosome or part of a chromosome to another, normal development can occur (as long as the correct amount of DNA is present), but reproductive issues often arise in the mature individual.

A **translocation** is a chromosomal abnormality in which all or part of a chromosome is transferred to another nonhomologous chromosome. (A nonhomologous chromosome is not part of the normal chromosome pair. For example, one number 13 chromosome and one number 15 chromosome are a nonhomologous pair, whereas two number 13s or two number 15s are homologous pairs.) A translocation can be balanced or unbalanced. Regardless of the balance status, a translocation is first described by the rest of the karyotype and then is described by a lowercase *t* and the chromosomes involved. For example, a female with a translocation of a number 21 chromosome onto a number 14 chromosome would be described as 45,XX,-14,-21,t(14q;21q). If the translocation involves only parts of chromosomes rather than whole chromosomes, the breakpoints also are listed (if known). For example, a male with a translocation between 12q14 and 22q21 would be described as 46, XY,t(12;22)(q14;q21).

Balanced Translocations

A **balanced translocation** is one in which the right amount of DNA is present (no more and no less) but is not located in its customary place. This type of translocation is very common in human development. Because this translocation is balanced, there is no specific risk either for abnormal development or miscarriage of the fetus, who is a balanced translocation carrier. This individual has the translocation on all cells, and neither phenotype nor physiologic function is affected. The two types of common balanced translocations are robertsonian and reciprocal translocations.

Robertsonian Translocations

A **robertsonian translocation** is a specific type of balanced translocation created by the fusion of the entire long arms (q arms) of two acrocentric chromosomes with loss of the short arms (p arms). (Recall from Chapter 1 that acrocentric chromosomes have the centromere near the very top end of the chromosome.) The acrocentric chromosomes are chromosome numbers 13, 14, 15, 21, and 22. A robertsonian translocation is the most common type of balanced translocation, occurring in about 1 out of every 900 live births. Because the very small p arms of acrocentric chromosomes carry no significant genetic material, their loss does not affect development and normal phenotypic appearance, even though the translocation is present in every somatic and germ cell. However, the person with such a translocation has a karyotype with only 45 chromosomes (Fig. 5–1). Whole chromosome translocations between acrocentric chromosomes are more common than between metacentric or submetacentric chromosomes. The reason for this is that the DNA of the centromeres of two acrocentric chromosomes attract each other, whereas the tips of whole chromosomes have no special attractive force. The presence of a robertsonian translocation can be diagnosed by analysis of plain stained karyotypes; however, identification of the specific chromosomes involved usually requires banding or other more precise chromosome identification techniques (see Chapter 14). Figure 5–2 highlights a t(13;21) robertsonian translocation.

Reciprocal Translocations

Reciprocal translocations are a specific type of balanced translocation in which segments of two nonhomologous chromosomes break and are equally exchanged. Such translocations can occur between any two chromosomes, not just between acrocentric chromosomes. Because there is no loss or gain of genetic material, the translocation is balanced, and the person's development and normal phenotypic appearance are not affected. Also, because this type of translocation involves only chromosome segments rather than whole chromosomes, the person's karyotype shows 46 chromosomes (Fig. 5–3). Although reciprocal translocations can be found incidentally among a small number of anyone's somatic cells, the individual is considered to be a translocation carrier only if the translocation is present in all cells. Identification of the specific chromosome segments involved in any reciprocal translocation requires banding or other more precise techniques for chromosome identification (see Chapter 14).

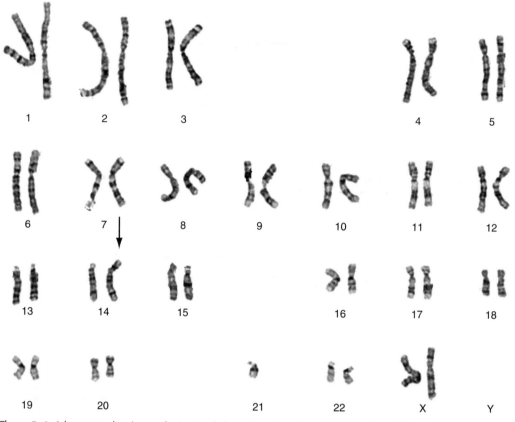

Figure 5–1. A karyotype showing a robertsonian balanced translocation; 45,XX,-der,t(14;21)(q10;q10).

Reproductive Consequences of Balanced Translocations

Although the person who has any type of balanced translocation does not suffer from abnormal development or physiologic function, there can be significant reproductive issues. Remember that the translocation is present in all of the person's somatic cells and in the cells that are or will become germ cells. The precursors to the germ cells were once diploid, having the balanced translocation in all the early germ cells. Formation of the germ cells and progression to gametes (gametogenesis) requires cell divisions known as *meiosis*, in which chromosomal reduction occurs to ensure that resulting gametes are haploid.

So, what are the possible outcomes for gametes from a person who is a balanced carrier of a robertsonian translocation? When the diploid precursor germ cells undergo meiosis, there are three possibilities. Figure 5–4 demonstrates these possibilities for the ova of a woman who has a t(14;21). In the precursor cells, she has one completely normal chromosome 14, one completely normal chromosome 21, and a whole chromosome 21 linked to a whole chromosome 14. This precursor egg is balanced with two normal 14s and two normal 21s. However, when her precursor eggs undergo meiosis, several different results can happen. She may produce a mature ovum that has one separate chromosome 14 and one separate chromosome 21. When this ovum is fertilized with a sperm that also contains one separate chromosome 14 and one separate chromosome 21, the resulting individual has the normal

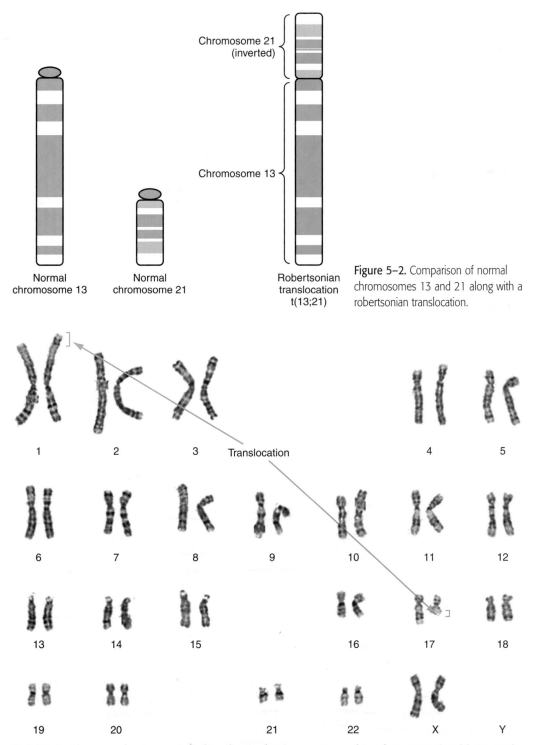

Chromosome 21
(inverted)

Chromosome 13

Normal
chromosome 13

Normal
chromosome 21

Robertsonian
translocation
t(13;21)

Figure 5–2. Comparison of normal
chromosomes 13 and 21 along with a
robertsonian translocation.

1	2	3	Translocation	4	5

6	7	8	9	10	11	12

13	14	15		16	17	18

19	20		21	22	X	Y

Figure 5–3. A karyotype showing a reciprocal translocation between segments of 1 and 17; 46, XX,t(1;17)(p36;q11.2).

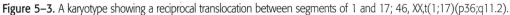

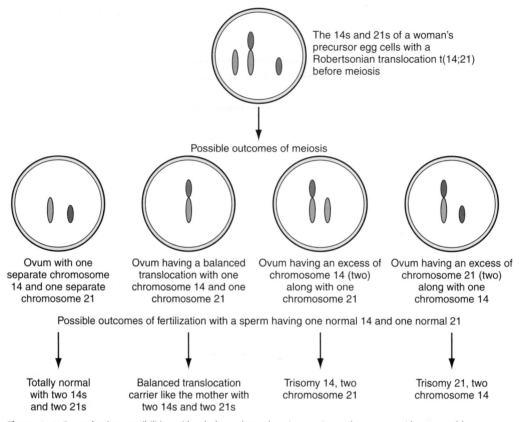

The 14s and 21s of a woman's precursor egg cells with a Robertsonian translocation t(14;21) before meiosis

Possible outcomes of meiosis

Ovum with one separate chromosome 14 and one separate chromosome 21

Ovum having a balanced translocation with one chromosome 14 and one chromosome 21

Ovum having an excess of chromosome 14 (two) along with one chromosome 21

Ovum having an excess of chromosome 21 (two) along with one chromosome 14

Possible outcomes of fertilization with a sperm having one normal 14 and one normal 21

Totally normal with two 14s and two 21s

Balanced translocation carrier like the mother with two 14s and two 21s

Trisomy 14, two chromosome 21

Trisomy 21, two chromosome 14

Figure 5–4. Reproductive possibilities with a balanced translocation carrier and a person with a normal karyotype.

number of chromosomes 14 and 21 and is not even a translocation carrier. For this person, there are no developmental, functional, or eventual reproductive consequences related to being the offspring of a person who is a balanced translocation carrier.

The translocation carrier may also produce a mature ovum with a balanced translocation of one normal chromosome 21 attached to a normal chromosome 14. When this ovum is fertilized with a sperm that contains one separate chromosome 14 and one separate chromosome 21, the resulting individual has the normal number of chromosomes 14 and 21 but is also a balanced translocation carrier. For this individual, there are no developmental or functional consequences related to being the offspring of a person who is a balanced translocation carrier, but the reproductive issues will be the same for this individual as for his or her mother.

The translocation carrier may produce a mature ovum containing a separate chromosome 14 and the additional one that has the chromosome 21 attached. When this ovum is fertilized with a sperm that contains one separate chromosome 14 and one separate chromosome 21, the resulting individual has the normal number of chromosomes 21 but also has trisomy 14, which is not compatible with life.

Lastly, the translocation carrier may produce a mature ovum that contains a separate chromosome 21 and one that is attached to chromosome 14. When this ovum is fertilized with a sperm that contains one separate chromosome 14 and one separate chromosome 21, the resulting individual has the normal number of chromosomes 14 but also has trisomy 21. For this person, there are significant developmental, functional, and reproductive consequences related to being the offspring of a person who is a balanced translocation carrier. (Trisomy 21 is discussed later in this chapter in the "Trisomy 21" section.)

For individuals who have reciprocal translocations, the reproductive issues are similar. If the germ cells created as a result of meiosis have the normal chromosomes rather than the ones containing the translocations, the resulting individual has no chromosomal problems with regard to development, function, or reproductive issues related to the translocation. When the germ cells contain only the chromosomes with the reciprocal translocations and not the normal nonhomologous chromosomes, the resulting individual is a balanced translocation carrier who has no developmental or functional consequences related to being the offspring of a balanced translocation carrier. However, the reproductive issues will be the same for this individual as for the parent who is the reciprocal translocation carrier.

When germ cells created during meiosis have only *one* of the reciprocal translocations along with the normal nonhomologous chromosome, the resulting zygote will be missing specific gene alleles. This can result in failure of the zygote to progress into an embryo, or, if pregnancy progression does occur, it will result in an individual with developmental problems, functional problems, and reproductive issues.

When germ cells created during meiosis have *both* of the reciprocal translocations along with the normal nonhomologous chromosome, the resulting zygote will have three copies of some specific gene alleles. This can result in failure of the zygote to progress, or progression will result in an individual with developmental problems, functional problems, and reproductive issues.

Unbalanced Translocations

An **unbalanced translocation** results when a child inherits more or less than two copies of a chromosome or part of a chromosome from a parent. Such inheritance represents a disproportionate or unbalanced inheritance of the gene alleles on that chromosome and results in abnormal anatomic development and abnormal physiologic function. These unbalanced translocations can lead to trisomy, monosomy, and other chromosomal disorders.

Common Chromosomal Disorders

Trisomy

Overview

Inheritance of an extra copy of one chromosome results in a condition called **trisomy.** For example, Down syndrome, or trisomy 21, results from the inheritance of three copies of chromosome 21 instead of just two copies. Most commonly, trisomies occur when one pair of chromosomes fails to separate properly during meiosis, a problem termed **nondisjunction.** Any chromosome pair can undergo nondisjunction, which results in a trisomy. However, trisomy 21 is the most common trisomic problem that results in a live birth. It is assumed that trisomy of most other chromosomes is not compatible with life.

Examples of Common Trisomic Disorders

The most common disorders of trisomy are trisomy 21, 18, and 13. It is theorized that the reason for these chromosomes to be involved in trisomic conditions that can result in a term pregnancy instead of an early miscarriage is that they contain relatively few gene alleles. Trisomy of chromosomes containing more alleles is more likely to be *embryo lethal*, and the pregnancy does not progress beyond the first trimester. The presence of extra sex chromosomes, especially the X chromosome, also is relatively common.

Most incidences of trisomy occur as a result of nondisjunction during the meiosis of ova, although this can occur during spermatogenesis as well. This condition is most often associated with advanced maternal age at the time of conception (age greater than 35 years is considered "advanced" with regard to pregnancy). Trisomy can also occur as a result of a robertsonian translocation (see earlier), or as a result of an unbalanced translocation of material from one chromosome to another. This condition is rarer and requires more careful or precise chromosome analysis or other genetic testing techniques to identify. The developmental and functional consequences of trisomy are the same regardless of the origin of the extra chromosome material.

TRISOMY 21

Trisomy 21, also known as *Down syndrome*, involves an extra number 21 chromosome in all or most of a person's cells. In the United States, it occurs as frequently as 1 in every 800 births, although the rate is decreasing as a result of prenatal diagnosis and pregnancy termination. The disorder is found among all races and ethnicities.

Developmental and functional abnormalities result from having three copies of all or most alleles on chromosome 21. Table 5–1 lists the common problems or abnormalities associated with trisomy 21. It

---

TABLE 5–1

Abnormalities Associated With Common Trisomic Conditions

Trisomy	Common Abnormalities
Trisomy 21 (Down syndrome)	Decreased intellectual development Congenital heart defects (especially cardiac cushion defects) Simian crease across palms Epicanthal folds with upslanting palpebral fissures Flat facies Widely spaced eyes Slightly low-set ears Small, short nose Brushfield spots (speckling) on iris Short neck with limited motion and extra skin folds Short little finger that curves inward Wide gap between first and second toes Intestinal obstruction Shorter stature than siblings Thicker lips with slightly protruding tongue Poor muscle tone and reflexes (at birth) More likely to have hearing and vision losses at earlier ages Cataract formation Hypothyroidism Premature aging Increased risk for leukemia
Trisomy 18 (Edward syndrome)	Small, strawberry-shaped head with receding chin, small jaw, and elongated occiput Low-set, abnormal ears Clenched fist with overlapping fingers Single palmar creases, arch-patterned fingerprints

TABLE 5–1

Abnormalities Associated With Common Trisomic Conditions—cont'd

Trisomy	Common Abnormalities
	Rocker-bottom feet with a prominent heel (toes may appear large and be fused)
	Severely reduced intellectual development
	Heart malformations (atrial-septal defects, ventricular-septal defects, coarctation of the aorta)
	Kidney malformations
	Esophageal atresia
	Omphalocele
	Inguinal and umbilical hernias
	Brain cysts
Trisomy 13 (Patau syndrome)	Small head (microcephaly)
	Small lower jaw (micrognathia)
	Cleft lip (with or without cleft palate)
	Clenched fist with overlapping fingers
	Single palm crease
	Extra digits on hands or feet (polydactyly)
	Fusion of digits on hands or feet (syndactyly)
	Rocker-bottom feet
	Severe reduction of intellectual capacity
	Low-set ears
	Abnormal iris (split, off-center, keyhole shaped)
	Small, close-set eyes (may even have eye fusion)
	Umbilical and inguinal hernias
	Heart malformations (heart on right side of body [dextrocardia], atrial septal defects, ventricular septal defects, patent ductus arteriosus)
	Abnormal rotation of internal organs
	Fusion of brain hemispheres (holoprosencephaly)
	Deafness
	Vision problems
	Seizures
	Apnea

is important to remember that not all problems or abnormalities are present in any one person who has trisomy 21. In addition, any one (or more) of these problems may be present in a person who has no chromosomal disorder (e.g., having a single palmar crease [simian crease] on one or both palms does not classify a person as having Down syndrome).

Individuals with Down syndrome do share many phenotypic features, such as hair color, eye color, skin tone, blood type, and other inherited characteristics with their family members. However, the classic facial features associated with Down syndrome are unique enough to allow Down syndrome individuals to look similar to each other. Although the life expectancy of individuals with Down syndrome has increased significantly as a result of better diagnosis and management of associated health problems, on average it is still lower than for the general population.

At one time, individuals with Down syndrome were all considered to have severely reduced cognitive ability. However, as a result of having such individuals remain part of a family and participate in all aspects of social interaction, the ultimate level of intellectual function now appears relatively high. Cognition and learning may require more intense interactions and a greater number of practice times, but many skills and cognitive abilities, and the psychosocial perception in people with Down syndrome, approach nearly "normal" levels. Some people who have Down syndrome hold jobs (even as actors who must memorize lines and assume the persona of another individual), drive cars, and have successfully completed college courses. Such individuals are termed *high functioning;* however, the actual intellectual potential for any person with Down syndrome is uniquely dependent on environmental stimulation. As with many disorders that impact cognitive development, the ultimate potential of any affected person to attain completely normal physical and psychosocial development or for less than fully normal development cannot be predicted.

Reproductive issues are also a concern. Males with trisomy 21 are sterile and do not produce off-spring. Females with trisomy 21 have an approximate 50% chance of producing a zygote with trisomy 21 as the result of any conception. However, many of these conceptions do not progress to term pregnancies. So, the actual percentage of children with trisomy 21 born to mothers who have trisomy 21 is considerably less than 50%.

TRISOMY 18

Trisomy 18, also known as Edward syndrome, involves an extra number 18 chromosome in all or most of a person's cells. It is the second most common trisomic condition, occurring in about 1 out of 3000 to 5000 births, affecting many more females than males.

Severe developmental and functional abnormalities result from having three copies of all or most alleles on chromosome 18, and most affected children are stillborn. Of those that are born alive, more than 90% die within the first year of life (Rasmussen et al., 2003). Table 5–1 lists the common problems or abnormalities associated with trisomy 18. Just as for trisomy 21, not all problems or abnormalities are present in any one person who has trisomy 18.

Although very few children with trisomy 18 survive childhood and have greatly reduced intellectual capacity, some are able to interact with family members. Skills such as social smiling, rolling over, and limited self-feeding have been reported (Trisomy 18 Foundation, 2010).

TRISOMY 13

Trisomy 13, also known as Patau syndrome, involves an extra number 13 chromosome in all or most of a person's cells. It occurs in about 1 out of every 10,000 to 16,000 births (National Institutes of Health, 2009).

Severe developmental and functional abnormalities result from having three copies of all or most alleles on chromosome 13, and both stillbirths and early neonatal deaths are common. Of those who are born alive, more than 90% die within the first year of life (Rasmussen et al., 2003). Some of the phenotypic features of trisomy 13 are similar to those of trisomy 18, although others are unique to the disorder. Table 5–1 lists the common problems or abnormalities associated with trisomy 13.

Although most children with trisomy 13 die before their first birthday, some survive into adulthood but are not independent in activities of daily living. In addition to greatly reduced intellectual capacity, physical growth is poor. These individuals are usually short. Depending on which skeletal malformations also occur, some are able to sit, stand, and walk. Those individuals who remain in loving and stimulating home environments tend to interact socially, although speech is extremely limited.

EXTRA X CHROMOSOMES

Having extra copies of the X chromosome is relatively common. This can result in trisomy X, tetrasomy X, pentasomy X, and Klinefelter syndrome.

TRISOMY X. Some women have three X chromosomes (trisomy X) and a karyotype of 47,XXX. This condition is estimated to occur as frequently as 1 in 300 to 400 births; however, because the physical phenotype is normal and the individual is fertile, few are ever diagnosed (Milunsky and Milunsky, 2010). Inactivation of two of the three Xs is most likely the reason for the normal phenotype. The most outstanding and consistent feature is that these women are taller than average and are taller than most family members. Additional associated features may include slight delays in language development and motor skills. An IQ slightly lower than siblings has also been reported, as has a higher incidence of shyness and a lack of self-confidence (Milunsky and Milunsky, 2010). Because these features are not unique to people who have an extra X chromosome and are influenced by both environmental and social factors, variation in the expression of these features is great. Most importantly, the ultimate potential of any affected person for completely normal physical and psychosocial development or for less than fully normal development cannot be predicted.

TETRASOMY X. Tetrasomy X (48,XXXX) and pentasomy X (49,XXXXX) are much rarer conditions than trisomy X, and both are consistently associated with phenotypic abnormalities. Females who are 48,XXXX are usually tall and have a greater reduction in intellectual capacity (IQs range between 35 and 70). The head is small and has minor changes in facial features, such as epicanthal folds and a depressed nasal bridge. There is an overall increased incidence in skeletal abnormalities and unstable behavior (Milunsky and Milunsky, 2010).

PENTASOMY X. Fewer than 40 females who have five X chromosomes have been reported (49,XXXXX). Among these individuals, consistent phenotypic features include greatly reduced intellectual function, short stature, cleft palate, hypotonia, coarse facial features, microcephaly, hypertelorism, and congenital heart defects.

KLINEFELTER SYNDROME. Men can have an extra X chromosome, resulting in a 47,XXY karyotype, also known as *Klinefelter syndrome*. This sex chromosome abnormality (SCA) is a common sex chromosome abnormality seen among live-born children and is estimated to occur in 1 out of every 600 male births (Milunsky and Milunsky, 2010). Fetal survival for this chromosomal abnormality is about 97%, and most individuals are not identified at birth. The cause is both maternal and paternal nondisjunction and is associated with both maternal and paternal aging.

No specific morphologic features are present at birth or through childhood except that the boy is taller than average, with long legs. Puberty usually begins at the expected time, with normal levels of testosterone and the presence of secondary sex characteristics. As the teen ages and becomes a young adult, testosterone levels decline and the gonadotrophin hormone (luteinizing hormone [LH] and follicle-stimulating hormone [FSH]) levels become very high. Changes in genitalia occur, including small testes and a small penis. *Gynecomastia* (breast development in men) is present in about 50% of individuals. Fertility problems include lack of sperm production (*azoospermia*) or greatly reduced sperm production (*oligospermia*) and decreased libido. Health problems that are more likely to develop during adulthood among men with Klinefelter syndrome include osteoporosis, systemic lupus erythematosus, thyroid disease, diabetes, breast cancer, non-Hodgkin lymphoma, and germ cell tumors.

Other features associated with Klinefelter syndrome include a slightly reduced IQ (lower than siblings), delayed or slower language skills and reading, delayed walking, decreased motor skills, and an increase in attention-deficit hyperactivity disorder (ADHD) and autism spectrum disorders (ASD). Again, because these features are not unique to people who have a 47,XXY karyotype and are influenced by both environmental and social factors, variation in the expression of these features is great. Most importantly, the ultimate potential of any affected person for completely normal physical and psychosocial development or for less than fully normal development cannot be predicted.

Although men with Klinefelter syndrome are not able to father children normally, pregnancy is possible through the process of aspirating sperm from the epididymis and then performing either in vitro fertilization (IVF) or intracytoplasmic sperm injection (ICSI). Because the spermatozoa of Klinefelter men may have an extra X chromosome, their offspring have a greater risk for a sex chromosome abnormality.

EXTRA Y CHROMOSOMES

Another sex chromosome abnormality is the presence of an extra Y chromosome, resulting in a 47,XYY karyotype. This karyotype is estimated to occur in 1 out of 1000 male births; however, because there are no phenotypic abnormalities, the actual incidence is not known. The origin of the extra Y chromosome is always paternal (your mother cannot give you a Y chromosome) and occurs as an error in meiosis II of spermatogenesis. This is not an age-related problem.

Most men with 47,XYY are never diagnosed. The only physical association is tall stature, with these men being typically taller than their parents and siblings. A wide variety of psychosocial issues have been associated erroneously with this karyotype as a result of biased data collection. Decades ago, prison populations and those in institutions for the criminally insane were often the source of much testing (without personal consent), and the 47,XYY karyotype was first discovered in these environments. Thus, early genetic papers warned of an excess of psychopathology and socially deviant behavior among people with this karyotype. More recent studies have shown the incidence of psychopathology among 47,XYY individuals to parallel that of the general population.

Other features reported with a 47,XYY karyotype include more severe teenage acne and slower motor and language development. These individuals are reported to have a higher incidence of learning disabilities; are more easily distracted; are hyperactive; are more easily frustrated; and have behavior that is impulsive, disorganized, and aggressive. However, these personal traits may only be present consistently in those individuals whose behavior warranted further study.

Men with a 47,XYY karyotype are fertile. Because the extra Y chromosome is likely to be present in approximately 50% of mature spermatozoa, there is an increased incidence of this karyotype in the male offspring.

Monosomy

Overview

Inheriting only one chromosome of a pair is a condition called **monosomy.** The most common cause of this condition is thought to be nondisjunction during meiosis in which one sex cell with 46 chromosomes should undergo a reduction division that results in two cells, each with half of each chromosome pair. When nondisjunction occurs, one cell will retain a full pair of chromosomes and the other cell does not have that chromosome at all. When this sex cell unites with the opposite sex cell, the resulting individual will have only 45 chromosomes instead of 46. Although in theory monosomy can occur among any pair of chromosomes, the only common incidence of monosomy is Turner syndrome, in which a female is missing one of the X chromosomes and has a karyotype of 45,X. In addition, a very few cases of monosomy 21 have been reported.

Turner Syndrome

The loss or partial loss of an X chromosome results in Turner syndrome and a 45,X karyotype. (Older references may term this *karyotype 45,XO;* however, there is no "O" chromosome.) Studies of early pregnancy losses indicate that this is by far the most common chromosomal abnormality conceived but that 99% do not survive the first trimester. In the United States, the frequency of Turner syndrome is 1 in 1500 to 2500 female live births (Milunsky and Milunsky, 2010).

Girls with Turner syndrome are often identified at birth (or even during pregnancy by ultrasound) because of the presence of "classic" phenotypic features. These include a smaller-than-expected size at full-term pregnancy, neck webbing, pedal edema, and cardiac abnormalities (Table 5–2). On ultrasound, many fetuses have a *nuchal hygroma,* which is a fluid-filled cyst that forms like a collar around the neck. In addition, the prenatal alpha (α) fetoprotein levels are not appropriate for gestational age. Although lower-than-normal levels are most common, higher-than-normal levels have also been reported.

The consistent features of this syndrome include short stature and a decreased childhood growth rate with no adolescent growth spurt. The average final adult height for girls with Turner syndrome who do not receive growth hormone supplementation is 57 inches (Milunsky and Milunsky, 2010). Most

---

TABLE 5–2

Common Features Associated With Turner Syndrome (45,X)

Body Area or System	Feature
Skeletal features	Short stature (few reach a final adult height above 60 inches) Wide chest Disproportionately large hands and feet Congenital dislocated hip Scoliosis Kyphosis Osteoporosis (adult)
Lymphedema	Pedal edema Hygroma
Facial features	High, arched, narrow palate Widely spaced eyes Poor dentition (short dental roots, thin enamel) Wide mandible with small chin Low posterior hairline
Cardiovascular problems	Coarctation of the aorta Bicuspid aortic valve Aortic dissection Hypertension Coronary artery disease Long Q-T syndrome Partial anomalous pulmonary connection
Endocrine problems	Hypothyroidism Diabetes mellitus type 1 Diabetes mellitus type 2
Renal problems	Collecting-system malformations Horseshoe-shaped kidney Malrotation of one or both kidneys
Eye and vision problems	Epicanthal folds Drooping eyelids Uptilted palpebral fissures Red-green color blindness Strabismus Hyperopia

Continued

TABLE 5–2

Common Features Associated With Turner Syndrome (45,X)—cont'd

Body Area or System	Feature
Ear and hearing problems	Malformed ears Unusual relationship between position of eustachian tube and middle ear Excessively high incidence of otitis media Conductive hearing loss Progressive sensorineural hearing loss (adults) Cholesteatoma formation
Cognitive function	Normal intelligence Good verbal skills Some difficulty with math, spatial perception, problem-solving
Secondary sexual features (without hormone supplementation)	Absent or delayed menses Poor breast development Infertility Ovarian dysgenesis with loss of ova and fibrotic changes Small, undeveloped uterus

people with 45,X have some degree of gonadal dysgenesis, although 5% to 10% do menstruate and a few have even become pregnant.

Health problems are common and can be significant for the person who has Turner syndrome (see Table 5–2). Many require careful management to prevent or reduce complications. Life expectancy is slightly less than average, generally as a result of the cardiovascular complications of the syndrome, especially long-term hypertension and hyperlipidemia, which may be present even in early childhood (Bondy, 2007).

Older references describe girls and women who have Turner syndrome to have less than average intelligence and poor social skills. Lower intelligence is not a consistent characteristic of this syndrome, and social interactions are more influenced by family and social environmental factors. Just as for many types of chromosome disorders, the variation in ability among girls and women with Turner syndrome is enormous and ultimate potential cannot be predicted.

Triploidy

Very rarely, triploidy occurs in human development. **Triploidy** is the inheritance of an extra copy of each chromosome, resulting in a person who has 69 chromosomes per cell instead of 46. Although the extra genetic material is balanced in all cells, this condition is usually lethal. Most triploidy conceptions are lost as spontaneous miscarriages, and only a few progress to term. Infants are usually stillborn or die within the first few days after birth. Although an extremely small number of infants with triploidy have survived a few months, none have reached the first birthday. The condition is considered incompatible with life.

The most common cause of triploidy conceptions is the fertilization of one ovum by two sperm. The result is one copy of all maternal chromosomes and two copies of all paternal chromosomes. It is also possible for an ovum to have failed to complete meiosis and have 46 chromosomes. When fertilization of this ovum occurs, the zygote and embryo have two copies of all maternal chromosomes and one copy of all paternal chromosomes. Triploidy is associated with numerous malformations and health problems. The specific problems vary somewhat based on whether the extra set of chromosomes is maternal or paternal in origin. For parents whose infant had triploidy, the risk for conception with another triploidy on future pregnancies does not appear to be increased.

Partial Chromosome Duplications and Deletions

Overview

In addition to having additional or missing whole chromosomes, it is also possible to have extra pieces of and deletions of chromosome material. This is essentially having a triple dose of some gene alleles or a single dose of some alleles. Both types of conditions are relatively uncommon in gene-coding regions. When the duplicated or deleted chromosome material of a gene-coding region is present in most or all of an affected person's tissues, they are usually accompanied by many anatomic and functional problems. Chromosomal analysis of duplications and deletions is usually not sufficient to determine how many copies of genes are affected, and other genetic testing methods are needed to precisely determine which chromosome pieces are involved. Remember that a duplication or deletion large enough to be visualized on chromosomal analysis usually contains a minimum of 200,000 bases.

Duplications represent amplified gene presence and expression. They are more likely to cause a change in phenotype and symptoms if the duplication is large. For example, a duplication of several genes on chromosome 21 provides a triple dose of those genes to the affected individual, and he or she expresses some degree of the Down syndrome phenotype.

Deletions represent a loss of alleles and reduced expression. Just like duplications, deletions are more likely to cause a change in phenotype and symptoms if the deleted area is large. Some children with congenital problems that include reduced intellectual capacity may have small deletions of specific gene alleles that have not yet been identified. For children who have syndromes associated with specific deletions, the functional potential may not truly be known for several reasons. First, because many of these children were predicted to be profoundly retarded, most were placed in institutional care where stimulation was limited and life spans were short. The syndromes were rare, and the need to determine possible functional potential was not considered important or likely to be fruitful. With a more modern approach toward keeping affected children at home in contact with other children and providing more than just custodial care, expectations of function and social interaction are increasing. Just as for many types of chromosome disorders, the variation in function of individuals who have duplications or deletions is great and ultimate potential cannot be predicted.

Unlike trisomy and monosomy, most partial chromosome duplications and deletions are random events that result from chromosomal breakage and structural rearrangement, usually during gametogenesis. They are not related to parental age and, because many individuals who have the duplication or deletion are not capable of reproduction, there is little risk for passing on the aberration. The exception is when the source of the ovum or sperm involved is the unbalanced haploid gamete of a balanced translocation carrier.

Examples of Syndromes of Deletion

A wide variety of deletions in autosomes and sex chromosomes have been found among tissues obtained from spontaneous and induced abortions. The examples presented here, although rare, represent autosome deletions found among live-born children.

WAGR SYNDROME

WAGR syndrome stands for Wilms' tumor, *a*niridia, *g*enitourinary malformations, and *r*etardation. It was noted that children born without an iris *(aniridia)* often had other consistent clinical features, including severely reduced cognitive function (mental retardation) and a variety of genitourinary (GU) tract malformations. The GU malformations can be as mild as first-degree hypospadias, in which the urethral opening on the penis is located off to one side rather than centered, or as severe as complete exstrophy of the bladder. About 40% of children expressing these symptoms at birth went on to develop a specific type of kidney cancer called Wilms' tumor (nephroblastoma), usually before age 5. The consistent expression of this phenotype suggested a chromosome problem; however, the specific deletion was not identified until the late 1970s. The deletion is a relatively small one located in the interstitial band region of 11p(13) on chromosome 11. This deletion can be seen on chromosomal analysis only when the metaphase chromosomes viewed are long and well banded.

It is interesting that the cancer occurs in only 40% of affected individuals, even though the other manifestations are always present. This suggests that the deletion increases the risk for the specific cancer but that actual cancer development requires additional factors. Chapter 12 discusses the genetic basis of cancer development in more detail.

RETINOBLASTOMA

Retinoblastoma is a rare malignant tumor of the retina that generally occurs in early childhood. Most often it is a sporadic cancer, and there is no history of any other family members who have the same type of cancer. In addition, there is an inherited type of retinoblastoma in which the incidence follows an autosomal dominant pattern of expression. Individuals at greatest risk for this type of retinoblastoma are missing the *RB* gene on at least one chromosome 13. The role of the *RB* gene product is to prevent transcription factors from enhancing cell division. In this sense, the *RB* gene is a cancer suppressor gene. When one allele of the pair for this gene is not present, the risk for retinoblastoma greatly increases. (Chapter 12 discusses the roles of transcription factors and cancer suppressor genes in more detail.)

Although retinoblastoma in general is a childhood cancer, individuals with the deletion in chromosome 13 develop the tumor at earlier ages. The tumor has been found in children during the first week after birth and has even been identified by ultrasound during the third trimester of pregnancy. Of note is the fact that other phenotypic features are not associated with this deletion, although the development of other cancers is more common.

CRI DU CHAT

Cri du chat translates from the French as "cry of the cat." It is a syndrome in which affected infants and children have a distinctive cry that sounds like that of a cat. The chromosomal deletion is a small part of 5p in either the terminal or interstitial region of chromosome 5. The manifestations of this disorder include microcephaly, cleft lip and palate, widely spaced eyes (hypertelorism), epicanthal folds, low-set ears with few folds, a small chin, a variety of heart defects, and moderately to severely reduced cognition. In general, the larger the deletion, the greater the degree of reduced cognition.

ANGELMAN SYNDROME

Angelman syndrome occurs as a result of a deletion in the maternally derived chromosome 15 from q11 to q13. The condition is estimated to occur in 1 out of 10,000 to 15,000 births. Children with this deletion commonly have a normal appearance at birth, with no obvious birth defects and some feeding difficulties. As the infant ages, there is developmental delay and a slow gain of head circumference so that the head is microcephalic compared with body size. Over time, the developmental delay and reduced cognition become more apparent. The child learns to walk but usually has an unsteady or clumsy gait with jerky motions. The child smiles and laughs frequently regardless of circumstances. (Very old textbooks describe this syndrome as the "happy puppet" syndrome because of the continual smiling and jerky gait.) This is accompanied by an easily excited personality and hand waving or flapping motions. Speech is usually greatly impaired, although the child can communicate using nonverbal cues and signals.

Most children develop seizure disorders that become less severe with aging but that do persist throughout adulthood. Other features that may or may not accompany the syndrome include the presence of an occipital groove; a tongue that protrudes; a large mouth with widely spaced teeth; drooling; strabismus; and skin, hair, and eye color that is lighter than those of other family members (Williams et al., 2006).

PRADER-WILLI SYNDROME

Prader-Willi syndrome (PWS) occurs as a result of a deletion in the paternally derived chromosome 15 from q11 to q13. It is estimated to occur in 1 out of every 10,000 to 30,000 live births worldwide and affects all races and ethnicities. The loss of alleles from chromosome 15 affects many parts of the body. At birth, infants with PWS have a normal appearance with no obvious birth defects. The face may be narrow and the infant may have skin, hair, and eye coloring that is lighter than those of other family members. The most notable problems in infancy are hypotonia, poor sucking reflex, and failure to thrive (Thomson, 2010).

As the child ages, other characteristic changes are observed. Most children have a short stature with disproportionately small hands and feet. Developmental delay and a mild to moderate reduction in cognition are present. In both males and females, the gonads are small. The most outstanding feature is an insatiable appetite that usually manifests by age 3 years. The food craving and overeating lead to obesity and all of the health problems associated with it. Behavioral problems, especially temper tantrums and poor impulse control, are common. For affected individuals of both genders, puberty is delayed or incomplete, and most are infertile. Without treatment with gender-specific hormones, secondary sex characteristics do not develop. When obesity and its associated health problems are controlled, people with PWS have life expectancies that are the same as the general population.

"How can the same chromosomal deletion result in two very different phenotypes?" If you are not asking yourself this question, go back and reread the Angelman syndrome and Prader-Willi syndrome sections. Then read the next section, which discusses genomic imprinting.

Genomic Imprinting

Genomic imprinting is an epigenetic event in which a gene (or gene allele) is inactivated by means other than mutation, so the DNA sequence of the gene remains normal but its expression is inhibited. This is an abnormal state, and we are unsure of how often it occurs. Usually, imprinting, when it occurs, happens during gametogenesis, which can allow identification of whether the allele is maternally inherited or paternally inherited. When a gene or genes have been imprinted during gametogenesis, the imprint remains in the cells of the conceived child throughout life. The effect of an imprinted gene allele from one parent means that only the nonimprinted allele from the other parent is expressed. For the most part, when the nonimprinted gene allele is normal, its sole expression is not a problem. Problems arise with sole expression of mutated nonimprinted gene alleles.

For example, suppose a couple has decided to have a baby, and they are concerned about the possibility of having a child with sickle cell disease in which there is an abnormality in the beta chain of hemoglobin. This disease is autosomal recessive and is expressed only in individuals who are homozygous for a mutation in the *HBB* gene (loci on chromosome 11). Testing of this couple finds that the husband is heterozygous for an *HBB* mutation and the wife is homozygous for normal alleles of the *HBB* gene. The possible outcome of a pregnancy for this couple is a child who is either homozygous for normal *HBB* gene alleles or is heterozygous with one mutated and one normal *HBB* allele (and would be a carrier of sickle cell disease). So, the couple goes ahead, gets pregnant, and has a daughter.

Shortly after birth, testing shows the daughter to have only one mutated *HBB* allele, and she is expressing only hemoglobin S. Further testing shows that the maternal normal *HBB* allele is not being expressed in this child as a result of imprinting.

Another cause for such a scenario is the loss of the mother's *HBB* allele and a duplication of the father's mutated *HBB* allele, so the child is homozygous for the sickle cell gene. This strange occurrence can be the result of **uniparental disomy (UPD)** in which both chromosomes of a pair (in this case, chromosome 11) come from just one parent. The gamete of the father contained two of his number 11 chromosomes instead of just one. For this to work out, the mother's ovum had to be completely missing chromosome 11. So in this case, two mistakes are still mistakes!

Now let's get back to how the same deletion of 15q can result in either Angelman syndrome or Prader-Willi syndrome, depending on which parent contributed the chromosomal deletion. For decades it was assumed that one chromosome of a pair that had all normal gene alleles was the same as a homologous chromosome with all normal gene alleles from another person, even one of the opposite gender. The Angelman and Prader-Willi issue tells us that something is different for at least chromosome 15 between men and women. When no maternal material from 15q(11–13) is present and only paternal material is expressed, Angelman syndrome results. When no paternal material from 15q(11–13) is present and only maternal material is expressed, Prader-Willi syndrome results.

When a child has uniparental disomy of chromosome 15 with both chromosomes being derived from the father, and there is no deletion of material on either chromosome, Angelman syndrome results. Even though no deletion exists, without maternal input, the result is the same as if one chromosome 15 had a deletion. The same situation occurs when both copies of chromosome 15 are inherited from the mother so that there is no paternal input, resulting in Prader-Willi syndrome.

Only a few other disorders have been found to be associated with uniparental disomy of other chromosomes, although instances of uniparental disomy have been documented for nearly all human chromosomes. These include Beckwith-Wiedemann syndrome (chromosome 11) and cystic fibrosis (chromosome 7). Although rare, the possibility of uniparental disomy needs to be considered when a person expresses an autosomal recessive disorder but only one parent is a carrier or is affected. This phenomenon can relieve the pressure placed on a mother when an infant demonstrates an autosomal recessive trait for which she is a carrier but the father is not. Obviously, this complicates genetic counseling and demonstrates that the "gray area" of genetics/genomics is getting larger rather than smaller as more is known.

Mosaicism

Mosaicism is a condition in which two (or more) different karyotypes are consistently present in one individual. This represents that some cells have an abnormal karyotype and others have a normal karyotype. There have been many misconceptions and "reconceptions" about mosaicism. For example, when parents are told that their baby boy has Down syndrome with mosaicism and the proportion of cells with 47 chromosomes (47,XY,+21) is 70% and the cells with 46 chromosomes (46,XY) is 30%, they sometimes assume that this child is "only 70% a Down syndrome individual" and will be at least 30% "smarter" than the average person who has "pure" Down syndrome. Years ago, such parental hopes were dashed as they were told that Down syndrome is Down syndrome. Now such beliefs and issues are less clear.

First of all, mosaicism can be tissue-specific, meaning that some tissues can express a mixture of normal and abnormal karyotypes, and other tissues may express all or nearly all of just one type.

Because most cytogenetic studies are performed on blood cells or skin cells, when mosaicism is found in these tissues, the percentage of cells with abnormal karyotypes may not represent the actual proportion of cells with the abnormality in other tissues. So, it is possible for a person to have 70% of his blood cells be 47,XY+21 and perhaps have the proportion of 47 chromosome cells be very small in the brain. Geneticists suggest that tissue-specific differences in mosaicism may be responsible for the extreme variation seen in behavior and cognition among people with the same chromosome disorder. After all, we do not biopsy brain cells to check the ratio of chromosomally normal to chromosomally abnormal neurons in living people.

One example of mosaicism is the birth of monozygotic twins diagnosed with trisomy 13 mosaicism by amniocentesis at 16 weeks gestation. The parents chose not to terminate the pregnancy, and the twin girls were born at 37 weeks gestation. Twin A had the classic phenotype of trisomy 13 and died within 12 hours after birth. Twin B had no observable features of trisomy 13, although her blood cells demonstrated 50% mosaicism.

Twin B is now 15 years old and still maintains 50% trisomy 13 mosaicism in her blood cells. She is very pretty, is an honor student, is on the varsity field hockey team, and is in the high school marching band. She has been counseled that her risk to conceive a child with trisomy 13 is likely to be greater than the general population based on statistical probability alone. (Her eggs have not been karyotyped to know what the mosaicism percentage is in that tissue, if any.)

What is the explanation for this huge difference between two identical twins? The most likely process is that the nondisjunction causing the trisomy 13 did not occur in one of the parental gametes before conception but occurred in one of the dividing embryonic cells after conception (Fig. 5–5). This had to occur before the original embryo split into two embryos. So, suppose at the 32 cell stage of the embryo, cell division resulted in 64 new cells; one contained 47 chromosomes with three number 13 chromosomes, and one contained only 45 chromosomes with just one chromosome 13. The remaining 62 cells had 46 chromosomes with two number 13 chromosomes. As this 64 cell stage embryo underwent another round of cell division, 127 cells resulted (124 with 46 chromosomes, two with trisomy 13, and the one monosomy 13 cell did not divide). By the time the embryo split to form two separate embryos, it contained perhaps 1008 cells, and only 16 of them had trisomy 13 (the cell with monosomy 13 died off). So, 504 cells go to each of the two new embryos, but the trisomic cells are not equally divided between these embryos. One embryo receives 15 trisomic cells and 489 normal cells, and the other receives 1 trisomic cell along with 504 normal cells. So embryo A has 15 times the dose of trisomic cells at this stage than embryo B. As development progresses and commitment occurs, it is possible that few, if any, trisomic cells are the precursor cells for any of embryo B's vital organs (and those trisomic cells may not continue to divide at the same rate as the normal cells). As a result, embryo B (eventually, twin B) has a very low percentage (if any) of trisomy 13 cells in her brain, heart, liver, and other vital organs, whereas embryo A (twin A) has a much higher percentage of trisomy 13 cells in all her tissues, leading to abnormal development.

The situation presented above is an actual but rare case. However, its existence complicates counseling issues and predictability for mosaicism. Many geneticists believe that low-level mosaicism for chromosome abnormalities is higher among the general population than first thought, but because such individuals have no functional problems, they are not diagnosed. Additionally, based on the very high rate of spontaneous pregnancy loss for embryos with Turner syndrome (99%), some geneticists purport that all living girls and women with Turner syndrome really are mosaic for 45,X, just not in the blood or skin tissues that are used for chromosome analysis.

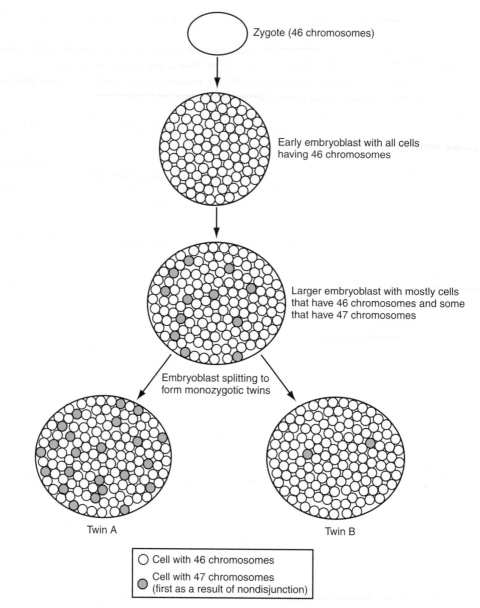

Figure 5–5. Possible mechanism for unequal mosaicism in monozygotic twins.

Genotype-Phenotype Gender Mismatch

Overview

After karyotyping became possible, some people were discovered to have the genotype of one gender and the phenotype of the opposite gender without undergoing surgery, hormonal manipulation, or any other form of artificial or intentional phenotype adjustment. These are not very common problems, but they do occur. So, there are phenotypic women who have a 46,XY karyotype and phenotypic men who have a 46,XX karyotype, conditions known as **sex reversal.**

When we are conceived, our genetic gender is determined by chromosome constitution. Usually, zygotes with a 46,XY genotype develop into phenotypic males, and those with a 46,XX genotype develop into phenotypic females. In addition to the sex chromosomes, many autosomal genes are needed to ensure an appropriate gender match between genotype and phenotype.

When the hollow ball of the early embryoblast cells begins to organize after commitment (see Chapter 3) into various early tissues that will become specific organs, a structure known as a **bipotential gonad** forms in both males and females. This development begins during the fifth week after conception in the urogenital ridge area of the embryo. The bipotential gonad, at one time known as an *indifferent gonad,* has the potential to develop into a testis or an ovary, depending on which hormones and other factors influence it. Usually, in a 46,XY embryo, this tissue forms a testis, and in an embryo with a 46,XX karyotype, it forms an ovary. In addition to this bipotential gonad, there are other tissues that develop into male or female sex organs, depending on the presence of genetic, hormonal, and some unidentified factors. The important concept to remember here is that these tissues are present in both XX and XY embryos.

Early embryonic tissue capable of developing into male sex organs, including the penis, scrotum, prostate, and the tubular system connecting the testis to the urinary system, is the mesonephric ductal tissue (wolffian glands). The tissue capable of developing into female sex organs is the paramesonephric ductal tissue (müllerian ducts). The mesonephric tissues have androgen (testosterone is one androgen) receptors on them, and the paramesonephric tissues do not.

Normal Gender Development

Initial Male Development

The Y chromosome has several genes that work in coordination to cause the bipotential gonad to organize early into a testis and begin secreting the androgen testosterone. One of these genes is the *SRY* gene, whose product is testis-determining factor (TDF). Other gene products with loci on the Y chromosome are the anti-müllerian factor (also known as *müllerian inhibition substance*) and the H-Y antigen. The H-Y antigen and TDF together organize the bipotential gonad into a testis, which then begins secreting testosterone as early as 6 to 7 weeks after conception. The testosterone binds to receptor sites on the mesonephric ductal tissue and causes it to undergo mitosis and differentiation into anatomic male sex structures. At the same time, anti-müllerian factor causes regression and degeneration of the paramesonephric ductal tissues so that anatomic female sex structures do not develop.

Initial Female Development

At one time, geneticists believed that complete female development associated with the 46,XX genotype occurred purely as a result of the absence of a Y chromosome, a theory called *default sex.* However, this is no longer the simple answer. Complete female development requires the input of maternal hormones, the absence of Y chromosome-associated gene products, the input of both X chromosomes, and the input of factors from autosomal gene products.

Without the presence of TDF, testosterone, and anti-müllerian factor, the mesonephric ducts regress and degenerate. Under the influence of maternal hormones, the bipotential gonad develops into an active ovary around 6 weeks after conception that almost immediately begins generating cells that will become future ova. The lack of anti-müllerian factor together with the genetic influence of autosomal gene products causes the development of the paramesonephric ductal tissues into complete anatomic female sex structures.

Sex Reversal

Multiple genetic mutations or rearrangements can be involved in sex reversal. The mechanisms presented here describe only the most common ones that have been identified as actual physiologic phenomena and are not merely theoretical.

XY Females

An identified genetic problem resulting in an XY genotype with a female phenotype is complete androgen insensitivity or androgen insensitivity syndrome (AIS), and appears to occur at a rate of 1 in about 50,000 live births. (This condition was originally known as *testicular feminization* before the actual mechanism had been elucidated.) In this condition, all tissues, including the masculine tissues (mesonephric ductal tissues), are missing androgen receptors. An interesting fact is that the androgen receptor gene (*AR*) is located on the X chromosome, not the Y (normal women do have some androgen receptors and can respond to both internal and external androgens).

In individuals who have complete androgen insensitivity, the presence of the Y chromosome starts the organization of the bipotential gonad into a testis at the appropriate time in embryonic life. This testis begins secreting testosterone; however, the testosterone has no developmental influence on the mesonephric ductal tissues, because they lack the receptors for binding and allowing the testosterone to change the gene activity of these cells. Thus, the mesonephric ducts regress and the paramesonephric ducts undergo partial growth. At birth, the child has female external genitalia.

Often, it is not until puberty that the individual and her parents begin to suspect something is not quite right. This girl does go through her adolescent growth spurt and starts to develop hip curves and breasts, but she does not begin menstruation. On physical examination, the girl is found to have a vagina that ends as a blind pouch, with no accompanying uterus and fallopian tubes. Although scalp hair is plentiful, all body hair, including axillary and pubic hair, is sparse. The once organized testicular tissue, often located within the abdomen or inguinal canals rather than in the correct ovarian position, may or may not continue to produce androgens that essentially have no target tissue. However, this gonad is at higher risk of developing testicular cancer.

A girl with complete AIS cannot become pregnant but is female in every other sense. The genitalia at birth appears clearly female, and this phenotype continues throughout life. The person may even have an enviably female figure. In fact, there is a well-known Hollywood actress who has complete AIS. This individual does not doubt her femininity and, now in her 50s, is a strikingly beautiful woman with a 46,XY karyotype.

When androgen insensitivity is partial, there is greater variation in phenotype, sexual identification, and sexual function. This problem is beyond the scope of this text.

XX Males

So, without a Y chromosome and its genes, which are important to male development, how can a person with an XX genotype naturally develop an XY phenotype? Remember that the Y chromosome contains relatively few genes. When the *SRY* gene is present, even if a complete Y chromosome is not, male sex structures can develop and result in a male phenotype.

The most common cause of this phenomenon is translocation of the *SRY* gene onto one of the X chromosomes (46,XX+SRY), which occurs in 1 out of every 20,000 to 25,000 live births. As a result, men with this genotype share many characteristics with men who have Klinefelter syndrome. Phenotype exceptions are that XX men tend to have a shorter-than-average final height, normal intelligence, and normal penile length. Just like men with Klinefelter, these men produce no sperm and are infertile. Some sexual development problems are more common in XX men, including some degree of *hypospadias* (abnormal location of the urethral opening) and *cryptorchidism* (undescended testicles).

Just like for AIS, there are varying degrees of expression of XX^{+SRY}. Discussion of these variations is not within the scope of this text.

Mitochondrial Gene Inheritance

Overview

Mitochondria are organelles (little organs) within a cell's cytoplasm that are responsible for generating most of a high-energy chemical substance used to power cellular work. In this sense, mitochondria are considered the "power plants" of cellular energy production. These organelles contain the very small amount of cellular DNA (extranuclear DNA) that is not located in the nucleus, which is known as *mitochondrial DNA* or *mtDNA*. There are many copies or sets of mtDNA in every mitochondrion.

Mitochondrial DNA differs from nuclear DNA in several ways. The shape of mtDNA is circular, and this circle is sometimes referred to as the *mitochondrial chromosome*. The mtDNA replicates separately from nuclear DNA during cell division. A critical difference is that both mtDNA replication and subsequent distribution are not as well regulated as nuclear DNA replication and distribution. Thus, there is no mechanism to ensure that each new daughter cell receives an equal amount of mitochondria and mtDNA. Because mtDNA has few, if any, DNA repair mechanisms, it is more prone to permanent mutations than is nuclear DNA. In addition, mtDNA appears to have only coding regions (exons) for 37 genes and no noncoding regions (introns). As a result, any mutation is much more likely to affect the expression of one or more mtDNA genes.

Function

Recall that all normal body cells perform at least one differentiated function that always requires energy. A common energy source used in cellular actions and reactions is that derived from the breakdown of the high-energy compound **adenosine triphosphate (ATP).** This compound contains two high-energy "squiggle" bonds that, when broken (hydrolyzed), release a large amount of energy within the cell to perform important functions. Although ATP and a few other high-energy substances can be generated outside of the mitochondria, the reaction that most efficiently generates large amounts of ATP without the buildup of toxic wastes is **oxidative phosphorylation.** This reaction occurs within the mitochondria and requires sufficient amounts of oxygen and hydrogen molecules that have been stripped from our essential foodstuffs, especially carbohydrates.

The process of oxidative phosphorylation is driven by a number of gene products, many of which are present only in the mitochondria. Each mtDNA chromosome contains the coding genes for 37 products that, together with an additional 74 small products from nuclear DNA genes, ensure proper activity of oxidative phosphorylation and the generation of ATP. The mtDNA gene products include 13 small proteins that are parts (subunits) of the enzymes needed for oxidative phosphorylation, along with two types of ribosomes and the 20 different types of transfer RNAs (tRNAs) needed for translation during the synthesis of enzymes used to drive the oxidative-phosphorylation process.

Different cells vary in the amount of mitochondria present in the cytoplasm. Those cells that are least active, such as mature red blood cells, have few, if any, mitochondria. Cells that continually work or perform multiple functions, such as liver cells, skeletal muscle cells, and cardiac cells, each contain thousands of mitochondria. When a mutation results in specific mtDNA product not being made, the cell's energy supply may be insufficient to perform its functions properly. Problems related to disorders of mtDNA appear first in cells that require a continuous supply of large amounts of ATP.

Parental Origin

An interesting feature of mtDNA is that it is all maternally derived. Maternal inheritance of mtDNA occurs because of the basic structures of the mature gametes, the ovum, and sperm. The mature ovum is the largest single cell in the human body and has a relatively small nucleus because it is haploid. Thus, the cell contains a large volume of cytoplasm and mitochondria that will be distributed to the new cells after fertilization for many rounds of cell division. New cytoplasm and new mitochondria are not generated for several days after fertilization. The actual size of the egg does not increase with many rounds of cell division because, with each division, the cells within the egg become smaller. Because the work of the ovum after fertilization is rapid cell division (a process that requires high energy), the cytoplasm of the mature ovum contains at least 100,000 mitochondria, each containing a lot of mtDNA. This amount represents close to one-third of the total DNA content of the mature ovum.

Mature sperm, on the other hand, are the smallest cells in the body and contain practically no cytoplasm. (The mature ovum is about 1000 times larger than a mature sperm.) In addition, the little cytoplasm with mitochondria that a sperm does have is located in the middle tailpiece, which drops off the sperm when it penetrates the ovum during fertilization. Thus, these mitochondria never become part of the zygote. Essentially, the mature sperm is a swimming haploid nucleus (Fig. 5–6). Its mitochondria are located outside the cell at the connection between the sperm head and the principal tailpiece. The purpose of these mitochondria is to generate the energy needed to move the tail for sperm propulsion.

At fertilization, the sperm head with its nucleus and no mitochondria enters the mature ovum to form a zygote. This zygote now is the large diploid mature ovum, complete with all its cytoplasm and approximately 100,000 maternal mitochondria, each containing thousands of copies of mtDMA. Figure 5–7 shows the first five rounds of cell division for this zygote in which nuclear DNA is replicated and the number of cells increased, but the initial size of the ball of cells does not enlarge.

Figure 5–6. Anatomy of a mature sperm.

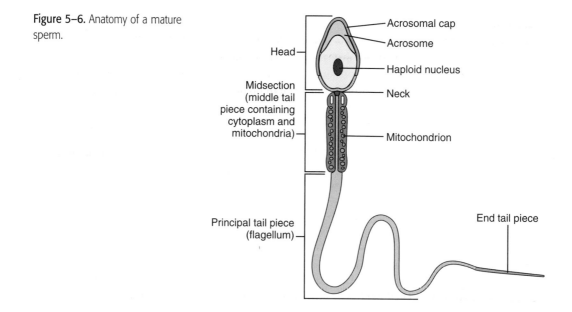

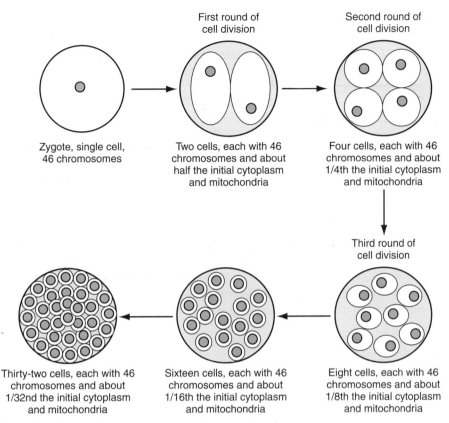

First round of
cell division

Second round of
cell division

Zygote, single cell,
46 chromosomes

Two cells, each with 46
chromosomes and about
half the initial cytoplasm
and mitochondria

Four cells, each with 46
chromosomes and about
1/4th the initial cytoplasm
and mitochondria

Third round of
cell division

Thirty-two cells, each with 46
chromosomes and about
1/32nd the initial cytoplasm
and mitochondria

Sixteen cells, each with 46
chromosomes and about
1/16th the initial cytoplasm
and mitochondria

Eight cells, each with 46
chromosomes and about
1/8th the initial cytoplasm
and mitochondria

Figure 5–7. Five rounds of cell division after the conception of a zygote.

Replication

Replication of mtDNA occurs only within the mitochondria, even in cells that will become mature ova. Within the ovum, mitochondrial and mtDNA replication does not occur at the same time that meiosis of the nuclear DNA occurs. Most mitochondrial and mtDNA replication in ova is a fairly rapid process. This means that replicated segments of mtDNA do not remain in close contact with each other, and there is no "crossing over" or swapping of chromosome material between segments. In addition, after replication, mtDNA is randomly sorted and distributed into the newly produced mitochondria. When mitochondrial reproduction is occurring during typical mitosis of somatic cells, the newly produced mitochondria are distributed randomly into the two new daughter cells. When the mtDNA remains unmutated, this random assortment and distribution has no particular meaning. However, when a mutation occurs within mtDNA, random assortment and distribution are responsible for variance in the extent of impairment and which tissues are involved or impaired.

Mitochondrial Disorders

Overview

More than 100 different point mutations in mtDNA have been observed to cause human disorders, some of which are apparent in childhood and some that do not manifest until adulthood. Mitochondrial disorders occur at a rate of about 1 out of every 10,000 live births (Scaglia et al., 2004). Some people with mutations of mtDNA have observable clinical and functional impairments, whereas others may have no manifestations of disease but do have either a specific mutation in mtDNA, reduced enzyme activity, changes in the appearance of some cells, or indicators of impairment in metabolism.

The majority of problems associated with mtDNA mutations and mitochondrial disease are present in the musculoskeletal, cardiovascular, and neurological systems. Why are the results of mtDNA mutations more apparent in these systems and tissues? Because these cells are highly dependent on the mitochondrial production of ATP and contain many thousands of mitochondria per cell. The significant reduction or loss of mitochondrial ATP production in these cells results in an observable reduction of function. The mechanisms for mtDNA mutations that cause mitochondrial disorders can include problems in transcription, translation, or post-translational modification of proteins and polypeptides coded for by mtDNA (Smits, Smeitink, and van den Heuvel, 2010). Table 5–3 lists examples of human diseases caused by mutations in mtDNA.

Some mitochondrial diseases affect only one tissue or organ and may become obvious only in adulthood, such as Leber's hereditary optic neuropathy (LHON), in which the person develops bilateral, painless, blurred vision followed by progressive vision loss during young adult life. Other mitochondrial diseases affect many tissues and organs and manifest in relatively early childhood. One such disorder is myoclonic epilepsy with ragged red fibers (MERRF). The first symptom is myoclonus and

TABLE 5–3

Examples of Mitochondrial Diseases

Disorder/Disease	Specific Mutation (When Known)
Chronic progressive external ophthalmoplegia (CPEO)	*tRNA^Asn*
Kearns-Sayre syndrome (KSS)	Large deletions of mtDNA
Leber's hereditary optic neuropathy (LHON)	*MT-ND1* *MT-ND2* *MT-ND4* *MT-ND4L* *MT-ND5* *MT-ATP6* *MT-CYB* *MT-CO3*
Leigh syndrome	T8993G and T8993C mutations of *MT-ATP6;* sequence variance in all mitochondrial genes
Mitochondrial encephalomyopathy, lactic acidosis, and strokelike episodes (MELAS)	3243A>G in *MT-TL1*
Mitochondrial neurogastrointestinal encephalopathy (MNGIE)	*TYMP* (on chromosome 22)
Myoclonic epilepsy with ragged red muscle fibers (MERRF)	8344A>G in *MT-TK;* 8356T>C in *MT-TK;* 8363G>A in *MT-TK;* 8361G>A in *MT-TK;* sequence variance in all mitochondrial genes
Neuropathy, ataxia, retinitis pigmentosa (NARP)	8993C>T in *MT-ATP6*

usually occurs in early childhood sometime after the toddler stage. This is usually followed by generalized epilepsy, ataxia, muscle weakness, and dementia. Other associated findings include hearing loss, short stature, optic atrophy, and cardiomyopathy. Another multisystem mitochondrial disease is **mitochondrial e**ncephalomyopathy, **l**actic **a**cidosis, and **s**trokelike episodes (MELAS) that usually begin in childhood. Early childhood development is usually normal, and the onset of initial symptoms (generalized tonic-clonic seizures, recurrent headaches, anorexia, weakness in arm and leg muscles, and recurrent vomiting) occurs before 10 years of age. After seizures, the person often has strokelike problems with brief periods of one-sided paralysis and blindness. By adolescence or young adulthood, most patients have impaired motor abilities, vision, hearing, and cognition. The eventual development of diabetes mellitus is common. For those mtDNA diseases that affect multiple organs and tissues, fatigue is the most prevalent early symptom.

Mechanisms of Variation in mtDNA Mutation Expression

Most mitochondrial diseases that result from point mutations usually are inherited from the maternal line as mutations in the germ cell mtDNA. Those that result from deletions or duplications may not be inherited but occur from somatic cell mtDNA mutations during the early embryoblast stage of development. So, how is there such variation in expression with regard to the tissues involved and the degree of impairment?

Three mechanisms are largely responsible for variation in expression of mitochondrial disease, whether the disease is maternally inherited or results from mtDNA deletions that occur after conception. These mechanisms are replication segregation, homoplasmy, and heteroplasmy.

REPLICATION SEGREGATION

Replication segregation is the random sorting of newly synthesized mitochondria to new daughter cells. When a mutation first occurs in mtDNA, it is present in only one mtDNA molecule of a single mitochondrion within one cell. As mtDNA within that single mitochondrion replicates, that mitochondrion eventually has multiple copies of mtDNA with the mutation along with multiple copies of normal mtDNA. The ratio of mutated mtDNA to normal mtDNA is relatively low. However, this is all still in one cell. If that cell is not capable of cell division, the mtDNA mutation does not affect the energy production of the tissue or organ, because the loss of one cell's function within a tissue of billions of cells is at too low a level to be problematic.

When this cell that contains a particular mixture of mitochondria with mutated mtDNA and mitochondria with normal mtDNA undergoes cell division, each mitochondrion replicates and the total number of mitochondria are divided between the two new daughter cells. However, because the mitochondria are randomly segregated (distributed) into the two new daughter cells, these two new cells each only contain approximately equal numbers (amounts) of mitochondria, but the ratio of mutated mtDNA to normal mtDNA is unlikely to be equal. When one daughter cell's cytoplasm contains mitochondria with either all normal mtDNA or all mutated mtDNA, the condition is termed **homoplasmy.** When one daughter cell's cytoplasm contains a mixture of mitochondria that have normal mtDNA and mutated mtDNA, the condition is termed **heteroplasmy.** (The actual unequal distribution of mutated mitochondria during cell division occurs in a manner similar to the unequal distribution of the extra chromosome in Fig. 5–5.)

HOMOPLASMY

When a daughter cell with homoplasmy of the mitochondria divides, all resulting new daughter cells will have the same mitochondrial population as this cell. If the original daughter cell is homoplasmic for mitochondria with normal mtDNA, the immediate new daughter cells will also be homoplasmic for mitochondria with normal mtDNA (providing there is no mutational event occurring in these cells). On the other hand, if the original daughter cell is homoplastic for mitochondria with mutated mtDNA, the immediate new daughter cells also will be homoplasmic for mitochondria with mutated mtDNA. As this cell reproduces, more cells that are homoplasmic for mitochondria with mtDNA are produced, eventually resulting in a tissue or organ that has a high concentration of cells with impaired energy generation and reduced function.

HETEROPLASMY

When a daughter cell with heteroplasmy of mitochondria divides, the resulting new daughter cells are likely to have heteroplasmy with a mixture of mitochondria with normal and mutated mtDNA. However, because of random segregation, the ratio of heteroplasmy will be different from the original daughter cell and will be different between the two new daughter cells. The progeny of the cell with a lower ratio of mutated mtDNA may continue to dilute this ratio through many rounds of cell division over time, resulting in a tissue or organ that has such a low concentration of cells with poor energy generation that overall function is minimally affected. On the other hand, the progeny of the cell with a higher ratio of mutated mtDNA could actually amplify the ratio of mutated mtDNA through random segregation, so that over time, homoplasmy of mitochondria with mutated mtDNA occurs. When the concentration of cells that are homoplasmic for mitochondria with mutated DNA increases within a tissue or organ, the function of that tissue or organ is reduced proportionately. Just as with mosaicism for nuclear chromosomal aberrations, tissues or organs that have more cells with high percentages of mitochondria that contain mutated mtDNA are more likely to express the phenotype.

Early in embryonic development, the randomness of the distribution of mitochondria that contain mtDNA with mutations during mitosis is largely responsible for variation in the expression of any mitochondrial disease. Added to this is the fact that some 74 nuclear DNA gene products are also involved in mitochondrial function. Products of these genes interact with and can modify the expression of mtDNA genes. A mutation in any of these nuclear genes involved in mitochondrial function can also affect energy generation and tissue or organ expression of mitochondrial disease.

Summary

Most individuals are genetically "normal," although very few humans are genetically perfect. Rearrangements of genetic material occur frequently during the process of gametogenesis. Fertilization and conception occur more frequently than does a live birth or even a detectable pregnancy. Some conceptions fail to develop beyond the earliest stages, and still others fail to implant in the uterus. Even when implantation occurs, pregnancy loss during the first trimester is significant. Both random and heritable genetic problems account for many of these losses.

GENE GEMS

- Although chromosome structure is temporary, the double-stranded DNA that makes up the chromosome is a permanent section of the total DNA within one cell's nucleus.
- Individuals who have balanced translocations do not have abnormal development or phenotypes as a result of the translocation; however, these translocations do have reproductive consequences.
- Individuals who have unbalanced translocations do have abnormal development or phenotypes as a result of the translocation.

- Robertsonian translocations occur only between acrocentric chromosomes.
- The most common sex chromosomal abnormality conceived is monosomy X (Turner syndrome, 45,X).
- The most common autosomal chromosomal abnormality among live-born infants is trisomy 21 (Down syndrome).
- Many specific phenotypic features are associated with various trisomies; however, few affected individuals express every feature.
- Individuals with an extra X chromosome or an extra Y chromosome are usually taller than other family members.
- Monosomy of autosomal chromosomes appears to be lethal.
- With any chromosome disorder, the variation in expression is great and the limitations or ultimate potential of any one affected person cannot be generalized or predicted.
- Children who have Angelman syndrome and children who have Prader-Willi syndrome have the same chromosomal deletion, but the parental origin of the chromosome with the deletion differs.
- Early tissues that are capable of developing into anatomical male sex structures (mesonephric ducts) and those that are capable of developing into anatomical female sex structures (paramesonephric ducts) are present in both XX and XY embryos.
- The most common mechanism for XY females is complete androgen insensitivity.
- The most common mechanism for XX males is translocation of the *SRY* gene to an X chromosome during crossover in gametogenesis.
- Heritable mitochondrial disorders that result from point mutations are usually transmitted by maternal inheritance only.
- Mitochondrial DNA deletions occur after conception and usually are random events that are not heritable.
- The most common symptom associated with mitochondrial diseases is fatigue.
- The mature ovum is the largest single cell in the human body, and the mature sperm is the smallest single cell in the human body.

Self-Assessment Questions

1. What is the best example of "genomic imprinting"?
   a. A child inherits a trait that his paternal grandfather expressed but that his father did not express.
   b. Boys can inherit only masculine traits from their fathers because women do not have a Y chromosome.
   c. There is a qualitative difference in some gene alleles based on whether they are inherited from the mother or the father.
   d. When the number of sex chromosomes is greater than normal, the resulting individual is most often infertile.

Continued

2. What is the difference between "triploidy" and "trisomy"?
   a. Triploidy involves an extra copy of every chromosome, and trisomy involves an extra copy of only one chromosome.
   b. Trisomy involves an extra copy of every chromosome, and triploidy involves an extra copy of only one chromosome.
   c. Triploidies are maternally derived, and trisomies are paternally derived.
   d. Trisomies are fatal more frequently than are triploidies.

3. Why do balanced translocation carriers have normal development and function?
   a. The extra chromosomal material is present only in germ cells and not in somatic cells.
   b. The extra chromosomal material is present only in somatic cells and not in germ cells.
   c. They have the correct amount of chromosomal material, and only its location is abnormal.
   d. Their translocations involve only DNA noncoding regions, with no involvement of actual gene-coding regions.

4. Which feature is common among people who have Klinefelter syndrome (47,XXY) or a karyotype with 47,XXX but not among people who have Down syndrome or Edward syndrome?
   a. Severe mental retardation
   b. Cleft palate
   c. Tall stature
   d. Infertility

5. Why does a person who has a deletion of the coding regions for five genes on one chromosome 15 have some manifestations or overt problems?
   a. The deletions occurred in an autosome and not in a sex chromosome.
   b. He or she has only one copy of the gene alleles, which results in reduced function.
   c. The overall expression of the deleted areas is the same as if trisomy 15 were present.
   d. The deleted areas are introns rather than exons, thus no compensation occurred on the homologous chromosome.

6. What is the most likely explanation for a baby boy to have Tay-Sachs disease when the child's mother is not a carrier for the problem but the father is a carrier?
   a. The mother is not really the biological parent of this child.
   b. The mother's normal gene allele is not expressed and the father's Tay-Sachs allele is expressed.
   c. A new mutation occurred in the father's sperm in which the Tay-Sachs gene has become dominant.
   d. The father's Tay-Sachs gene has been translocated from its usual locus to the Y chromosome and thus is expressed in any male child.

7. What is the best explanation for a person whose karyotype from blood cells shows nearly all cells to have trisomy 21 to have 10 clinical manifestations of Down syndrome and an above-average intelligence?
   a. The trisomy was a result of nondisjunction of paternal gametes instead of maternal gametes.
   b. The person has pseudo–Down syndrome, in which environmental conditions caused the person to have development that mimics only the physical manifestations.
   c. The person has genomic imprinting, in which the paternal number 21 chromosome is not expressed and both maternally derived number 21 chromosomes are expressed.
   d. The person has mosaicism of trisomy 21, with blood cells having a high proportion and neurons having a low proportion of cells, with three number 21 chromosomes.

8. Why does injection of testosterone fail to induce male secondary sex characteristics in females who are 46,XY with complete androgen insensitivity?
   a. Their target tissues for testosterone lack testosterone receptors.
   b. The injected testosterone is destroyed just as rapidly as their own naturally produced testosterone.
   c. Their production of estrogen far exceeds the amount of testosterone that can be administered safely.
   d. The injected testosterone inhibits the gonadotrophin hormone feedback loops, decreasing production of testosterone by the remaining testicular tissue.

9. A 21-year-old soldier disappeared in Vietnam. Forty years later, bones are discovered that may include his remains. Which available living relative's mitochondrial DNA would be the most accurate sample to obtain for comparison to determine whether the bones belong to this soldier?
   a. Father
   b. Daughter
   c. Sister's son
   d. Brother's son

CASE STUDY

The firstborn child of a mother who is 25 years old and a father who is 28 years old is diagnosed with Down syndrome at age 6 months. The karyotype is 47,XY,+21. Both parents have college degrees in business administration. One works at a facility that manufactures cosmetics, and the other works in a large computer call center. No other family members have ever had Down syndrome. The child is meeting all of his developmental milestones at this time and is taking part in an early childhood stimulation program daily. How would you respond to the following questions from the parents?

1. Could this have occurred as a result of environmental exposure to chemicals or radiation at work? Why or why not?

2. What are the possibilities that any other children they conceive may have Down syndrome? (Consider whether this child is likely to have trisomy 21 as a result of nondisjunction or as a result of an unbalanced translocation.)

3. What can they expect this child to achieve?

4. What are the chances that this child could have a child with Down syndrome?

References

Angelman Foundation (2009). Retrieved August 2010 from www.angelmanfoundation.org.

Bondy, C. (2007). Clinical practice guideline: Care of girls and women with Turner syndrome: A guideline of the Turner syndrome study group. *Journal of Clinical Endocrinology and Metabolism, 92*(1), 10–25.

Milunsky, J. Prenatal diagnosis or sex chromosome disorders. In Milunsky, A., and Milunsky, J. *Genetic disorders and the fetus: Diagnosis, prevention and treatment,* 6th ed. Oxford: Wiley-Blackwell, 2010, 273–352.

Milunsky, A., and Milunsky, J. *Genetic disorders and the fetus: Diagnosis, prevention and treatment,* 6th ed. Oxford: Wiley-Blackwell, 2010.

National Institutes of Health (2010). Facts about Down syndrome (updated March, 2010). Retrieved August 2010 from www.nichd.nih.gov/publications/pubs/downsyndrome.cfm.

National Institutes of Health (2008). Genetic Home Reference: Prader-Willi Syndrome. Retrieved August 2010 from http://ghr.nlm.nih.gov/condition/prader-willi-syndrome.

National Institutes of Health (2009). NIH Genetics Home Reference: Your guide to understanding genetics conditions. Retrieved August 2010 from http://ghr.nim.nih.gov/condition/trisomy-13/.

Rasmussen, S., Wong, L., Yang, Q., May, K., and Friedman, J. (2003). Population-based analysis of mortality in trisomy 13 and trisomy 18. *Pediatrics, 111*(4 part 1), 777–784.

Scaglia, F., Towbin, J., Craigen, W., et al. (2004). Clinical spectrum, morbidity, and mortality in 113 pediatric patients with mitochondrial disease. *Pediatrics, 114*(4), 925–931.

Smits, P., Smeitink, J., and van den Heuvel, L. (2010). Mitochondrial translation and beyond: Processes implicated in combined oxidative phosphorylation deficiencies. *Journal of Biomedicine and biotechnology, 2010* (article ID 737385), 1–24.

Thomson, A. (2010). The transition between the phenotypes of Prader-Willi syndrome during infancy and early childhood. *Developmental Medicine and Child Neurology, 52*(6), 506–507.

Trisomy 18 Foundation (2010). Retrieved March 2011 from www.trisomy18.org/site/PageServer.

Verity, C., Winstone, M., Stellitano, L., Krishnakumar, D., Will, R., and McFarland, R. (2010). The clinical presentation of mitochondrial diseases in children with progressive intellectual and neurological deterioration: A national, prospective, population-based study. *Developmental Medicine & Child Neurology, 52*(5), 434–440.

Westly, E. (2010). When powerhouses fail. *Nature Medicine, 16*(6), 625–627.

Williams, C., Beaudet, A., Clayton-Smith, J., et al. (2006). Angelman syndrome 2005: Updated consensus for diagnostic criteria. *American Journal of Medical Genetics Part A, 140*(5), 413–415.

Self-Assessment Answers

1. c 2. a 3. c 4. c 5. b 6. b 7. d 8. a 9. c

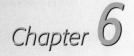

Family History and Pedigree Construction

KEY TERMS

Pedigree

Proband

Punnett squares

Risk stratification

Introduction

A major nursing assessment responsibility is collecting data for an accurate patient and family history. One way to organize family information to help identify individual and family risks for specific disorders is by constructing a pedigree. A **pedigree** is a pictorial or graphic illustration of family members' places within a family and their medical history. Being able to organize a family history into a pedigree is an important skill for all health professionals and is an expectation for registered nurses with a bachelor of science in nursing (BSN) degree. The American Association of Colleges of Nursing has included in its document *Essentials of Baccalaureate Education for Professional Nursing Practice 2008* that all BSN graduates must be able to "generate a pedigree from a three-generation family history using standardized symbols and terminology."

Completing a family history is an easy and affordable way to begin genetic screening; however, family history is not a stable thing. On the day you take your patient's family history, there may be no one with cardiac problems. The next day, your patient's 35-year-old brother or sister could have a myocardial infarction, changing your patient's genetic risk for cardiovascular disease from low to high. Sometimes family history changes depending on who provides the information. For example, Uncle Charles may remember more about the family's health problems than your patient, and sometimes family members will remember things differently. Perhaps one relative says that a grandmother died because of a heart problem, but a different relative remembers that she died from cancer. It can be difficult for the health-care worker to tease out what actually happened.

Family History

The best way for a family history to be as complete and as accurate as possible is for several family members to construct it together. A study has found that about 96% of Americans believe that knowing one's family history is important, but sadly, only about one-third of those responding reported having made any effort to collect their family's health history. The U.S. Department of Health and Human Services provides a Surgeon General's Family Health History Initiative with all the tools needed for a family to complete and update the family health history (www.hhs.gov/familyhistory/). Easy-to-follow directions are provided at the Web site in both English and Spanish, and families can develop their family histories alone or under the guidance of a health-care professional. Instructions include what questions to ask, as well as what documents could help provide important information and should be on hand when the information is gathered and recorded. A family gathering during the holidays is a great time for people to collect their family's health history because, for many, this is a time when most of their relatives are together. Having family members know about the plan for putting the history together and bringing any documents or pictures to the gathering that can enhance memory are helpful to the process. Once the history is generated, each family member should have a copy. Encourage your patients to collect and frequently update their family health histories and to bring them along when visiting any health-care provider.

Genetics Referral

Risk stratification is the process of identifying whether a person is at a high, moderate, or low risk of developing a genetic disorder. It is an important step in deciding whether or not a patient or family would benefit from genetics referral. However, there are no clear and specific guidelines for just when a patient and/or family should be referred. It is important that the nurse or allied health professional not attempt to provide genetic counseling, as this is beyond the scope of practice; however, it is helpful to have a good sense of when referral should be considered. Whelan and colleagues (2004) have assembled a list of conditions that are "red flags" for genetic referral, meaning that an individual or family with one or more of these conditions should be referred to a genetics specialist (Table 6–1). Referral to a genetics specialist (as defined in Chapter 16) should be considered by the health-care team if the patient has a group of problems or malformations present since birth (congenital anomalies), extreme or exceptional presentation of common conditions, neurodevelopmental delay or degeneration, extreme or exceptional pathology, or surprising laboratory values.

Table 6–2 provides a list of questions for the health-care provider to use with a patient to ensure important points are included when obtaining a family history. These are easy to remember by using the acronym *SCREEN*, which stands for *Some Concern* about diseases that might run in the family, especially problems with *Reproduction*, *Early* disease or death in family members, *Ethnicity* (some genetic diseases are more common in people who are from certain ethnic groups), and *Nongenetic* risk factors for disease. The questions are simple and can be added to a general health assessment to make it likely that genetic risk will be identified (Hinton, 2008).

TABLE 6–1

F-Genes Mnemonic for Red Flags of Genetic Disease

Family history. Multiple affected siblings or individuals in multiple generations. Remember that lack of a family history does *not* rule out genetic causes.

G: group of congenital anomalies. Common anatomic variations are, well, common, but two or more anomalies are much more likely to indicate the presence of a syndrome with genetic implications.

E: extreme or **exceptional presentation of common conditions.** Early onset cardiovascular disease, cancer, or renal failure. Unusually severe reaction to infectious or metabolic stress. Recurrent miscarriage. Bilateral primary cancers in paired organs, multiple primary cancers of different tissues.

N: neurodevelopmental delay or **degeneration.** Developmental delay in the pediatric age group carries a very high risk for genetic disorders. Developmental regression in children or early onset dementia in adults should similarly raise suspicion for genetic etiologies.

E: extreme or **exceptional pathology.** Unusual tissue histology, such as pheochromocytoma, acoustic neuroma, medullary thyroid cancer, multiple colon polyps, plexiform neurofibromas, multiple exostoses, most pediatric malignancies.

S: surprising laboratory values. Transferrin saturation of 65%, potassium of 5.5 mmol/L, and sodium of 128 mmol/L in an infant; cholesterol greater than 500 mg/dL and unconjugated bilirubin of 2.2 mg/dL in an otherwise healthy 25-year-old; phosphate of 2 mg/dL and glucose of 35 mg/dL in a 6-month-old child.

Developed by the Red Flags Working Group of the Genetics in Primary Care (GPC) project (Alison Whelan MD, Chair). Reproduced with permission. Whelan, A. J., Ball, S., Best, L., et al. (2004) Genetic red flags: Clues to thinking genetically in primary care practice. *Prim Care*, 31, 497–508, viii.

TABLE 6–2

Abbreviated Family History: SCREEN for Familial Disease

SC	Some Concern	Do you have any concern about diseases that run in the family?
R	Reproduction	Have there been complicated pregnancies, infertility, or birth defects?
E	Early disease/death	Has anyone in your family become sick or died at an early age?
E	Ethnicity	How would you describe your ethnicity?
N	Nongenetic	Are there risk factors that run in your family?

Hinton, R. B., Jr. (2008). The family history: Reemergence of an established tool. *Critical Care Nursing Clinics of North America, 20*(2), 149–158, v. Reproduced with permission.

Pedigree Construction

Pedigree Symbols and Conventions

As described earlier, a pedigree is a pictorial or graphic illustration of members' positions within a family and their medical history. It allows health-care providers to view the health history of multiple generations and makes is easier for genetics professionals to identify persons who are at risk. Once you become familiar with the symbols and conventions used to construct pedigrees, they are easy to read. A well-constructed pedigree makes communicating the medical issues of extended family to health-care team members quicker and easier.

By using the standard pedigree symbols presented here, the family's history can be sketched out as it is provided, and whether a disease "runs in the family" may become clear. You may even be able to identify possible modes of transmission, such as autosomal dominant or autosomal recessive.

The symbols have been standardized so that all clinicians use the same symbols for the same things. In this way, the information is communicated from one clinician or facility to another without confusion. Circles are used to represent women, and squares represent men. Lines depict relationships, with horizontal connecting lines indicating mating, not necessarily marriage (Fig. 6–1).

Vertical lines are called *lines of descent* and are drawn between biological parents and children. The symbols for all children born to a couple are drawn from the same line. So a mating couple with a son and two daughters would look like the depiction in Figure 6–2.

A horizontal slash through a symbol indicates that the person is deceased, and the age of death is indicated beside the symbol. If the mother in the family in Figures 6–1 and 6–2 had been married before and had one son with her previous husband before he died, the pedigree would look like the depiction in Figure 6–3.

Figure 6–1. Mating between a man and a woman.

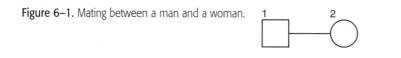

Figure 6–2. Lines of descent and sibship lines.

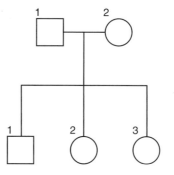

Figure 6–3. Deceased mate and second mating with both matings producing offspring.

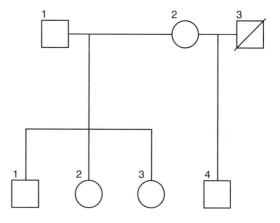

When a pedigree is being used to record the history of one particular trait, such as hypertension, the circle or square representing every affected person is shaded (Fig. 6–4).

When multiple traits are being recorded, the list of health problems is commonly written next to each person's symbol. Sometimes the symbols have color-coded segments that correspond to different traits. When these are present, they must be explained in a legend because these symbols are not standardized. In Figure 6–5, a blue upper-left quadrant indicates coronary artery disease and a black upper-left quadrant indicates hypertension, so the father, who has both hypertension and coronary artery disease, has blue in the upper left and black in the upper right. On the pedigree depicted in Figure 6–5, the proband is indicated by an arrow in the lower left corner. (The **proband** is usually defined as the person in a family who brought the potential genetic issue to the attention of a health-care professional.) The proband has both diabetes mellitus type 1 and asthma, while his brother has only asthma.

Although it is useful for nurses and other health-care professionals to have the ability to construct and analyze pedigrees, communicating the information about transmission patterns is best left to genetic professionals. These professionals may be physicians with specialty work in genetics, certified genetics counselors, PhD-educated geneticists, or advanced practice nurses with a specialization in genetics. These roles are discussed in detail in Chapter 16. As part of their scope of practice, bedside nurses and other nongenetics professionals are expected to identify patients and families who may be at an increased risk for genetic problems; however, it is in the scope of practice for genetic professionals to quantify and communicate that risk.

Figure 6–4. Person affected with the trait of interest.

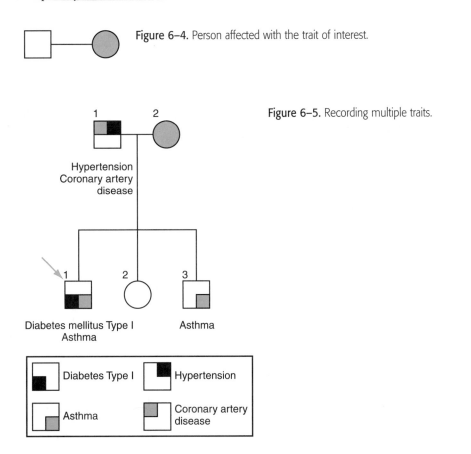

Figure 6–5. Recording multiple traits.

For a pedigree to provide useful information regarding the potential of a genetic disorder within a family, it must contain at least three generations. The generations are identified by Roman numerals, so in the three-generation pedigree, the grandparents would be generation I, the parents would be generation II, and the children would be generation III. If a pedigree shows more than three generations, the oldest generation is designated as generation I, with each succeeding generation numbered in order after the first generation. Within each generation, individuals are designated by Arabic numerals, and all persons in the pedigree are numbered from left to right. The goal is for each family member to have a distinct identifying number. Figure 6–6 shows the correct numbering of a three-generation pedigree.

Additional information should be included on the actual pedigree to increase its usefulness in identifying a heritable genetic problem. One type of especially important information is family ethnicity. It is helpful to note the ethnicity (or ethnicities) of each side of the family, because genetic risk varies with the geographic origin of ancestors. For example, it is very helpful to know if a patient's grandparents were Ashkenazi Jews (from Eastern Europe), because that particular ethnic group is at higher risk for a number of recessive traits, such as Gaucher disease, Tay-Sachs disease, some types of breast cancer, and cystic fibrosis.

Remember to sign and date the pedigrees you construct so that those who view them later will know when the data were collected and if the pedigree needs to be updated. It is also helpful to work in pencil so that you can make adjustments as you collect the family history data. If you are constructing this pedigree as a family history, it is important to identify the proband of the family. He or she is often the first person in the family who is affected or identified. Sometimes the proband does not have the actual problem him- or herself but is just worried because there is a possibility of a genetic issue. If you are generating a pedigree as part of your patient assessment and no specific problem is known, the proband is the patient whose family history you are obtaining.

Punnett Squares

Punnett squares are diagrams that are used to determine the risk of offspring being affected when the mode of transmission and the parents' carrier status are known. The maternal and paternal genotypes are represented by uppercase letters to indicate dominant alleles, and lowercase letters represent recessive

Figure 6–6. Three-generation pedigree with appropriate Roman and Arabic numbering.

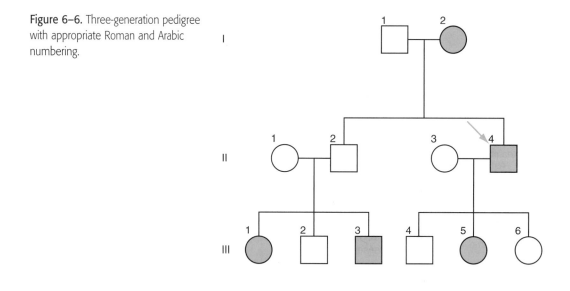

alleles. A homozygote would be either BB or bb, and a heterozygote would be Bb. Remember that Punnett squares represent genotypes and not phenotypes, and whether a person is ill may depend on other factors, such as incomplete penetrance or whether the trait is likely to result in pregnancy loss if the embryo is a homozygote.

In Figure 6–7, the probability of each pregnancy resulting in a child with the genotype *BB* is 25%, *Bb* is 50%, and *bb* is 25% (Fig. 6–7A). If this Punnett square represented a recessive trait such as cystic fibrosis, we could estimate the risk of an unaffected child being a carrier. An unaffected child would not be *bb* (homozygous recessive), which is blackened out in Figure 6–7B. She or he could be either BB (not affected and not a carrier—risk 25%) or Bb (not affected but a carrier—risk 50%). Therefore, the risk that an unaffected child in this family is a carrier would be 2 out of 3 or 2/3.

There are other limitations to the use of Punnett squares. Things get a bit more complicated when you consider genotype for two different traits (dihybrid cross). For the Punnett square to work, the genes being considered must be located on different chromosomes. Some alleles may affect the expression of other alleles, and some genes can be imprinted so that it makes a difference when the allele was inherited from the mother or the father (imprinting). What you figure out by doing a Punnett square may be unrelated to what you see in the phenotype. Things get confusing when the genes of interest are located on the X or Y chromosomes, because most men have only one X chromosome and most women have no Y. There are also variations in dominance, such as codominance seen in the ABO system of human blood type, which can make it more confusing. Remember when the gene for a trait

		Mother	
		B	**b**
Father	**B**	BB	Bb
	b	Bb	bb

A

Figure 6–7. (A) Punnett square of the possible offspring of two heterozygous parents. (B) The trait is expressed in the offspring with two recessive alleles.

		Mother	
		B	**b**
Father	**B**	BB	Bb
	b	Bb	

B

is found in the mitochondrial DNA, virtually all transmission will be maternal. Doing a Punnett square analysis can be helpful to determine the likelihood of having an affected or carrier child when transmission follows a standard mendelian pattern.

Pedigree Analysis

This chapter provides some guidelines to follow when analyzing a pedigree to identify possible transmission. When analyzing a pedigree, proceed in the following organized manner:

1. Make sure that you have collected all the relevant information from the family and that you construct your pedigrees according to conventions presented in this chapter.
2. Look at the pedigree and test it against the possible interpretations. Use the guidelines for each mode of inheritance that were provided in Chapter 4. See what fits and what does not. For example, if you have male-to-male inheritance, you can not have X-linked transmission.
3. Test against possible hypotheses:
   a. Autosomal dominant
   b. Autosomal recessive
   c. X-linked dominant
   d. X-linked recessive
   e. Y-linked
   f. Maternal (mitochondrial)
4. Discard all hypotheses that do not fit the pedigree.
5. If only one remains, accept it as your working idea.
6. If two or more remain, which is the more likely? For example, which is the more likely explanation for the pedigree in Figure 6–6?
   A. Person II-2, who comes from a family with several affected members and has affected children, has the genotype (but not the phenotype) for the trait (i.e., the trait is passed in an autosomal dominant fashion but has incomplete penetrance).

   OR

   B. Person II-2 is a carrier for a rare trait and selected a mate (person II-1) from the general population who is also a carrier for the same rare trait, *and* persons I-1 and II-3 are also carriers (i.e., the trait is passed in an autosomal recessive fashion).

   Hint: Option A is way more likely!

Examples of Pedigree Analysis

In Figure 6–8A, the following conditions apply:

- Males are represented by *squares.*
- Females are represented by *circles.*
- A person who has died has a *diagonal line* drawn through his or her symbol.
- A vertical line is called a *line of descent* and indicates the connection between parents and their offspring.
- The *proband* is indicated by an arrow.
- A mating (not necessarily a marriage) is represented by a solid horizontal line, called the *relationship line*, between the partners.
- If the relationship is *casual,* not a formal marriage or a committed partnering, the relationship line can be *dashed* (Fig. 6–8B).

- The horizontal line connecting siblings is called the *sibship line.* Each person in each generation is given an Arabic numeral starting from the left (Fig. 6–8C).
- Person 4 in generation II was adopted into the family. The vertical dashed line indicates that there is no biological relationship (Fig. 6–8D).
- This pedigree indicates that person 4 in generation II was adopted out of the family (Fig. 6–8E). She no longer lives with them, but there is still a biological relationship with her siblings and birth parents.
- This pedigree indicates that person 4 and person 5 in generation II are *dizygotic (fraternal) twins* (Fig. 6–8F).
- The addition of a horizontal line connecting the twins' lines of descent indicates that they are *monozygotic (identical) twins* (Fig. 6–8G).
- When a symbol is made small, it indicates a *pregnancy loss.* When the sex of the fetus or embryo is unknown, the diamond (or sometimes a triangle) symbol is used (Fig. 6–8H).
- When the relationship line is double, it indicates consanguinity (these individuals are biologically related). For example, a double line would be used if two cousins were in a mating relationship (Fig. 6–8I).
- A double (or sometimes single) diagonal line through the relationship line indicates that the couple is divorced (Fig. 6–8J).
- A short horizontal line at the end of a line of descent indicates that a couple has no children. They may be infertile or they may have chosen not to have children. The short horizontal line can be doubled to indicate known infertility (Fig. 6–8K).

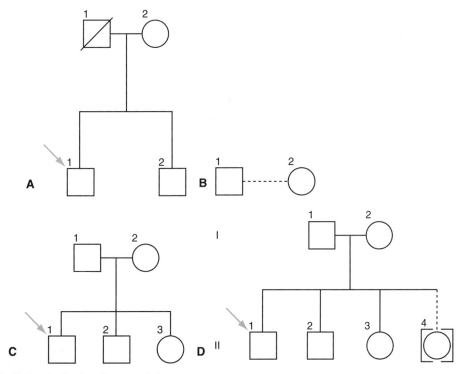

Figure 6–8. (A–K) Standardized pedigree symbols.

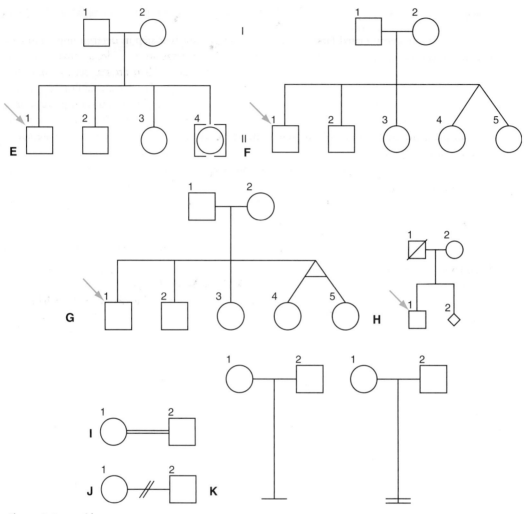

Figure 6–8. cont'd

Summary

Collecting an accurate and updated family history is an important first step in determining a family's genetic risk. Constructing a pedigree with a minimum of three generations provides a convenient way to communicate a family's health history to other health-care providers. There are standard symbols for pedigree construction and standard conventions that help to make this communication easier. Conducting a step-by-step analysis of a pedigree can reveal the most likely transmission pattern of a single-gene genetic disorder. Pedigree analysis is more difficult for multifactorial (complex) disorders, because multiple genes or combinations of genes and the environment are involved. There are some traits that are considered important triggers or "red flags" for referral to genetics professionals, such as groups of congenital anomalies and neurodevelopmental delay. Identifying a family history that should be evaluated by genetics professionals is an important role for all health-care providers.

GENE GEMS

- Encourage your patients to complete an accurate family history when their family members are gathered together.
- Teach your patients the importance of bringing an updated family history with them when they meet with a health-care professional.
- Record a three-generation pedigree using Roman numerals to indicate generations and Arabic numerals to indicate individuals.
- Include ethnicity for each side of the family.
- When analyzing a pedigree, test it against assumptions for each transmission pattern.

Self-Assessment Questions

Which of the following best describes the inheritance pattern in the pedigree illustrations?
- **a.** Autosomal dominant
- **b.** Autosomal recessive
- **c.** X-linked dominant
- **d.** X-linked recessive
- **e.** Y-linked dominant
- **f.** Y-linked recessive
- **g.** Mitochondrial

1. First Pedigree (Fig. 6–9A) *a*   autosomal dominant
2. Second Pedigree (Fig. 6–9B) *b*
3. Third Pedigree (Fig. 6–9C) *d*
4. Fourth Pedigree (Fig. 6–9D) *g*
5. Fifth Pedigree (Fig. 6–9E) *b*

Continued

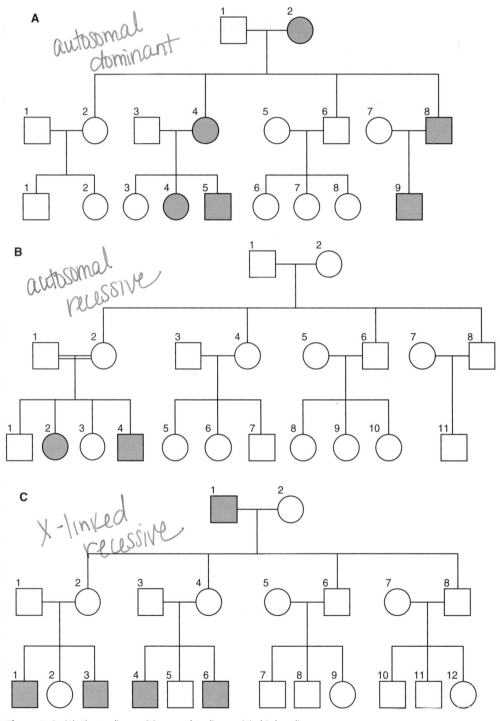

Figure 6–9. (A) First pedigree, (B) second pedigree, (C) third pedigree,

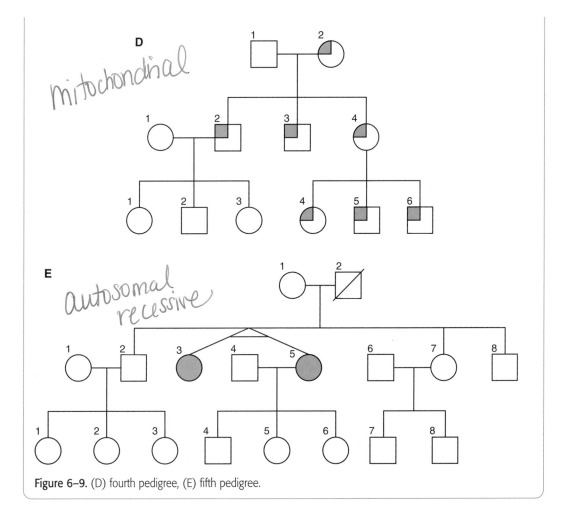

Figure 6–9. (D) fourth pedigree, (E) fifth pedigree.

CASE STUDIES

Family Histories

Family A

Doug and his maternal grandfather, Brad, are color-blind. Neither Doug's brother (Dick) nor his sister (Donna) is color-blind. His father, Carl, who is the youngest of three sons (Charles and Caleb) has normal color vision, but his oldest brother, Caleb, is also color-blind. Caleb has two sons (David and Dennis) who have normal color vision and one daughter, Darlene, who also has normal color vision. Carl's mother, Brenda, reports that one of her parents (Doug's paternal great-grandparents, Albert and Adele) was color-blind but does not remember which one. Doug's partner is his paternal uncle's daughter, Darlene. Doug and Darlene have two sons, Ethan and Elliot, and two daughters, Emma and Elise. Ethan, Elliot, and Emma all are color-blind. Elise has normal color vision.

   Draw the pedigree, indicating affected individuals and probable carriers (see the correct pedigree in Fig. 6–10A).

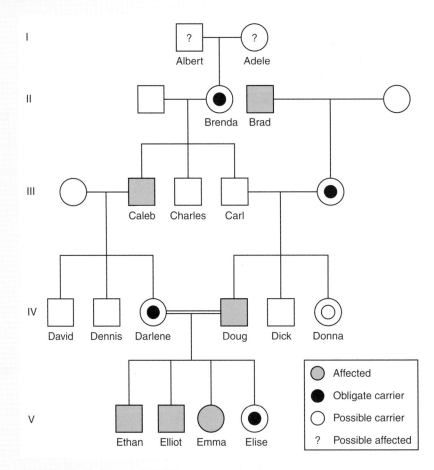

Figure 6–10A. Pedigree for Family A.

1. Which of Brenda's parents is most likely to have been color-blind?
2. What is the probability that Elise could have a son who is color-blind?
3. What is the probability that Elise could have a daughter who is color-blind?
4. Is it possible for Ethan or Elliot to have children who are not color-blind? Explain why or why not.
5. Is it possible for Emma to have children who are not color-blind? Explain why or why not.

Family B

A couple, Jack and Jill, are both deaf, and each has one parent who also is deaf. Jack and Jill have eight children: six boys and two girls, four of whom (one daughter and three sons) are also deaf.

Draw the pedigree for the family (see the correct pedigree in Fig. 6–10B. See the correct Punnett square in Fig. 6–10C).

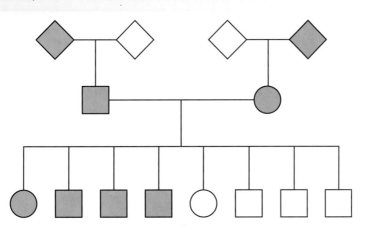

Jack and Jill

Autosomal dominant
Males and females about equally affected
Affected individuals have affected children
Transmitted down to all generations

If the deafness were autosomal recessive, all of Jack and Jill's children would be deaf. If it was x-linked recessive, again all of their children would be deaf. If it was X-linked dominant, all of their daughters would have it.

Figure 6–10B. Pedigree for Family B.

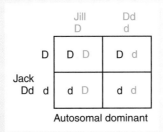

Autosomal dominant

Figure 6–10C. Punnett square for Family B.

Continued

1. Identify the specific pattern of inheritance (if any) indicated for this family.

2. Indicate what criteria the pedigree presents that supports the correct pattern of inheritance for this health problem.

Family C

Belinda is 52 years old and has just been diagnosed with a "recurrence" of ductal carcinoma of the breast, previously treated by lumpectomy and radiation 8 years ago. Her father is still living at age 80, and her mother died of ovarian cancer at age 38 (diagnosed at age 36). Her sister, Bonnie, was diagnosed with breast cancer 9 years ago at age 35 and has just undergone a bone marrow transplant. Her brother, now age 43, was treated 3 years ago with surgery and chemotherapy for breast cancer. She tells you that both of her parents' families are rather small. Her mother had one sister, Adele, who died of some kind of female cancer when she was 34, and one brother, Arthur, who died of bone cancer at age 40. Her father's only sibling, a brother, died in the Holocaust. Belinda's daughter, Caroline, is 30 and was recently diagnosed with ovarian cancer.

Draw the pedigree for the family (see the correct pedigree in Fig. 6–10D).

1. Identify the specific pattern of inheritance (if any) indicated for this family.

2. Indicate what factors in the pedigree support your choice for the correct pattern of inheritance for this health problem.

Figure 6–10D. Pedigree for Family C.

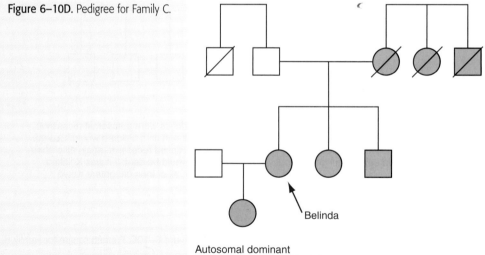

Autosomal dominant
Males and females affected
Affected individuals have affected offspring
Transmitted from one generation directly to the next

References

Hinton (2008). The family history: Reemergence of an established tool. *Critical Care Nursing Clinics of North America, 20*(2), 149–158.

Whelan A. J., Ball, S., Best, L., et al. (2004). Genetic red flags: Clues to thinking genetically in primary care practice. *Primary Care, 31*, 497–508, viii.

Self-Assessment Answers

1. a **2.** b **3.** d **4.** g **5.** b

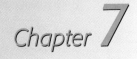

Congenital Anomalies, Basic Dysmorphology, and Genetic Assessment

Learning Objectives

1. Use genetic terminology associated with dysmorphology assessment.
2. Compare the classifications of congenital anomalies, including dysmorphic features.
3. Differentiate among syndromes, sequences, and associations.
4. Distinguish between major and minor congenital anomalies.
5. Compare the processes that result in malformation, disruption, deformation, and dysplasia.
6. Identify common congenital anomalies.
7. Describe assessment strategies that are important in determining if a patient has dysmorphic features.

KEY TERMS

Associations	Dysmorphology	Macrocephaly
Brachydactyly	Dysplasia	Major anomaly
Canthus	Epicanthic folds	Malformation
Cleft lip/palate	Frontal bossing	Microcephaly
Clinodactyly	Gestalt	Micrognathia
Congenital anomalies	Hypertelorism	Midface hypoplasia
Craniofacial anomalies	Hypotelorism	Minor anomaly
Craniosynostosis	Lip pits	Oligohydramnios
Deformation	Long fingers/toes	Palpebral fissure
Disruption	Low-set ears	Philtrum

Plagiocephaly	Retrognathia	Syndrome
Polydactyly	Sequence	Teratogen
Ptosis	Syndactyly	

Introduction

Dysmorphology (*dys* = "painful"; *morph* = "shape") is the study of **congenital anomalies** in the anatomical form or body parts of a person, or abnormal patterns of development. These are sometimes called *birth defects* or *malformations,* even though the term *malformation* has a specific definition, which we will discuss later in this chapter. The term *dysmorphology* was coined in the 1960s by Dr. David Smith, so it is a relatively new area of study. *Smith's Recognizable Patterns of Human Malformations* remains the classic text on dysmorphology (Jones, 2006). This text, and others like it, helps clinicians to match dysmorphic features with the disorders associated with them.

Terminology has been inconsistent over time, so an international group of experts published a series of articles in 2009 to standardize the definitions of terms used to describe dysmorphic features. We have made every effort to define this chapter's key terms so that they are consistent with the definitions published by these experts: Allanson, Biesecker et al., 2009; Biesecker et al., 2009; Carey et al., 2009; Hall et al., 2009; Hunter et al., 2009. We suggest that you review these articles if you are interested in learning about dysmorphic features in more detail.

It is useful to identify the associated disorder or syndrome of a particular anomaly or pattern of anomalies for a variety of reasons. For one, a correct diagnosis can guide medical management. For example, if a child's collection of dysmorphic features indicates that he has Noonan syndrome, the clinical geneticist will know that the child must also be seen by a cardiologist, because congenital heart defects (CHD) and hypertrophic cardiomyopathy (HCM) are common features of Noonan syndrome (Tartaglia et al., 2010). Some head and neck features that are characteristic of Noonan syndrome include a triangular-shaped face, **hypertelorism** (widely spaced eyes), downward-slanting eyes, **ptosis** (drooping eyelids), **low-set ears,** a high nasal bridge, and a short webbed neck. Without knowing something about Noonan syndrome, a clinician observing this collection of features might not look for heart involvement. It is also important to remember that every person with a syndrome does not have every symptom found in that syndrome. For example, about 80% of people with Noonan syndrome have short stature, but that means that 20% of people with Noonan syndrome are of average height. Although short stature is common in Noonan syndrome, not everyone has it.

Identifying the syndrome can also help determine the probable progression of the disorder and can assist genetic professionals in guiding parents with future reproductive decision making. Sometimes treatment is available that will have an enormous impact on the future of an affected child. For example, knowing that a child has Gaucher disease, which is a lysosomal storage disease like those discussed in Chapter 8, means that enzyme replacement therapy can be started immediately. Starting enzyme replacement early can prevent the grossly enlarged liver and/or spleen that are characteristic of this disorder.

Major and Minor Anomalies

Congenital defects are often classified as either major or minor anomalies. **Major anomalies** are serious and usually require medical or surgical attention. They can have life-threatening implications or have a

serious cosmetic effect. For example, while a cleft lip may not put a child's life at risk, the child's physical appearance and self-esteem may be seriously affected; therefore, cleft lip is considered a major
anomaly. Serious concerns such as cognitive impairment, heart defects, or renal agenesis are also considered major anomalies.

A **minor anomaly** does not have serious functional or cosmetic consequences and may or may not
be surgically corrected. Minor anomalies are found in less than 4% of the general population. Most dysmorphic features are classified by clinicians as minor anomalies. However, when several minor anomalies appear in a child, they can help lead the clinician to a correct diagnosis. An example of a minor
anomaly is **clinodactyly,** which is a laterally curved digit. This is most commonly found when the fifth
finger is curved inward toward the other fingers (Fig. 7–1). It probably happens because of an unusual
shape or positioning of the growth plate in the small bones of the fingers. This can result in abnormal
positioning of the finger joints. While clinodactyly can be found in approximately 10% of the general
population, it is also common among people who have Down syndrome.

One of the authors of this textbook has clinodactyly of her right fifth finger. She first noticed it in
the third grade when she was putting on gloves to march in a parade. She found that her right glove
did not fit like her left glove fit. The knuckle of her right fifth finger is positioned lower on that finger
than on any of her other fingers, making it appear to be a joint shorter than her left fifth finger. This is
an example of a minor anomaly with no clinical significance.

One important part of the definition of *minor anomaly* is that it has no serious significance to
the person affected with it. However, clinicians must remember that a person may be very upset
about a seemingly insignificant abnormal feature. There is an old joke about minor surgery that
defines minor surgery as the kind of surgery that is done on someone else! Any surgery seems
major when you are the person having it. When people are personally affected, a small difference in
appearance can be frightening. New parents can be very distressed by something they perceive as
abnormal in their infant that seems minor to health-care providers. It is important that the family's
concerns be taken seriously.

In most cases, a single dysmorphic feature does not mean that a child has a disorder. Between 13%
and 39% of healthy newborns have one minor anomaly, but less than 1% of healthy newborns have
two minor anomalies. Some sources suggest that if a child has three minor anomalies or one major
anomaly, chromosome studies should be done to help determine the cause of the problem (Jones,
2006). In practice, it is more complicated than this. For example, genetic studies would be done on a

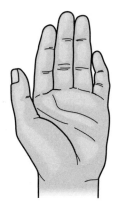

Figure 7–1. Clinodactyly of the fifth finger.

child with a cleft lip only if he or she also had developmental delay, growth delay, or a speech problem such as apraxia (difficulty coordinating mouth movements or difficulty saying what is intended). Decisions about whether to order genetic studies are made by genetic professionals who can consider all the elements of what is going on with a child.

It is important that minor anomalies are considered within the context of family history. Do any of the minor anomalies seen in the child appear in other family members? Sometimes what seem to be minor anomalies may not be caused by any disorder but may simply reflect an inherited group of unusual features. The familial contribution to a child's minor anomalies, along with other conditions (such as malformations) that might appear in other family members, could provide clues to potential single gene or submicroscopic chromosome imbalances.

The risk of a child having a major anomaly that is not immediately obvious increases dramatically with the number of minor anomalies identified. For example, if a child has three or more minor anomalies, the risk of that child having a major structural defect is about 20%. While a single minor anomaly is usually of no significance, finding an unusual feature should alert the clinician to look carefully to see if there are other abnormalities that may have been missed.

Classification of Congenital Anomalies

Congenital anomalies can be classified in many ways. They might be classified according to the mechanism that caused them or according to whether they affect a single body part or multiple body parts. Remember that many people have normal variations that are not associated with disease. These are defined as variations that are found in more than 4% of the population. For example, Mongolian spots, the flat blue or blue-gray spots on the back, buttocks, the base of the spine, or other body areas of people with dark skin, are not found in everyone, but they are also not associated with disease. Thus, Mongolian spots represent a normal skin pigment variation.

Specific terms are used to characterize anomalies by their type. The major categories are malformation, deformation, disruption, and dysplasia.

A **malformation** is caused by a primary problem in the growth or development of a particular tissue. For example, a **cleft lip,** a feature caused by the failure of the lip and/or palate tissues to fuse during development, is considered a malformation because it is due to a developmental problem in the formation of the face. The tissues making up the lip do not fuse properly, leaving a gap (or cleft). While a cleft lip, with or without cleft palate, is usually caused by a combination of genetic and environmental factors, it is the result of an abnormal developmental process. Chromosome problems account for about 25% of malformations, but others, such as *achondroplasia,* are inherited as single gene disorders.

A **deformation** is caused by the effect of a physical or mechanical force that prevents the proper growth of a structure that would have developed normally. The embryo or fetus may be perfectly fine, but something is preventing it from growing properly. Constriction in the uterus is one possible cause. The correction of deformations often occurs after the mechanical stressor is removed. If removing the stressor does not correct the problem, clinicians start to consider the possibility that the structure was not properly formed.

Sometimes deformations are caused by a disease process that results in constriction, but the direct cause of the problem is always mechanical. For example, anything that reduces the size of the uterus can cause a deformation. With **oligohydramnios,** which is the state of not having enough amniotic fluid, fetal growth is restricted because the lesser amount of amniotic fluid keeps the uterus from expanding enough to accommodate normal fetal growth. Also, having twins, triplets, or larger numbers of multiples can cause the physical restriction of intrauterine space. Any of these conditions can lead to contractions in the joints or other signs of deformation.

A **disruption** is a bit more difficult to understand. In a disruption, a normal developmental process is "disrupted" by some event that leads to the destruction of normal tissue. For example, exposure to certain drugs can cause a disruption, as can trauma or vascular insufficiency. It is different from a malformation because everything started out normally. For example, the formation of amniotic bands, which are fibrous strands of amniotic sac tissue, can restrict the proper growth of fetal body parts, including fingers, toes, arms, and legs. Amniotic band disruptions are rare, but the result can be mild to life-threatening, depending on what part of the body is being constricted and how tightly it is entrapped. Some infections, such as rubella, cytomegalovirus (CMV), and toxoplasmosis, can also cause disruptions.

Whereas these classifications are useful clinically, they do sometimes overlap. Here is where it gets a bit complicated. Let us go back and look at oligohydramnios; remember that it can be a mechanical cause of deformations, but the oligohydramnios may be caused by a primary genetic problem, such as Potter sequence. In Potter sequence, the embryo does not develop functional kidneys (a malformation called *renal agenesis*). The fact that the fetus has no kidneys means that it cannot make urine. Because the fetus cannot make urine, there will be less amniotic fluid. The low level of amniotic fluid is the direct mechanical cause of fetal growth restriction, which makes it a *deformation*. In this case, we have an abnormality in fetal growth that can be looked at as both a malformation and a deformation.

Dysplasia is an alteration in the size, shape, and organization of cells. Single gene disorders are the most common genetic cause. An example of a genetic disorder that is caused by dysplasia is ectodermal dysplasia, where there is abnormal cell growth in the skin, hair, nails, or sweat glands.

Syndrome or Sequence

The difference between a syndrome and a sequence can also be confusing. Sometimes the words are used incorrectly, and there are a number of sequences that are commonly referred to as syndromes. A **syndrome** is a collection of features that occur together and have a consistent pattern. They are thought to have the same cause. The word *syndrome* comes from the Greek words for "running together." Down syndrome is caused by an extra chromosome 21, and it results in a collection of symptoms that are easily recognized by the clinician. (See Chapter 5 for more information about Down syndrome.) Syndromes are more likely to be caused by chromosomal inheritance than are single anomalies.

A **sequence** is a little different. In a sequence, one anomaly starts a chain reaction that causes another problem that then causes another, and then sometimes another. One example is Pierre-Robin sequence. The anomaly that starts out Pierre-Robin is **micrognathia** (a small jaw, which is caused by shortening and narrowing of the mandible) in the developing fetus (Fig. 7–2). Sometimes the word **retrognathia** is used to indicate that the jaw is moved posteriorly (and may be accompanied by micrognathia). This small jaw causes the tongue to be positioned backward into the pharynx (glossoptosis). The posteriorly positioned tongue can cause a cleft palate and sometimes respiratory obstruction. It is a sequence of events that started with the poorly formed jaw (Fig. 7–3). Although all of these features (small jaw, posteriorly displaced tongue, respiratory obstruction, and cleft palate) occur together, they were all caused by the chain of events that started with the jaw problem (Allanson, Cunniff et al., 2009).

Potter sequence (mentioned earlier in the explanation of disruptions) is another example. The renal agenesis caused the low amniotic fluid level, which then led to growth restriction. The chain of events makes it a sequence. To make it a bit more complicated, sometimes a sequence is part of a syndrome. For example, Pierre-Robin sequence can be found in velo-cardio-facial syndrome, Stickler syndrome, and trisomy 18. The primary malformation, which is micrognathia (with or without retrognathia), leads to the cascade of anomalies within these syndromes.

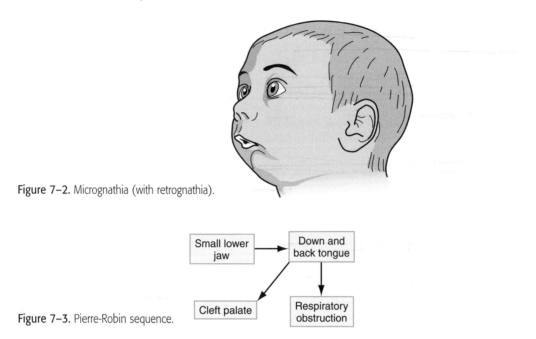

Figure 7–2. Micrognathia (with retrognathia).

Figure 7–3. Pierre-Robin sequence.

When a collection of features occurs together but the relationship is not clear, the term **association** is used. Sometimes disorders are called *associations* until more is learned about how they happened. Then the name is changed to *syndrome* or *sequence*.

Dysmorphology Assessment

When clinical geneticists or genetics nurse practitioners approach a new patient, they look for the overall pattern of anomalies. Sometimes, particularly when looking at facial and developmental features, experts in clinical genetics talk about getting a sense of the whole pattern or picture of the patient. The term **gestalt** is used to convey this overall impression. Being able to appreciate the gestalt comes from much experience working with patients who have anomalies and with their families.

Sometimes dysmorphic features are caused by prenatal exposure to drugs known as **teratogens**, which are substances that can alter development and cause a birth defect. This word has an unfortunate derivation (*terata* = "monstrosities"). For example, there is a particular set of dysmorphic features associated with fetal alcohol spectrum disorder (FASD) (CDC, 2010). While being exposed to alcohol as a fetus may not, at first, appear to be a genetic problem, there are certainly people who have a genetic predisposition to abuse alcohol and other drugs, so in some ways, this can be considered a genetic problem. Furthermore, if FASD were completely environmental, you would expect a dose/exposure response. That would mean that developing fetuses who were exposed to the most alcohol in utero would be the sickest. However, this is not the case and some babies who are born to mothers who are known alcoholics have no detectable phenotype at all. Both maternal genes and fetal genes related to alcohol metabolism and clearance probably contribute to how susceptible a fetus will be to the harmful effects of alcohol exposure. FASD is a good example of a disorder with dysmorphic and developmental features in which an affected child will benefit from an early and correct diagnosis (Fig. 7–4). FASD is also an example of a disruption.

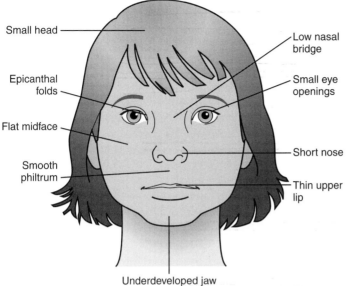

Small head

Low nasal bridge

Epicanthal folds

Small eye openings

Flat midface

Smooth philtrum

Short nose

Thin upper lip

Underdeveloped jaw

Figure 7–4. Dysmorphic features in fetal alcohol spectrum disorder (FASD).

People often think that every set of abnormalities they see clinically must have a name. More than 3500 nonchromosomal syndromes have been cataloged in the London Dysmorphology Database (Winter and Baraitser, 2005). Only about 50% of rare patterns of anomalies actually have been named (Jones, 2006). This is sometimes difficult for families to understand, because they want very much to know what is wrong with their child. Having a name for the problem could make a difference to their sense of control. Parents often want to know if the same problem will happen to future children. Sometimes doing a chromosome study or microarray will identify a chromosome imbalance that is not linked to a recognized named disorder. In these situations, further testing of parents may be necessary to determine if the chromosome imbalance is likely to be associated with the child's condition or if it is merely a benign inherited imbalance from an unaffected parent. Once a cause is established, genetics professionals can often help parents understand the recurrence risk; however, when no genetic abnormality can be found, even the best genetics professionals cannot provide the parents with an accurate idea of how likely it is that the problem will reoccur in future children.

Assessment Through a Genetic Lens

The physical assessment skills you use for general assessment do not vary when you are considering whether a child or adult has a genetic disorder. It is still important to follow a head-to-toe pattern and to use general assessment skills, including inspection, palpation, and auscultation. What is different is the consideration of findings that vary from what is normal. The presence of both major and minor anomalies must be carefully considered and documented to inform decisions for referral to genetics professionals. Unfortunately, most dysmorphic features are not specific for only one disorder. For example, low-set or malformed ears are features of many genetic disorders, including Beckwith-Wiedemann syndrome, Potter syndrome, Rubinstein-Taybi syndrome, Smith-Lemli-Opitz syndrome, Treacher Collins syndrome, trisomy 13, and trisomy 18. So, while finding that a child has low-set ears is important, this finding must be combined with other observations before one can attribute it to a specific genetic disorder. Finding low-set ears in a child does signal the need for further careful evaluation. However, it is important to remember that the presence of low-set ears also occurs in people who have no other dysmorphology, major anomalies, or cognitive impairment.

Another important consideration is to always view an individual in the context of his or her family. Sometimes features that may appear dysmorphic are simply family traits. For example, a tall, thin person with **long fingers and toes** (formerly called *arachnodactyly*) may have Marfan syndrome. However, she or he may also just come from a family that includes many healthy members who are tall and thin and have long fingers. Being able to meet or see photographs of other family members can help genetics specialists decide what is and isn't a cause for concern. Of course, remember that many traits are heritable, and if only a few family members share a trait, the possibility that they each carry the genetic variation must be considered.

Cognitive Impairment

Cognitive impairment (CI) is one reason for evaluation by a genetics professional. Please note that the term *cognitive impairment* is being used here to indicate a condition found in people who have limitations in their mental abilities, with IQs measured at 70 or less. They may have difficulty communicating, developing social skills, and solving problems. They may need assistance with activities of daily living (Chelly et al., 2006). Some professionals prefer to use the term *developmentally delayed* when referring to people who have these problems with thinking. The older term, *mentally retarded*, is considered derogatory by many people who specialize in caring for those who are cognitively impaired. Specialists differ in what they believe is the most appropriate terminology. Some believe that mental retardation is a diagnosis and the term should still be used when referring to this collection of cognitive symptoms, while others prefer *intellectual disability*. In this text we are using the term *cognitive impairment* to indicate the difficulty some people have in thinking and processing information from the world around them.

CI can be attributed to genetics in a significant number of affected people. More than 500 genetic disorders can cause CI, but most of these are very rare. Extra chromosome material, as in Down syndrome; microdeletions, as in cri du chat or Williams syndrome; and copy number variants, as in some cases of Charcot-Marie-Tooth disease (NINDS, 2010), can all result in CI. Table 7–1 lists selected disorders in which cognitive impairment is a feature. It is often difficult to find the specific cause of CI; some people are affected due to environmental issues during the pregnancy, such as exposure to alcohol, infections, or malnutrition. Nevertheless, between 25% and 50% of severe cognitive impairment is due to a genetic problem.

Of course, cognitive impairment is not itself a dysmorphic feature, but it does often coexist with dysmorphology and can be considered a major anomaly. Therefore, it is an important finding that can contribute to a clear understanding of what is wrong with a person. Cognitive impairment is often classified as *syndromic*, meaning it occurs with other clinical features, or *nonsyndromic*, meaning that the impairment is the only feature of the disorder. One of the by-products of understanding more about the biological and chemical changes of disease is that the line between syndromic and nonsyndromic disorders is beginning to blur. Less obvious clinical features are being identified along with cognitive impairment for most cases that were once considered nonsyndromic (Chelly et al., 2006).

TABLE 7–1

Selected Named Genetic Disorders That Can Cause Cognitive Impairment and Associated Common Dysmorphic Features

Named Disorder	Classification	Locus	Common Dysmorphic Features
Angelman syndrome	Imprinting or deletion	15q11	Distinctive "coarse" facial features, microcephaly, scoliosis
Down syndrome	Large chromosome problem	Trisomy 21	Distinctive facial features, epicanthic folds, palmar creases, upslanting palpebral fissures, flat nasal bridge, open mouth with tendency of tongue protrusion, and small ears with overfolded helix
Cri du chat	Microdeletion	5p15.2	Distinctive facial features, microcephaly, widely set eyes (hypertelorism), low-set ears, a small jaw, and a rounded face
22 q deletion syndrome (includes DiGeorge syndrome)	Deletion	22q11	Cleft palate and some mild variation in facial features
Rubinstein-Taybi	Single gene	16p13.3	Distinctive facial features, broad thumbs and first toes, eye abnormalities, dental problems, obesity
Coffin-Lowry syndrome	X-linked	Xp22.2	Distinctive facial features and skeletal anomalies. Prominent forehead, widely spaced and downslanting eyes, a short nose with a wide tip, and a wide mouth with full lips
Williams syndrome	Single gene	7q11.23	Distinctive facial features, including a broad forehead, a short nose with a broad tip, full cheeks, and a wide mouth with full lips and small, widely spaced teeth that may be crooked or missing
Fragile X syndrome	Trinucleotide repeat (expansion mutation)	Xq27	Distinctive facial features with long and narrow face, large ears, prominent jaw and forehead, unusually flexible fingers, macro-orchidism

Data for this table are from these sources:
Chelly, J., Khelfaoui, M., et al. (2006). Genetics and pathophysiology of mental retardation. *Eur J Hum Genet, 14*(6), 701–713; NLM. (2010). Genetics Home Reference. Retrieved August 2010 from http://ghr.nlm.nih.gov/condition/down-syndrome.

Measurement

Not too long ago, dysmorphic features were evaluated only qualitatively. Clinicians looked at patients and described what they saw. Perhaps a child's eyes looked like they were too wide apart (**hypertelorism**) or the **philtrum** (the groove or depression that lies midline between the upper lip and the nose) looked too long. These qualitative descriptions made it difficult for other clinicians to judge the severity of the condition or to compare one child's features to another child's. Comparing the features of one affected child to another child affected with the same condition can help document how much variability there is among people with the same genetic problem. Now a system of precise measurements has been developed so that features can be compared against an age-related norm, and changes in a child's features can be recorded as the child grows and develops. For example, we can clearly establish whether a child's head circumference, height, or weight conforms to published normal growth curves and remains in the same percentile over time.

Figure 7–5 shows standard ways to measure various facial features. For example, the **canthus** is the angle formed by the meeting of the upper and lower eyelids. The inner canthus is closer to the nose, and the outer canthus is closer to the ear. The inner canthus distance is measured as the space between the inside of each eye, while the outer canthus distance is measured as the space between the outside of each eye. The philtrum length is measured from the top of the lip to the nose.

When a primary clinician refers a patient to a medical geneticist, the structure and growth of the entire body and specific body parts is documented (Hall et al., 2007). This is a complex process, and to do it well requires advanced training. However, the nurse or allied health professional at the bedside can recognize basic dysmorphic features and structural anomalies that should trigger referral.

When considering the possibility that the patient may have a genetic disorder, attention is focused on clinical features that could indicate the need for further evaluation. This chapter includes a brief overview of selected dysmorphic features that are of particular interest in determining whether a person

Figure 7–5. Standard facial measurements.

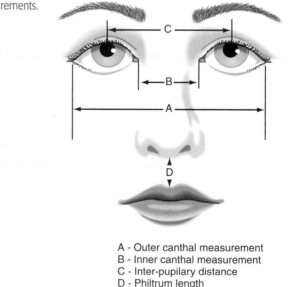

A - Outer canthal measurement
B - Inner canthal measurement
C - Inter-pupilary distance
D - Philtrum length

has a genetic disorder. There are many, many more! Targeted resources will provide a more comprehensive picture of dysmorphology, and these are included in the reference list.

Dysmorphic Features and General Appearance

It is important that the clinician begin the genetic assessment with observation of the general appearance of the patient. Unusual features are often photographed for future reference. Having a photograph also allows review by specialists, who may not be able to see the patient in person. The use of technologies such as telemedicine can allow a genetics specialist located in another geographic area to complete a physical examination with the assistance of local clinicians who are physically with the patient.

Some genetic disorders result in variations in normal height and/or weight. It must be determined whether the patient's height and weight are in the range of normal for his or her age and are consistent with those of family members. Growth curves are available to help with this determination. If a child's height or weight falls outside of the normal range, possible causes can be considered, but this is only one piece of evidence. For example, in Prader-Willi syndrome (PWS), failure to thrive is common during infancy due to hypotonia and feeding difficulties, so babies with PWS may be underweight. However, children with PWS may have an increased body weight or obesity due to *hyperphagia* (excessive eating). This is thought to be caused by an abnormality in the hypothalamus, which limits the ability to feel satisfied after eating. However, not all obese children have PWS. There are other characteristics associated with PWS, such as cognitive impairment and hypogonadism.

Another example is that people with achondroplasia have short stature with disproportionately short arms and legs and a relatively large head because of a bone growth problem. However, their short stature does not appear in isolation. There are also characteristic facial features, including midface hypoplasia and frontal bossing. In **midface hypoplasia,** the central part of the face, including the upper jaw, cheeks, and eye region, are small in proportion to the rest of the face. **Frontal bossing** describes a very large forehead with bilateral bulging of the frontal bone prominences.

Tall stature is seen in people who have Marfan syndrome (MFS). This connective tissue disorder causes patients to be tall and thin, but the problem with connective tissue also causes a weakening of the blood vessel walls, which can lead to an aneurysm. It is particularly important that young people with MFS avoid strenuous physical activity that might lead to rupture of an undiagnosed aneurysm and possible death. Identifying young people who are at risk for serious or life-threatening injury during athletics and referring them for follow-up evaluation are important reasons for a thorough presports physical examination.

Dysmorphic Features of the Skull

Craniofacial anomalies are variations from the usual formation of the skull and face. The head is assessed for its size, shape, and the symmetry of features. The head size should be compared to the size of the rest of the body to determine whether it is in proportion. **Plagiocephaly** exists when there is significant asymmetry of the skull. It can be caused by the way a newborn is positioned during sleep, which is called *positional molding*. This kind of molding is benign and has become more common since the American Academy of Pediatrics recommended that newborns sleep on their backs to reduce the incidence of sudden infant death syndrome (SIDS). Molding is more likely to be the cause when the deformity is in the posterior skull. Plagiocephaly may also be caused by an early fusion of one of the lambdoid cranial sutures. When the anterior skull is asymmetric, an underlying problem is more often the cause. **Craniosynostosis** occurs when more than one of the cranial sutures fuses together earlier than it should. If several sutures close too early, the brain may not have room to grow and intracranial pressure will increase (Reardon, 2008). This is a serious medical problem that requires urgent surgical attention.

Scalp defects may or may not involve the skull. However, most scalp defects are not associated with a problem within the brain, and they usually do not signify that there is a more complicated syndrome involved. Sometimes scalp defects do result in severe bleeding. For example, aplasia cutis congenita (ACC) is a scalp defect that usually involves a single lesion on the scalp. For 86% of people with a single lesion, there are no other accompanying features. Some people have several lesions that are circular, oval, or form a line or a star. The lesions tend to be between 0.5 cm and 10 cm in size and often heal before birth, leaving behind a hairless area covered by thin, parchment-like skin. Of course, having accompanying dysmorphic features makes it more likely that an affected person has a genetic syndrome. For example, when ACC is accompanied by limb anomalies, the child may have Adams-Oliver syndrome, which can be either inherited (usually in an autosomal dominant manner) or sporadic, and often includes heart involvement.

Macrocephaly means "enlarged head," and even though it is easy to define, exactly what makes one consider that a head is unusually large is much less clear. The technical definition is a cranium whose occipitofrontal circumference is greater than the 97th percentile compared to others of the same age and gender (Allanson, 2009). Head circumference is the largest measurement around the head. It is also called *occipitofrontal circumference* because measuring from the frontal region, just above the eyebrow ridge, to an area near the top of the occipital bone produces the largest head measurement. Measurements always must be considered in terms of a child's age and general body size. Charts are available to help clinicians determine if a child is macro- or microcephalic. The term *macrocephaly* is just descriptive and does not imply a cause for the finding. Again, some families have large heads as a familial trait, but there are also a large number of pathologic conditions that include macrocephaly as a feature. Whenever there is variation in the size of the skull, there is concern about whether or not the brain is growing normally.

Microcephaly means that the head is smaller than expected. It is generally defined clinically as having a head circumference that is more than two standard deviations below what is expected for the child's age and gender (Ashwal et al., 2010). Microcephaly is an important finding, suggesting that the brain has grown abnormally. This may be caused by structural abnormalities or by a neurodegenerative process in the brain, or the small head circumference could just run in the family and have no consequence. Microcephaly can occur alone, with no other abnormal features, as an autosomal recessive condition. *Consanguinity* may be involved in these cases. A small head is also a feature of several rare genetic disorders, and a thorough physical assessment is essential when this is seen. For example, in Smith-Lemli-Opitz syndrome, there is microcephaly along with narrowing of the head at both temples and **syndactyly** (partial fusing of the digits) of the second and third toe. Microcephaly can also occur in chromosomal disorders, such as Down syndrome, or it may be due entirely to environmental factors, such as exposure to teratogens or maternal malnutrition (Ashwal et al., 2010).

Dysmorphic Features of the Face

Coarse facial features are seen in a number of genetic problems, including mucopolysaccharide (MPS) disorders like MPS type IV (a lysosomal storage disease). You can read about biochemical diseases like MPS IV in Chapter 8. Before deciding that someone has coarse facial features, her or his appearance should be compared with that of other family members. If coarse features are a family trait, they may not be associated with disease. It is difficult to describe what is meant by *coarse face*, except to say that the features are quite prominent and are not refined, sharp, or finely sculpted. It is an example of a *bundled term* that conveys an overall impression or gestalt. In MPS IV, patients have macrocephaly, enlarged tongues, prominent foreheads, and often a coarse texture to the hair. These large and broad features give a coarse appearance to the face. Figure 7–6 shows a man with a prominent nose, deep-set eyes, broad lips, and deep nasolabial folds. This man has a coarse face.

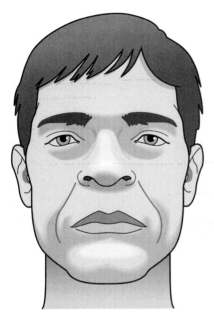

Figure 7–6. Coarse features.

The length of the philtrum can vary with the size of the nose, leading to a wide range of normal. The philtrum is smooth (no groove or depression) in a number of syndromes, including fetal alcohol spectrum disorder, but by itself, a smooth philtrum does not necessarily mean there is a genetic problem. On the other hand, if additional signs of dysmorphology have been documented, finding a smooth philtrum can help to support or refute a diagnosis. In Figure 7–4 you can see a smooth philtrum as one of the characteristic features in FASD.

Abnormal nasal bridge refers to an unusual appearance of the bony area between the eyes. There is a wide variation in what is considered normal for this feature, across age groups and populations, and this makes drawing conclusions a bit tricky. As we have mentioned before, the presence of additional dysmorphic features can make finding a raised or depressed nasal bridge more significant. A high nasal bridge is seen in Wolf-Hirschhorn syndrome, which is a chromosome deletion problem that often involves seizure activity and general hypotonia. A depressed nasal bridge can be seen in families with Stickler syndrome, which is transmitted in an autosomal dominant manner and often includes micrognathia and Pierre-Robin sequence.

Micrognathia is the term used to describe the appearance of a recessed chin caused by an unusually small mandible. If it is severe, micrognathia can result in feeding problems for affected infants and can also be the cause of Pierre-Robin sequence (described earlier). If the small jaw is not too severe, the child may outgrow the unusual appearance. Always remember that a dysmorphic feature may simply be a common family trait. But then again, family members who share one or more dysmorphic features may have an unrecognized genetic condition, such as Stickler syndrome or velo-cardio-facial syndrome. For this reason, the healthcare professional may best serve the family by having a low threshold for making a genetics referral based on dysmorphology. In other words, if you are concerned that something might be wrong, it is always best to have someone skilled in dysmorphic assessment evaluate the patient.

Dysmorphic Features of the Eyes

Hypertelorism is the term used to describe widely spaced eyes (Fig. 7–7). Several facial features can make the eyes look like they are spaced widely apart, when in fact the distance between them is perfectly normal. This can happen when a child has **epicanthic folds** or a depressed nasal bridge. It is also possible that the distance between the inner canthi is abnormally wide, but the intrapupillary and outer canthi distances are within normal range. While this situation appears to be hypertelorism, it is not. Rather, it is called *telecanthus*. While some families have wide-spaced eyes as a benign family trait, hypertelorism can be a feature in a number of genetic disorders, so, again, it is important that a thorough physical assessment follow this observation. Hypertelorism is seen in Aarskog syndrome, an X-linked disorder that has a number of other characteristic features, such as a wide philtrum, a fold in the top of the ears, and, in males, a shawl scrotum (a condition in which the scrotum surrounds the penis and looks very much like a shawl).

In **hypotelorism**, the eyes are much closer together than would be expected for the body size and age of the child (see Fig. 7–7). Hypotelorism raises suspicion about central abnormalities in the brain, such as holoprosencephaly (a condition in which the brain does not grow properly and the embryonic forebrain does not divide as it should). For this reason, neuroimaging is often recommended when an infant or young child with developmental delay has measured hypotelorism. It can also be a feature of a number of genetic disorders. One example is Kallmann syndrome, which is a hypogonadotropic hypogonadism that includes an impaired or absent sense of smell (anosmia). It is transmitted as an X-linked recessive trait.

The **palpebral fissure** is the space between the eyelids of each eye. When the outer canthus of the eye lies above an imaginary line that connects the two inner canthi, the palpebral fissure is considered to be upward slanting. An upward slant can be related to ethnic origin, or it may be simply a familial characteristic. Upslanting palpebral fissures are seen in many genetic disorders, particularly chromosome aneuploidies like Down syndrome. When the outer canthus of the eye lies below the imaginary line, the palpebral fissure is considered to be downward slanting. Downslanting palpebral fissures are common in Noonan syndrome, which also affects the heart and can result in bleeding disorders. It is important to do a careful cardiac assessment and look for other signs of dysmorphology when a child has downslanting palpebral fissures (Fig. 7–8).

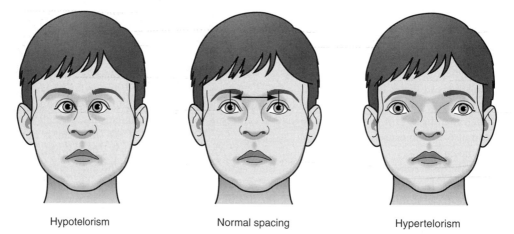

Hypotelorism   Normal spacing   Hypertelorism

Figure 7–7. Hypotelorism, normal spacing, and hypertelorism. Left = hypotelorism; middle = normal spacing; right = hypertelorism.

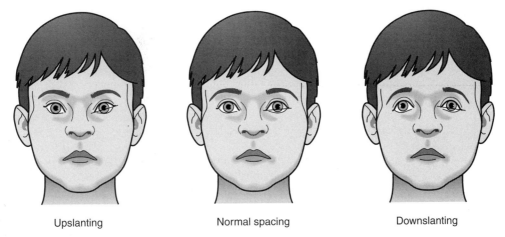

Upslanting   Normal spacing   Downslanting

Figure 7–8. Palpebral fissures. Left = upslanting; middle = normal; right = downslanting.

The epicanthus is a vertical fold of tissue that lies between the eye and the nose. It extends upward and merges with the upper eyelid. Sometimes the fold is so deep that the inner canthus cannot be seen on inspection. Epicanthic folds can be a normal variation in people of Asian descent. They can also be present in a young infant with a low nasal bridge, but this feature is typically gone by 2 years of age. Epicanthic folds are seen in a number of genetic disorders, including Down syndrome, Stickler syndrome, Williams syndrome, fetal alcohol spectrum disorder, and connective tissue disorders such as Ehlers-Danlos syndrome. Figure 7–9 shows an eye with a very prominent epicanthic fold, as might be seen in a child with Down syndrome.

Dysmorphic Features of the Ears

Low-set ears are a relatively common but highly nonspecific finding when assessing for dysmorphology. Many genetic disorders include low-set ears as a feature. When just looking at a face, it is easy to mistakenly conclude that ears are low-set, so using physical measurement to see whether they actually are low-set is essential. Ears are considered low-set when the root of the helix of the ear lies below an imaginary line drawn through the inner canthus of the eye and back to the ear. Figure 7–10 shows where this line is drawn, although the ears depicted in the figure are normally positioned.

There are many dysmorphic variations in the appearance or position of the ears. Ears can be rotated forward or backward. There can be auricular pits, which are shallow indentations that are usually seen just in front of where the helix inserts into the ear. Auricular pits can be seen in people who have

Figure 7–9. Prominent epicanthic fold.

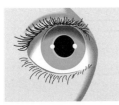

Prominent epicanthic fold

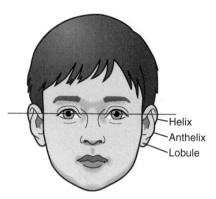

Figure 7–10. Measuring to determine if ears are low-set.

Beckwith-Wiedemann syndrome and in some people who have Treacher Collins syndrome. There are many variations in earlobe structure as well. Some people with Ehlers-Danlos syndrome do not appear to have any earlobes at all, while earlobes can be very prominent in people who have Kabuki syndrome. Of course, there is also a wide range of normal variations in earlobe configuration.

Dysmorphic Features of the Mouth

Cleft lip (CL), with or without cleft palate, is a relatively common anomaly that is associated with more than 400 different syndromes. (*CL* is the acronym that designates cleft lip without cleft palate, and *CLP* is used to indicate cleft lip with cleft palate.) These include Van der Woude syndrome, Stickler syndrome, and Patau syndrome (trisomy 13). The process of forming the structure of the mouth during embryonic development is very complex, and there are many opportunities for things to go wrong. For example, when the embryo is about 5 to 6 weeks old, the tissue that will become the upper lip is supposed to meet and fuse. At about 7 weeks, the tissue that will become the palate should also meet and fuse. If growth is inhibited and the tissues of the upper lip and/or palate do not meet, a gap (or cleft) results. In addition to genetic causes, CL/CLP can be caused by a number of environmental factors related to the lifestyle of the pregnant woman. These include having a diet that is low in vitamin B and folic acid, consuming alcohol, taking certain drugs, and smoking cigarettes.

Lip pits are symmetrical depressions in the lip, usually in the part of the lower lip called the *vermillion* (the area that is somewhat redder than the skin surrounding it). Lip pits are commonly associated with Van der Woude syndrome (VWS); VWS is a common, single-gene disorder associated with CL, CP, or CLP. VWS is an autosomal dominant trait with about 80% to 90% *penetrance*. Remember that 80% to 90% penetrance means that out of 100 people who have the gene variant that causes the disease, between 10 and 20 of them will show no clinical signs. About 70% of people who have VWS with lip pits also have CL or CP. Some family members with the same gene variant can have only lip pits, while others have CL/CP and others have just CP. This is an example of the genetic phenomenon called *variable expressivity* (Ziai et al., 2005).

Dysmorphic Features of the Hands and Feet

There are a number of variations in the development and formation of the hands and fingers. The Greek word for *digits,* meaning "fingers and toes," is *dactylos,* and you see this root word used in most names of finger and toe anomalies. **Polydactyly** refers to having an extra finger or toe. If the extra digit is on the thumb (radial side) or big toe side, it is *preaxial,* and if it is near the fifth finger (ulnar side) or fifth toe, it is *postaxial.* Postaxial polydactyly can run in families and can be transmitted in isolation as an autosomal dominant trait; however, it can also be a sign of a genetic disorder such as Ellis-van Creveld syndrome. Preaxial polydactyly is uncommon but can also be transmitted as an autosomal dominant trait in some families or can be part of a genetic condition, such as Nager syndrome.

Long, slender fingers (also called *arachnodactyly*) are often seen in people who have Marfan syndrome, but remember that long, slender fingers could just be a normal familial trait. It does make it much easier to play the piano. Short fingers or toes that are not in proportion to the rest of the body are called **brachydactyly**. While brachydactyly may occur as part of a syndrome, there is also a type that occurs in isolation, with no other anomalies present, and is transmitted in an autosomal dominant manner. We discussed clinodactyly earlier. It refers to curving of one or more digits.

When fingers (or toes) are partially or completely fused together, it is called *syndactyly*. It can affect only the skin and soft tissues (simple) or it can involve the bone as well (complex). Syndactyly occurs when the fingers or toes do not separate into individual digits during embryonic development. It is seen in at least 28 different syndromes, such as Apert and Holt-Oram syndromes.

Dysmorphology of the Joints

Joints are considered hypermobile or hyperextensible when they have a greater range of motion than what is commonly seen at a given age. About 5% of the population is hyperextensible. Women are twice as likely as men to be hyperextensible. However, hyperextensibility is also associated with disorders like Ehlers-Danlos syndrome and is an important assessment finding. Ehlers-Danlos syndrome refers to a group of connective tissue disorders that can include fragile blood vessels; soft, velvety, very elastic skin; abnormal scar formation; and hypermobility.

The extent of hypermobility can be quantified by using the Beighton and Wolf scale. On this scale, a person would get one point if she or he can bend forward with the knees straight and rest the palms of the hands on the floor. Other scale components evaluate hyperextension of the elbows, knees, thumbs, and fingers. A score of 5 out of the 9 items indicates that a person is hypermobile (Hall et al., 2007).

Summary

Dysmorphology assessment is a key tool for syndrome/disorder identification by genetics professionals. While it takes lots of practice and bedside experience to thoroughly assess for dysmorphic features, nurses can use their assessment skills to screen and refer people who may have a genetic condition. This chapter provides a brief overview of important concepts in dysmorphology and some of the more frequently recognized dysmorphic features. It is essential that the health-care professional not specializing in genetics be objective and accurate in describing anatomic variations and referring concerns to those professionals with the education and experience to complete a comprehensive assessment and make an accurate diagnosis.

GENE GEMS

- Dysmorphology focuses on the identification of abnormal features and their connection to genetic conditions.
- Congenital anomalies can be classified as major anomalies, which usually require intervention, and minor anomalies, which usually do not require intervention.
- Having one minor anomaly does not mean a person has a genetic problem.

Continued

- Causes of congenital anomalies are:
  - Malformations, which are caused by an abnormal developmental process
  - Deformations, which are caused by compression from mechanical forces
  - Disruptions, which are caused by a disturbance in the normal developmental process
  - Dysplasia, which is an alteration in the size and shape and organization of cells
- While a syndrome is a collection of symptoms that all come from the same cause, a sequence is a chain of symptoms in which each one causes the next.
- Pierre-Robin is an example of a sequence that begins with micrognathia and often results in cleft palate and airway obstruction.
- In addition to individual features, the clinician's overall impression of the patient's appearance (gestalt) is important.
- It is important to view the individual within the context of the family, because some dysmorphic traits could just be benign family characteristics or could give further support of a possible genetic condition that has gone unrecognized in the family.
- More than 300 genetic disorders can cause cognitive impairment.
- Standard ways of measuring features have allowed clinicians to compare suspected dysmorphology against age-related norms.
- Some features, such as low-set ears, are seen in a large number of different genetic disorders as well as in people who do not have a genetic disorder. They are considered nonspecific.

Self-Assessment Questions

1. What mechanism results in the malformation of cleft lip?
   a. An abnormal developmental process
   b. An abnormal organization of cells
   c. A mechanical process
   d. The breakdown of an originally normal developmental process

2. How is a congenital anomaly that requires intervention or management categorized?
   a. A dysmorphology
   b. A major anomaly
   c. A minor anomaly
   d. A disruption

3. What type of problem is Pierre-Robin, in which micrognathia begins a series of events that can result in an obstructed airway?
   a. A syndrome
   b. An association
   c. A sequence
   d. A dysplasia

4. Which of the following is *not* true regarding low-set ears?
   a. The ear position should be measured from the inner canthus.
   b. They may be normal or abnormal in appearance.
   c. They are found in only a small number of specific genetic problems.
   d. They can occur in Down syndrome or Turner syndrome.

5. You are working in a clinic and a 4-year-old child is brought in with a history of cleft palate repair. His parents say they want to have another child and ask you if their other children will have the same problem. They mention that Mom's uncle Bob had a cleft lip. What do you say?
   a. "There is a 3% to 5% risk that your next child will be affected."
   b. "Looking at your family history, I can tell that there is a 20% risk that your next child will be affected."
   c. "Let's make an appointment with a genetic counselor who will help determine your next child's risk."
   d. "You should have carrier testing to find out if your next child is at risk."

6. Naomi and her sister have the same allele for the gene of interest; however, Naomi has cleft lip, while her sister has only lip pits. What genetic process explains this difference?
   a. Genomic imprinting
   b. Decreased penetrance
   c. Genetic heterogeneity
   d. Variable expressivity

7. When geneticists assess dysmorphology, what do they consider?
   a. The "gestalt"
   b. The general feel and overall appearance of the patient
   c. Specific dysmorphic features, such as the shape of the face and the position of the ears
   d. All of the above

CASE STUDY

Sam appeared to be a healthy, normal newborn. His mother noticed that he had two small depressions on his lower lip when she was breast-feeding. At first, she thought these depressions were what her friends called "nursing blisters." Sam's pediatrician knew that lip pits occurred in about 2% of newborns, and because no one else in the family had them, she wasn't concerned. As Sam grew, the depressions did not disappear, but they weren't particularly upsetting to his parents. Sam looked quite normal, so his mother believed that they had been caused by pressure on his lower lip from his teeth and perhaps their presence earlier had been due to nursing. By this time, Sam's mom was pregnant again. When Sam's sister was born, she had an obvious cleft lip. The pediatrician seeing Sam and his sister began wondering if Sam's lip depressions and his sister's cleft lip might be connected and referred the family for genetic evaluation. Genetic testing revealed that both Sam and his sister carried a deletion in the 1q32-41 region. Both parents were tested, and Sam's mom also carried the deletion. Van der Woude syndrome was diagnosed.

1. Why do you think it took so long for this family to be diagnosed with Van der Woude syndrome?

2. What might you do if you wanted to determine (without genetic testing) if anyone else in the family might have had Van der Woude syndrome?

3. How could Sam's mom have the deletion that causes Van de Woude syndrome but not have any clinical signs?

4. What is the health-care professional's role in caring for this family?

References

Allanson, J. E., Biesecker, L. G., et al. (2009). Elements of morphology: Introduction. *American Journal of Medical Genetics Part A,149A*(1), 2–5.

Allanson, J. E., Cunniff, C., et al. (2009). Elements of morphology: Standard terminology for the head and face. *American Journal of Medical Genetics Part A, 149A*(1), 6–28.

Ashwal, S., Michelson, D., et al. (2010). Practice parameter: Evaluation of the child with microcephaly (an evidence based review): Report of the Quality Standards Subcommittee of the American Academy of Neurology and the Practice Committee of the Child Neurology Society Reply. *Neurology, 74*(13), 1079–1079.

Biesecker, L. G., Aase, J. M., et al. (2009). Elements of morphology: Standard terminology for the hands and feet. *American Journal of Medical Genetics Part A, 149A*(1), 93–127.

Carey, J. C., Cohen, Jr., M. M., et al. (2009). Elements of morphology: Standard terminology for the lips, mouth, and oral region. *American Journal of Medical Genetics Part A, 149A*(1), 77–92.

CDC. (October 21, 2010). Fetal alcohol spectrum disorder. Retrieved November 2010 from www.cdc.gov/ncbddd/fasd/index.html.

Chelly, J., Khelfaoui, M., et al. (2006). Genetics and pathophysiology of mental retardation. *European Journal of Human Genetics, 14*(6), 701–713.

Hall, B. D., Graham, Jr., J. M., et al. (2009). Elements of morphology: Standard terminology for the periorbital region. *American Journal of Medical Genetics Part A, 149A*(1), 29–39.

Hall, J. G., Allanson, J. E., et al. *Handbook of physical measurements.* New York: Oxford University Press, 2007.

Hunter, A., Frias, J. L., et al. (2009). Elements of morphology: Standard terminology for the ear. *American Journal of Medical Genetics Part A, 149A*(1), 40–60.

Jones, K. *Smith's recognizable patterns of human malformation.* Philadelphia: Elsevier, 2006.

NINDS. (May 12, 2010). Charcot-Marie-Tooth disease fact sheet. Retrieved November 2010 from www.ninds.nih.gov/disorders/charcot_marie_tooth/detail_charcot_marie_tooth.htm#156213092.

NLM. (2010). Genetics home reference. Retrieved August 2010 from http://ghr.nlm.nih.gov/condition/down-syndrome.

Reardon, W. *The bedside dysmorphologist.* New York: Oxford University Press, 2008.

Tartaglia, M., Zampino, G., et al. (2010). Noonan syndrome: Clinical aspects and molecular pathogenesis. *Molecular Syndromology, 1*(1), 2–26.

Winter, R. M., and Baraitser, M. *London Dysmorphology Database.* London, England: Oxford University Press, 2005.

Ziai, M. N., Benson, A. G., et al. (2005). Congenital lip pits and van der Woude syndrome. *J Craniofacial Surgery, 16*(5), 930–932.

Self-Assessment Answers

1. a 2. b 3. c 4. c 5. c 6. d 7. d

Genomic Health Problems Across the Life Span

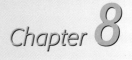
Enzyme and Collagen Disorders

Learning Outcomes

1. Use the genetic terminology associated with enzyme and collagen disorders.
2. Discuss the role of enzymes in normal physiologic function.
3. Describe the genetic defect, pattern of inheritance, pathophysiology, and the consequences of phenylketonuria.
4. Describe the genetic defects and patterns of inheritance for type 1 Gaucher disease, Hurler syndrome, Hunter syndrome, and Fabry disease.
5. Explain the pathophysiology, signs and symptoms, and consequences of type 1 Gaucher disease, Hurler syndrome, Hunter syndrome, and Fabry disease.
6. Explain the basis of enzyme replacement therapy for specific lysosomal storage diseases.
7. Discuss the role of collagen in normal physiologic function.
8. Describe the genetic defects and patterns of inheritance for osteogenesis imperfecta, Ehlers-Danlos syndrome, and Marfan syndrome.
9. Explain the pathophysiology, signs and symptoms, and consequences of osteogenesis imperfecta, Ehlers-Danlos syndrome, and Marfan syndrome.

KEY TERMS

Collagen

Ehlers-Danlos syndrome

Enzyme

Enzyme replacement therapy (ERT)

Executive functions

Fabry disease

Fibrillin

Gaucher disease

Hunter syndrome

Hurler syndrome

Hyperaminoacidemia

Lysosomal storage disease

Lysosomes

Marfan syndrome (MFS)

Osteogenesis imperfecta (OI)

Phenylketonuria (PKU)

Pleiotropy

Tay-Sachs disease

Introduction

Human body function is a dynamic and interactive process in which many proteins are produced, maintained, and often recycled daily. This huge "housekeeping" task requires the cooperation of many tissues and organs working in concert and responding appropriately to changes in body conditions to keep every body function in balance. Inappropriate overreactions in any part of the process can disrupt this balance. However, overreactions are rare. More commonly, a genetic mutation can disrupt just one specific area of the process, which then has a negative impact on overall physiologic function in some way. Two categories of inherited genetic problems are enzyme disorders and collagen disorders.

Although the gene coding for any enzyme could have a mutation or variation that affects the function of its product as a random occurrence, specific disease-causing mutations have been identified, and genetic testing is available for prenatal diagnosis. In addition, disease management strategies can reduce the negative outcomes for some of these genetic enzyme disorders. Genetic collagen disorders tend to have more pleiotropic effects, because collagen is a substance that is part of almost all body tissues. A pleiotropic effect, or **pleiotropy,** is one in which a single gene disorder results in problems expressed in many tissues and functions.

Neither inherited enzyme disorders nor inherited collagen disorders are common. This chapter focuses on those disorders that are more common or that can be managed to slow the rate of disease progression and complications or to exemplify a specific disorder type.

Enzyme Disorders

Overview

An **enzyme** is a biological catalyst that causes a biochemical reaction to occur or that increases the rate of a biochemical reaction within a cell, body tissue, or organ. Enzymes are common proteins used in many biochemical processes that change the composition of various body substances and proteins. These reactions often combine substances and form a larger compound, break compounds down into their individual components, add or remove side chains to activate or deactivate a compound, and prepare compounds for storage or elimination. All enzymes are gene products. A mutation in a gene coding for a specific enzyme usually reduces the enzyme's activity and results in a physiologic problem. The results of an ineffective enzyme, or one that is deficient, is that the expected action does not occur or occurs to only such a small degree that the final product is not present in sufficient quantities. On the other hand, the substance the enzyme should act on can build up to excessive levels, which can be toxic.

Most genetic enzyme disorders are inherited as recessive conditions, usually autosomal recessive, and many have serious adverse effects on a specific metabolic pathway or process. Some are **hyperaminoacidemias** in which one particular amino acid accumulates in the blood to toxic levels. Some of the excess amino acids are also present in the urine, which can be used to diagnose the disease. Table 8–1 lists some hyperaminoacidemias. Other genetic enzyme disorders are **lysosomal storage diseases** in which the enzyme within lysosomes is defective or deficient, causing the buildup of a precursor substance that becomes toxic to the cell. (**Lysosomes** are intracellular vesicles that contain many enzymes to degrade the protein and lipid by-products of metabolism.) Table 8–2 lists examples of the lysosomal storage diseases.

Usually in a genetic enzyme disorder, neither parent has an obvious problem, and the newborn does not have symptoms at birth. The reason that symptoms often are not apparent in the newborn is that the maternal enzymes cross the placenta and perform their specific functions in the cells of the fetus. When the child is born, its access to effective maternal enzymes stops, and the enzyme deficiency

---

TABLE 8–1

Examples of Hyperaminoacidemias

Disease	Specific Amino Acid	Involved Gene(s)
Alkaptonuria	Phenylalanine, tyrosine	*HGD*
Cystinuria	Cystine	*SLC3A1, SLC7A9*
Homocystinuria	Homocystine	*CBS, MTHFR, MTR, MTRR*
Maple syrup urine disease	Leucine, isoleucine, valine	*BCKDHA, BCKDHB, DBT, DLD*
Phenylketonuria	Phenylalanine	*PAH*

TABLE 8–2

Lysosomal Storage Diseases

Disease (% of Category)	Deficient Enzyme	Accumulated Product
Gaucher (14%)	Beta-glucosidase (glucocerebroside)	Glucosylceramide
Hurler (9%)	Alpha-L-iduronidase	Mucopolysaccharides (glycosaminoglycans)
Metachromatic leukodystrophy (8%)	Arylsulfatase A	Sulfatide sphingolipids
Sanfilippo A (7%)	Sulfamidase	Mucopolysaccharides (glycosaminoglycans)
Fabry (7%)	Alpha-glucosidase A (ceramide trihexosidase)	Globotriaosylceramide (GL-3)
Hunter (6%)	Iduronate sulfatase	Mucopolysaccharides (glycosaminoglycans)
Krabbe (5%)	Galactosylceramidase	Galactolipids
Pompe (5%)	Acid alpha-glucosidase	Glycogen
Tay-Sachs (4%)	Beta-hexosaminidase A	Ganglioside GM2

---

begins to affect the child's metabolism. Interestingly, sometimes the tissues and organs that are most affected are not those in which the enzyme is usually synthesized. As with other recessive disorders, the incidence of the problem is often higher in specific populations that have been either geographically or socially isolated, although the disorder can occur in anyone.

Phenylketonuria

Phenylketonuria (PKU) is a disorder in which the enzyme phenylalanine hydroxylase (PAH) is deficient, and the amino acid phenylalanine cannot be enzymatically converted to tyrosine, resulting in an excess of phenylalanine and a deficiency of tyrosine. Thus, it is an example of a problem that leads to hyperaminoacidemia. As discussed in Chapter 2, a protein is synthesized by connecting individual amino acids in the order coded for by the protein's gene. This process requires that the person has sufficient amounts of each of the individual amino acids. Some amino acids are classified as *essential amino acids,* meaning that they must be included in the diet because the human body cannot generate them from other substances. Tyrosine is critical for protein synthesis but is not an essential amino acid because, even when it is not ingested in the diet, it can normally be generated from phenylalanine.

The gene for phenylalanine hydroxylase is located on chromosome 12q24.1. More than 400 different types of mutations that cause the disease have been identified in this gene, which account for some differences in disease severity. The incidence of PKU in the United States is about 1 in 10,000 live births (OMIM, 2010). It is more common among people whose ancestors came from northern Europe, particularly Ireland and Scotland, and is rare in those whose ancestors came from Africa. Both genders are affected equally.

Pathophysiology

People who have phenylketonuria have a genetic deficiency of the enzyme phenylalanine hydroxylase (PAH). As a result, immediately after birth, the person starts to build up excessive amounts of phenylalanine in the blood and other body fluids. Some of this excess phenylalanine is metabolized by other enzymes and pathways into phenylpyruvate, a ketoacid that lowers the pH of the blood. Both phenylalanine and phenylpyruvate are found in the urine of patients with the disease.

The excess phenylalanine causes major problems in the developing nervous system, although the exact mechanism or mechanisms of brain damage are not completely identified. Problems also occur in skin pigmentation.

Signs and Symptoms

Tyrosine is an important amino acid for the production of thyroid hormones, melanin, and neurotransmitters, such as dopamine and the catecholamines (epinephrine and norepinephrine). When the level of phenylalanine is not managed, brain dysfunction results in severe cognitive deficiencies and diminished motor skills. Growth retardation is present and the skin, eyes, and hair color are lighter than those of parents or unaffected siblings. Additional symptoms usually include:

- Small head size
- Uncoordinated motor movement
- Seizure activity
- Tremors
- A musty or mousy odor, especially of the sweat, breath, and urine

PKU is now a part of newborn blood screening in every state. Depending on whether the infant is breast-fed or formula-fed, the disorder can be detected as early as 48 hours after birth. (Testing in breast-fed infants may not show positive results for 7 to 10 days.)

Management Strategies

Once the disorder has been identified in an infant, most of the developmental issues can be avoided with strict dietary management of phenylalanine levels. Some phenylalanine must remain in the diet because it is an essential amino acid; however, too much phenylalanine leads to problems. The specific management involves first feeding the infant a "medical food" that is a low-phenylalanine infant formula.

Throughout childhood and adolescence, the amount of phenylalanine consumed must be carefully controlled, usually less than 300 to 500 mg daily, although adjustments are needed for body size and during growth periods. After brain development is complete, less restriction of phenylalanine is needed but this is controversial. Most experts agree that the restriction should be lifelong. Even with good control over phenylalanine levels, most patients display somewhat lower cognitive abilities than siblings, hyperactive behavior, and below-normal executive functions (DeRoche and Welsh, 2008). **Executive functions** are those behavioral functions associated with prefrontal lobe brain activity and include solving problems, controlling impulses, planning, and making goal-directed actions.

A new drug recently approved for limited use in patients with PKU is sapropterin hydrochloride (Kuvan) (MD Consult, 2010). This drug is not a replacement enzyme but is a synthetic form of a cofactor needed for PAH activity. One theory for why it works in some people with PKU is that it is possible that the mutated form of PAH requires much more of the cofactor to be effective in converting phenylalanine to tyrosine. This oral drug, when used with a low-phenylalanine diet, reduces the blood levels of phenylalanine in some patients below what can be expected by dietary phenylalanine reduction alone.

With increasing life spans and cognition among people with PKU, a newer issue is the problem of an increased incidence of a variety of health problems and birth defects among infants born to women with PKU (Wright and Roberts, 2007). The infants do not have PKU; however, abnormal blood levels of amino acids, especially during embryonic life, result in a wide variety of birth defects, most commonly of the cardiovascular system. The best pregnancy outcomes for women with PKU are achieved when phenylalanine levels are well controlled before and during pregnancy.

Gaucher Disease`

Gaucher disease is a genetic lysosomal storage disease in which there is a deficiency of the enzyme beta-glucosidase, which results in the accumulation of glucosylceramide (also called *glucocerebroside*) in macrophages and some other mononuclear white blood cells (Chen and Wang, 2008). The gene for beta-glucosidase is located on chromosome 1q21, and the disease is transmitted in an autosomal recessive pattern. Gaucher disease is the most common of the lysosomal storage diseases and occurs most often among the Ashkenazi Jewish population (incidence of approximately 1 in 450 births) compared with non-Jewish populations (incidence of approximately 1 in 40,000 to 100,000 births). It is also more common among French Canadians in the Quebec area. About 20,000 individuals are living with Gaucher disease in the United States (OMIM, 2010).

Pathophysiology

Macrophages, which are mononuclear white blood cells, are present within most tissues and organs; however, there are three distinct forms of Gaucher disease that affect organs differently. The most common form of the disease is Gaucher type 1, which is also known as *non-neuronopathic* because central nervous system cells are not affected. Cells and tissues that are affected include macrophages in the liver, spleen, bone marrow, and lungs. Huge amounts of glucosylceramide collect in the macrophages of these tissues, resulting in organ enlargement. Gaucher type 2 is known as *acute neuronopathic-infantile disease* because neurons are severely affected, and death usually occurs within the first 2 years of life. Gaucher type 3, known as *chronic neuronopathic*, is less common than type 1 and not as severe as type 2. This discussion of Gaucher disease focuses on type 1.

Although the glucosylceramide accumulates in tissue macrophages rather than in actual organ cells, the excessively large macrophages exert pressure on nearby organ cells. In addition, as organs enlarge from the continually increasing size of macrophages, perfusion and oxygenation to the organs decrease. Both the increased pressure and poor organ perfusion greatly reduce organ function and shorten life.

Signs and Symptoms

The main signs and symptoms of Gaucher type 1 are related to the specific organs in which the macrophages enlarge. These include the liver and spleen, which can increase many times their normal sizes, resulting in a large protruding abdomen and abdominal pain. The bone marrow is infiltrated with enlarged macrophages, preventing the adequate production of red blood cells and platelets (thrombocytopenia). As a result, the person bruises easily with minimal trauma and is anemic (causing fatigue). Bone marrow infiltration also causes bone pain and osteoporosis. This condition can lead to pathologic bone fractures. Overall growth can be reduced as well, possibly as a result of liver compression and poor production of various somatomedins and other factors that influence growth. Although more people are affected in childhood, some people do not show signs and symptoms of the disease until adulthood.

Management Strategies

Some management strategies focus on the problems caused by the disease. For example, at one time, the management of anemia and thrombocytopenia was based on iron and vitamin supplements coupled with transfusions of blood and platelets. Growth factor therapy with epoetin alfa (Epogen, Procrit) can increase the production of red blood cells. Therapy with oprelvekin (Neumega) can increase the production of platelets (Workman, LaCharity, and Kruchko, 2011). The effectiveness of these drugs on bone marrow decreases as active marrow cells are replaced with glucosylceramide-filled macrophages.

An enlarged spleen can rupture and lead to death. A partial or total splenectomy can prevent this problem, but it also reduces the antibody-generating responses of the person when infection, especially viral infection, occurs.

Bone involvement can be managed with analgesics to help bone pain, calcium supplementation or drug therapy with bisphosphonates to prevent bone density loss, and trauma precautions to prevent fractures. Additional management involves removing cells from the marrow (core compression). Damaged joints can be replaced with partial or total joint prostheses.

Another management strategy is the actual replacement of the missing or malfunctioning enzyme with one that has been generated artificially, a process known as **enzyme replacement therapy (ERT).** Gaucher type I is a disorder that responds well to this type of therapy. The drug is imiglucerase (Cerezyme), which is infused intravenously every 2 weeks once a blood level has been achieved. Some patients have a dramatic reduction in liver size, spleen size, and bone pain within a few weeks of beginning the therapy, although each patient's response is variable. This therapy is very expensive and represents only a disease-management therapy, not a cure.

Currently, the only cure for Gaucher type 1 is a hematopoietic stem cell transplantation (HSCT) from a donor who does not have the disease. This process is successful because the healthy stem cells transplanted into the patient take up residence in the patient's bone marrow. These new cells produce a healthy version of the deficient enzyme, which then can be taken up and used by many cells. Not only is this procedure very expensive and often not covered by insurance, but it is also very dangerous. The main use of HSCT is in the treatment of some types of cancers. Under the best of circumstances, HSCT has a mortality rate that approaches 50% from the complications of the procedure. The cost of the treatment and the uncertainty of the outcome limit its utility as a management strategy for Gaucher or any other lysosomal storage disease.

Hurler Syndrome

Hurler syndrome, also known as *mucopolysaccharidosis I,* is a genetic lysosomal storage disease in which there is a deficiency of the enzyme alpha-L-iduronidase (IDUA), resulting in the accumulation of mucopolysaccharides (MPS) in the lysosomes of most cells. The gene for IDUA is transmitted in an autosomal recessive pattern and is located on chromosome 4p16.3. The disorder occurs in about 1 out of 100,000 births and affects males and females equally. More than 100 different mutations have been identified and are responsible for variation in disease severity (NIH, 2010).

Pathophysiology

Mucopolysaccharides (MPSs) are also known as *glycosaminoglycans* (GAGs). These substances are large molecules of sugar and protein that make up a major part of tissue basement membranes. There are many different types of MPSs, with each type having a slightly different chemical composition and requiring a different enzyme for degradation. These acellular substances are "recycled" almost daily to maintain basement membranes. Recycling involves enzymatically breaking down a formed MPS into its constituent parts within cellular lysosomes. When the enzyme responsible for degrading a specific type of MPS is either deficient or nonfunctional, the large MPSs accumulate within the lysosomes. With MPS I, the lysosomes of almost all cells are affected over time by the progressive accumulation of MPSs.

Signs and Symptoms

Infants with Hurler syndrome appear normal at birth, although a higher incidence of umbilical hernia in these children has been reported. The physical appearance begins to change within the first 6 months of life. Facial features become more coarse, with a large head, prominent forehead, flat face, short and wide nose, thick lips, heavy eyebrows, and a short neck. Physical growth is poor, resulting in a short stature. Combined with the facial changes, spinal deformity, and stiff joints, this gives the child a "dwarf" or "gargoyle" appearance. Skin is thicker and less flexible. Enlargement of the liver and spleen causes abdominal distention. The brain and surrounding structures are involved, often progressing to hydrocephaly. Development is delayed and intellectual functioning is limited. Over time, intellectual functioning deteriorates to a profound degree. As MPSs increase in cardiac tissue, this organ's function also deteriorates.

As the disease progresses, the respiratory structures are affected and airway obstruction is common. Poor cough and excessive nasal secretions increase the incidence of respiratory infections. Death commonly occurs as a result of pneumonia or cardiac dysfunction between the ages of 5 and 10 years.

Management Strategies

At one time, only supportive or comfort care was available for children with Hurler syndrome. Drug therapy was used to prevent or treat respiratory infections and to improve cardiac function. Currently, two additional management strategies are available, ERT and HSCT. The drug for ERT is laronidase (Aldurazyme), which is administered as weekly infusions. Although it prevents disease progression in many tissues and reverses liver and spleen enlargement, it does not prevent central nervous system deterioration because the drug does not cross the blood-brain barrier. Therefore, this expensive drug is used to reduce disease progression until HSCT can be performed (Bijarnia et al., 2009). Although HSCT is the standard of care for children with Hurler syndrome and should be performed before 2 years of age, it remains a costly and dangerous option (see the discussion in the "Management Strategies" section of "Gaucher Disease").

Hunter Syndrome

Hunter syndrome is a genetic lysosomal storage disease in which there is a deficiency of the enzyme iduronate sulfatase, which results in the accumulation of MPSs within the lysosomes of many tissues and organs. It is also known as mucopolysaccharidosis II (MPS II). Unlike Hurler syndrome, Hunter syndrome is an X-linked recessive disorder with the iduronate sulfatase gene *(IDS)* located on Xq28. The disorder occurs in about 1 out of 100,000 to 1 out of 170,000 births and affects males almost exclusively. Females are carriers. More than 300 different mutations have been identified and are responsible for variation in disease severity (NIH, 2010).

Pathophysiology

The actual pathophysiology of Hunter syndrome with regard to poor degradation of MPSs is identical to that of Hurler syndrome. Major differences are that people with Hunter syndrome have a slower onset of symptoms, and the effect on intellectual ability is more variable. In mild forms, loss of intellectual ability is minimal. In more severe forms, the loss of intellectual ability is more severe but occurs at a much later age than in Hurler syndrome.

Signs and Symptoms

The clinical picture of a person with Hunter syndrome looks very similar to that of the person with Hurler syndrome. In fact, the phenotype is so similar that, except for the slower onset and less frequent reduction of intellectual ability found in people with Hunter syndrome, at one time the two were considered to be the same disorder; however, the deficient enzyme is different. Additional symptoms of Hunter syndrome include gradual hearing loss and vision problems. People with the more severe form of the disease usually live for 10 to 20 years. People with the milder form of the disease usually live 20 to 60 years.

Management Strategies

Currently, two management strategies are available: ERT and HSCT. The drug for enzyme replacement is idursulfase (Elaprase), which is administered as weekly infusions. HSCT is a costly and dangerous option (see the discussion in the "Management Strategies" section of "Gaucher Disease"). For patients who have a mild form of Hunter syndrome, the benefits of this therapy may not be worth the associated risks.

Fabry Disease

Fabry disease is a genetic lysosomal storage disease in which there is a deficiency of the enzyme alpha-galactosidase A (also known as *ceramide trihexosidase*), which results in the accumulation of globotriao-sylceramide (GL-3) within the lysosomes of many tissues and organs. It is an X-linked recessive disorder, and the alpha-galactosidase A gene *(GLA)* is located on chromosome Xq22. The disorder affects about 1 in 40,000 to 60,000 males (NIH, 2010). Although much more common among males, female carriers may have significant symptoms of the disorder as a result of skewed X chromosome inactivation in different tissues (see Chapter 4; Schaefer et al., 2009).

Pathophysiology

The enzyme normally degrades GL-3, which is composed of three sugar molecules attached to a lipid molecule. Degradation of GL-3 is a part of the recycling of old red blood cells and other types of cells. When the enzyme is deficient, large amounts of GL-3 and one of its toxic metabolites, globotriao-sphingosine, build up within the blood and within the lysosomes of many tissues and organs (Schaefer, 2009). This lysosomal storage of GL-3 causes changes and damage within the blood vessels. As blood vessels become less efficient, chronic inflammatory responses start, leading to poor tissue perfusion, ischemia, and eventual tissue or organ failure.

Signs and Symptoms

Although the biochemical changes can be identified in early childhood, the onset of signs and symptoms of Fabry disease usually begin later in childhood. At first, symptoms are related to poor perfusion and include cold intolerance, insufficient sweating in hot environments, and pain episodes of unknown origin. In adolescents, the symptoms worsen with opacities developing in the eye. Episodic numbness and tingling in the fingers and toes also occurs. Angiokeratomas of the skin are common. Blood vessels are affected everywhere, but the more vascular organs, such as the heart, kidney, and brain, as well as those that are very oxygen-dependent, such as peripheral nerves, develop more damage earlier. In general, males begin to have symptoms about 3 to 5 years earlier than females. By adulthood, the person usually has some degree of renal insufficiency or failure. Strokes and hearing problems (deafness and tinnitus) are common. Cardiac problems develop, including angina, myocardial infarction, and heart failure. Without treatment, death usually occurs prematurely.

Management Strategies

After identification of the disorder, symptomatic and preventive strategies for kidney, brain, and cardio-vascular health are employed. These have limited effect because they do not address the cause of the problems associated with the disease.

ERT is now the standard of care for a person with Fabry disease. The two drugs are agalsidase alfa (Replagal) and agalsidase beta (Fabrazyme). Currently, only agalsidase beta is approved for use in the United States. It is administered intravenously every 2 weeks. A number of randomized controlled clinical trials indicate that this drug is able to normalize GL-3 levels in many tissues. The drug has not been available long enough to determine its overall effectiveness in preventing organ failure and premature death (Schaefer et al., 2009).

Tay-Sachs Disease

Tay-Sachs disease is a genetic lysosomal storage disease in which there is a deficiency of the enzyme beta-hexosaminidase A, which results in the accumulation of GM2-ganglioside in brain cells. The gene for beta hexosaminidase A is located on chromosome 15q23 to q24, and the disorder is transmitted in an autosomal recessive pattern. Three specific mutations are responsible for nearly all of the cases of the classic type of Tay-Sachs disease. The incidence of Tay-Sachs disease is highest among people of Ashkenazi Jewish ethnicity worldwide, about 1 in 3900 births. The incidence among non-Jewish populations is much less frequent, about 1 in 320,000 births (OMIM, 2010).

Pathophysiology

The precursor product or target of the enzyme beta-hexosaminidase A is a glycoprotein fat (lipid) substance known as a *ganglioside* (GM2). Without adequate levels of the enzyme, GM2 builds up in many cells but particularly in brain cells. The buildup increases neuronal size, causing them to have a ballooned and distorted appearance. Over time, brain cells accumulate large amounts of GM2 and their function is destroyed. When enough brain cells have been destroyed, death occurs. The most common cause of death is pneumonia related to respiratory muscle weakness and the inability of the child to swallow effectively (leading to aspiration).

Signs and Symptoms

At birth, an infant with Tay-Sachs has a completely normal appearance and reflexes. He or she has normal muscle tone and intellectual potential. During the first few months of life, the infant progresses normally, usually learning to control the head, recognize parental faces, socially smile, and roll over. At this point, normal development slows or stops. Over the next few months, physical development and cognitive development regress. One hallmark of the disease is seen when the retina is examined with an ophthalmoscope. The retinal cells have become filled with GM2 and are pale. This makes the fovea centralis stand out as a cherry-red spot against the pale retinal background.

Over time, the child's muscles become weaker and most reflexes diminish. One reflex continues—the startle response to sounds. All physical movement decreases and paralysis eventually occurs. Other signs and symptoms include blindness and seizure activity. Most children with Tay-Sachs disease die between 2 and 4 years of age.

Although the disorder is diagnosed on the basis of history and manifestations, blood testing can confirm the diagnosis by assaying blood enzyme levels. DNA analysis can determine which mutation is present. Carrier status also can be identified on the basis of enzyme levels and DNA analysis.

Management Strategies

Currently, no therapy exists to cure Tay-Sachs disease or prevent its progressive brain degeneration. Management strategies focus on delaying muscle weakness with passive exercise and preventing aspiration. Parents and siblings require much emotional support. Genetic counseling can be very beneficial in helping family members assess risk and make decisions regarding reproduction.

Summary

Although the gene defect for enzyme disorders is present from conception, the manifestations of the disorders usually are not present until after birth. Enzyme replacement therapy is available to help manage some, but not all, enzyme diseases. Hematopoietic stem cell transplantation can result in a cure for many enzyme disorders, even though bone marrow cells are not usually the cells affected by the disorder. The complications associated with this procedure and its cost must be considered when assessing the benefits versus the risks of pursuing this therapy.

Collagen Disorders

Overview

Collagen is a group of glycoprotein fibers that forms the major component of the connective tissue found in nearly all body tissues. It starts put as procollagen and is the most abundant protein in humans and other mammals. Procollagen is processed or modified in a variety of different ways to form different types of mature collagen fibers that work with other fibrous tissues to form cables that add strength and structure to most tissues (McCance et al., 2010). In addition, collagen fibers are part of the extracellular matrix between cells and tissues that function to hold tissues together and to promote communication between and among cells.

The production of different types of procollagen and the modification steps are genetically controlled. Gene mutations can affect the production and composition of any collagen type or interfere with its proper modification, assembly, or association with other molecules. Any of these problems can result in the phenotypic expression of a collagen disorder.

There are five main types of collagen within the human body, as well as many minor types:

- Type 1 collagen is the most common and is a major component of bones, the dermal layer of skin, tendons, ligaments, corneas, intervertebral disks, and the walls of arteries and other blood vessels. It is coded for by the *COL1A1* gene located on chromosome 17q21.33.
- Type 2 collagen is the major type of collagen found in cartilage and is coded for by the *COL2A1* gene located on chromosome 12q13.11.
- Type 3 collagen is a major component of connective tissue in the skin, lungs, intestinal walls, and the walls of blood vessels. It is coded for by the *COL3A1* gene located on chromosome 2q31.

- Type 4 collagen is a major component of connective tissue in the kidney and inner ear. There are several subgroups of type 4 collagen coded for by the *COL4A* genes 1-6, which are located on chromosomes 2, 13, and the X chromosome.
- Type 5 collagen works with other collagen types to provide strength to connective tissues in the skin, ligaments, bones, tendons, muscles, and the extracellular matrix. It is coded for mainly by the *COL5A1* gene located on chromosome 9q34.2-q34.3 (NIH, 2010).

Genetic mutations in any of the collagen genes usually affect more than one type of tissue (pleiotropy) and are involved in many genetic disorders (Table 8–3). The collagen disorders discussed in this chapter are the osteogenesis imperfecta and Ehlers-Danlos syndromes. In addition, another disorder, Marfan syndrome, which is a problem of fibrillin production that normally interacts with collagen for connective tissue strength and flexibility, is also discussed.

Osteogenesis Imperfecta

Osteogenesis imperfecta (OI) is a group of genetic disorders in which collagen formation is impaired, resulting in bones that fracture easily. Many different mutations, especially in the genes for type 1 collagen, result in great variation in disease severity. With some mutations, bone fractures occur in the fetal period and are lethal (osteogenesis imperfecta type II). Other mutations result in a more mild disease expression in which bones are brittle and fracture more easily, but bone deformity does not occur.

There are four major types of osteogenesis imperfecta that occur as results of mutations in a gene for type 1 collagen. All follow an autosomal dominant transmission pattern, although spontaneous mutations are responsible about 35% of the time (Osteogenesis Imperfecta Foundation, 2007). The most common

TABLE 8–3

Examples of Genetic Collagen Disorders

Collagen Type	Disorder/Health Problem
Type 1 collagen	Arthrochalasia
	Caffey disease
	Ehlers-Danlos (classical)
	Osteogenesis imperfecta
	Osteoporosis
Type 2 collagen	Achondrogenesis
	Czech dysplasia
	Hypochondrogenesis
	Kniest dysplasia
	Osteoarthritis (early onset, familial)
	Stickler syndrome
Type 3 collagen	Ehlers-Danlos (vascular, formerly type IV)
Type 4 collagen	Alport syndrome
Type 5 collagen	Ehlers-Danlos (classical)

type of the disease, osteogenesis imperfecta type I, occurs in about 1 out of 15,000 to 30,000 births. It affects males and females equally. The most severe form that occurs without lethality is type III. It is rare in the United States and occurs most commonly in central and southern Africa.

Pathophysiology

The primary problem with OI is failure to produce at least one functional chain of procollagen that is needed to associate with other molecules and form functional collagen in bone tissue. As a result, the developing bones have less structural integrity and strength, increasing the risk for fractures. The severity of the phenotype is related to both the degree of normal collagen reduction present in the bone and whether abnormal collagen is produced.

Signs and Symptoms

The clinical manifestations of osteogenesis imperfecta type I can easily be missed, because the collagen produced is normal but the amount is reduced. Usually, the person has no increase in fractures during infancy. Fractures do occur in response to relatively minor trauma throughout childhood, adolescence, and adulthood. In women, more fractures are seen after menopause. A common feature is the blue-tinged coloration of the sclera.

Osteogenesis imperfecta type II is the most severe. Essentially, no normal collagen is produced. Bone fractures and skeletal malformations, including skull deformities, occur in the prenatal period and are lethal. The infant, often born prematurely, has multiple fractures and bone malformations that can be seen on fetal x-rays or ultrasound images.

Osteogenesis imperfecta type III may produce fractures in prenatal life that are present at birth and result in skeletal deformities. The bone collagen produced is abnormal, and fractures continue throughout the life span. Linear growth is limited and fractures result in bone deformities. Other signs and symptoms may include muscle weakness, hearing loss, fatigue, joint laxity, curved bones, scoliosis, blue sclerae, and brittle teeth. With repeated spinal fractures that lead to spinal deformities, restrictive pulmonary disease occurs because the rib cage does not expand appropriately.

Osteogenesis imperfecta type IV is less severe than types II and III, because the collagen produced is abnormal but functions better than that produced in types II and III. The sclera coloration is normal (white), and fractures result in less deformity.

Currently there is no cure for OI. For individuals with mild or moderate disease, life expectancy is not shortened. For OI type III, the progressive deformities reduce life expectancy.

Management Strategies

Initial management strategies focus on preventing fractures, especially of the spine. Calcium supplementation is not helpful because the genetic defect does not make the bone calcium deficient. Other strategies involve physical therapy and safe exercise (primarily swimming); broken bone management with casts, splints, or wraps; braces to support legs, ankles, knees, and wrists; surgical implantation of rods to support the long bones; and the use of bisphosphonate-based drugs to maintain or improve bone strength. Canes, walkers, or wheelchairs are used to promote mobility and reduce stress on weight-bearing bones.

Ehlers-Danlos Syndrome

Ehlers-Danlos syndrome is a group of six different inherited disorders that occur as a result of mutations in the genes responsible for collagen formation or modification (Ehlers-Danlos National Foundation, 2008). These disorders vary in severity and the tissues most involved. *Classical Ehlers-Danlos* (formerly known as type I or type II) is caused by gene mutations for type 1 or type 5 collagen and is transmitted in an autosomal dominant pattern. *Hypermobility Ehlers-Danlos* (formerly known as type III) is transmitted as an autosomal dominant disorder, although no specific collagen mutation has been identified. *Vascular Ehlers-Danlos* (formerly known as type IV) is caused by a gene mutation for type 3 collagen and is transmitted in an autosomal dominant pattern. *Kyphoscoliosis Ehlers-Danlos* (formerly known as type VI) is caused by a mutation in a gene responsible for modifying collagen and is transmitted in an autosomal recessive pattern. Classical Ehlers-Danlos syndrome is the mildest form. Vascular Ehlers-Danlos and kyphoscoliosis Ehlers-Danlos syndrome have more severe complications and are associated with early death. The incidence of all types of Ehlers-Danlos syndrome collectively is about 1 in 5000 births. Males and females are affected equally.

Pathophysiology

The major pathology associated with all types of Ehlers-Danlos syndrome is the presence of abnormal collagen in many different connective tissues. The exact problems that develop depend on which type of collagen is affected and how much of the abnormal collagen is present in a specific type of connective tissue.

Signs and Symptoms

In classical Ehlers-Danlos, the skin and joints are most commonly involved. These tissues are hyperextensible and more stretchy as a result of abnormal collagen. Wide scars develop in areas of injury or skin stress. The skin is fragile and bruises easily.

The major symptom of hypermobility Ehlers-Danlos is hypermobile joints, especially the knees, elbows, fingers, toes, and the temporomandibular joint. These joints frequently become subluxated and dislocated. Joint pain is common and chronic. The skin is more extensible and fragile than normal but not as severely as in classical Ehlers-Danlos.

Vascular Ehlers-Danlos is severe and leads to premature death. The individual has very thin, fragile skin and short stature. Facial features include a small, triangular face, large eyes, and a thin nose. The bigger problems are associated with the thin connective tissue in midsized and large arteries. In addition, the intestinal connective tissue is very thin. All of these tissues become thinner as the child grows. Scars from any skin injury heal poorly. Although the fingers and toes may be hyperextensible, most other joints are not. The most common causes of death are hemorrhage from arterial rupture and sepsis from intestinal rupture, often before the age of 30.

The major features of kyphoscoliosis Ehlers-Danlos include laxity of nearly all joints and significant muscle weakness, even at birth. Motor development is delayed and a scoliosis-type spinal curvature usually develops in infancy and progresses as the child grows. The muscle weakness also progresses, and most individuals are unable to walk by adolescence or early adulthood. The sclera of the eye is thin and ruptures easily with minor trauma. Premature death is associated with respiratory problems.

Management Strategies

No type of Ehlers-Danlos syndrome can be cured. Management techniques vary, depending on which manifestations are most prominent. Patient and family education are critical to delaying complications. Learning how to protect the joints while maintaining mobility is important in preventing injury and reducing pain. Activities that cause pain are avoided, and physical therapy can help the afflicted person learn how to avoid overextending or locking the joints. Trauma, especially falls, needs to be avoided. Children are instructed to use knee and elbow pads. Keeping pathways clear and free of objects such as throw rugs can help, as can wearing well-fitting shoes during ambulation.

The use of vitamin C has been recommended to reduce symptom severity, especially for vascular Ehlers-Danlos. However, there is little evidence showing the effectiveness of this therapy.

Marfan Syndrome

Marfan syndrome (MFS) is an inherited genetic connective tissue disorder in which the gene for the glycoprotein fibrillin is mutated. Although MFS is not a collagen disease, it is similar in that fibrillin interacts with collagen and elastin to provide recoil strength to tissues during and after stretching. **Fibrillin,** like collagen, is a glycoprotein that assembles into long strands of microfibrils and is an essential component of specific connective tissues, especially those that respond by stretching when a force is applied. It is most abundant in tendons, muscles, the connective tissue that surrounds large arteries, and heart valves. In addition, this protein plays a role in eye and skin development. The gene for fibrillin is *FBN1,* located on chromosome 15q21.1. Although MFS is inherited as an autosomal dominant disorder, spontaneous mutations also have occurred and result in a more mild disease expression. MFS is relatively common, occurring at a rate of 1 out of 5000 births. Males and females are affected equally, and the disorder may be underdiagnosed (NIH, 2010).

Pathophysiology

Within those connective tissues that must "give" or stretch somewhat when a force is applied, three interacting components allow the stretch to occur without breaking and then return the tissue to the shape and size it was before the force was applied. These components are collagen, elastin, and fibrillin. Static strength is provided by collagen, and the give or stretch is provided by the elastin. A significant role of fibrillin is that of limiting the stretch to help ensure a return to the original resting shape of the connective tissue when the force is removed. So, in a sense, fibrillin adds dynamic strength to connective tissue.

Three major types of fibrillin have been identified. Most cases of MFS result from mutations in type 1 fibrillin. The *FBN1* gene is large, and many mutations occur. This mutation variability is most likely associated with the wide variations seen in the phenotype. As a result of mutations, fibrillin can fail to form at all, can form in low amounts, can form as abnormal microfibrils, or can form as a truncated, nonfunctional microfibril. Regardless of the mechanisms, connective tissue without sufficient amounts of healthy fibrillin is unstable, weaker, and becomes overstretched over time. In addition to *FBN1,* mutations in other genes *(FBN2, TGFBR2)* also affect the final function of fibrillin.

Signs and Symptoms

The phenotypes of people with Marfan syndrome vary. Because fibrillin is an important component of many tissues, the effects are widespread (pleiotropic). Although most people do not manifest all signs and symptoms, even within one family, the most common ones affect the skeletal, ocular, and cardiovascular systems (Iams, 2010). Most are not recognizable at birth and become more pronounced as the individual ages. These include:

- Tall, lanky stature
- "Wingspan" (arm-spread width) greater than height
- Loose or lax joints
- Very long fingers (arachnodactyly) that are hyperextensible
- Spinal curvatures
- Chest deformities
- Narrow, arched palate
- Crowded teeth
- Small or regressed chin
- Downward-slanting palpebral fissures

- Flat cornea
- Displaced or detached lens
- Myopia
- Small iris
- Mitral valve prolapse
- Widened aorta
- Aortic aneurysm
- Left ventricular enlargement
- Cardiomyopathy

The cardiovascular problems can significantly shorten life span. Dissecting aortic aneurisms and death can even occur in childhood. Without management, the average life expectancy for the person with MFS is 37 years (Gonzales, 2009).

Management Strategies

Marfan syndrome cannot be cured, and management is based on physical changes or symptoms. The first step in management is identifying the diagnosis. This can be a problem because the phenotype can be subtle and the person resembles other family members. In addition, some of the physical changes are similar to those of other disorders. Genetic testing is not practical for initial diagnosis because the large number of possible mutations make testing expensive. Testing is best used when a person is diagnosed based on phenotype and family history and has a specific mutation. This information can be used to determine whether other family members carry the mutation.

Although skeletal and ocular management are important, the primary management focuses on monitoring and protecting the cardiovascular system. Patients are encouraged to achieve and maintain a healthy weight appropriate for height and to avoid excessive weight gain. A balance of physical activity is needed to be physically fit without placing strain on the cardiovascular system. Strenuous exercise and heavy lifting must be avoided, as should any activity in which the chest could be hit. Thus, contact sports and those that involve running or catching a ball should be avoided. Walking is encouraged, as are less physically aggressive sports, such as golfing, bowling, recreational swimming, or low-intensity bicycling. These recommendations may be difficult, particularly during late childhood and early adulthood, when the focus on physical prowess and participation in team sports is emphasized. Think about the 6-foot-7-inch-tall 15-year-old who is pressured by the basketball coach to join the team. Also consider that a taller-than-average person might be expected by friends to help move furniture or carry a heavier load.

The health-care provider needs to evaluate the patient's cardiovascular status at least yearly. Tests are needed to assess left ventricular function and ejection fraction, mitral valve function, and aortic width. Maintaining blood pressure within the normal range is critical and may require pharmacologic management. Surgical intervention is needed when aortic dilation reaches a critical point and when heart valve function falls below an acceptable level.

Summary

At the present time, collagen disorders and connective tissue diseases cannot be cured. Thus, accurate diagnosis and early preventive intervention strategies are needed to delay complications and promote quality of life. Many of these disorders are inherited in an autosomal dominant fashion; however, some also have a relatively high rate of occurrence as a result of spontaneous new mutations. Health oversight by a knowledgeable health-care professional and appropriate genetic counseling are essential components of patient and family care.

GENE GEMS

- A mutation in a gene coding for a specific enzyme usually reduces the enzyme's activity and results in one or more physiologic problems related to toxic accumulation of the precursor substance.
- People with phenylketonuria must adhere to a low phenylalanine diet to prevent or slow the central nervous system complications of the disease.
- Enzyme replacement therapy for lysosomal storage diseases reduces the progression of the disease and must be continued on a regular basis for life.
- Of the three types of Gaucher disease, type I is most common, does not affect the central nervous system, and can be managed with enzyme replacement therapy (ERT).
- Signs and symptoms of Gaucher disease type 1 may not be present until adulthood.
- The phenotypes of Hurler syndrome and Hunter syndrome are very similar, although Hunter syndrome has a slower onset and a less detrimental effect on intellectual function.
- The incidence of Tay-Sachs disease is 100 times greater among Ashkenazi Jewish populations than among most non-Jewish populations.
- Many enzyme disorders can be cured by hematopoietic stem cell transplantation (HSCT), but the procedure is both costly and dangerous.
- There is no therapy to prevent progression of Tay-Sachs disease.
- Collagen is the most abundant protein found in humans and provides both structure and strength to many tissues.
- In mild forms of osteogenesis imperfecta, collagen is normal but is present in reduced amounts.
- In moderate and severe forms of osteogenesis imperfecta, the type 1 collagen produced is abnormal.
- About 35% of the cases of osteogenesis imperfecta occur as a result of a new spontaneous mutation.

Self-Assessment Questions

1. Which clinical situation best demonstrates the concept of pleiotropy?
   a. Congenital deafness is usually bilateral.
   b. The problem caused by a single gene mutation appears at an earlier age in each succeeding generation.
   c. A specific, single gene mutation results in the phenotype of mental retardation, absent iris, and exstrophy of the bladder.
   d. Huntington disease, caused by a single gene mutation present at birth, does not show manifestations until later in life.

2. Which normal physiologic process usually requires an enzyme?
   a. Degradation of glycosaminoglycans into sugar and proteins for recycling
   b. Propagation of a nerve action potential from the point of stimulation to the axon terminal
   c. Exfoliation (shedding) of dead skin cells from the stratum corneum of the epidermal layer
   d. Movement of water across a cell's plasma membrane from an area of high hydrostatic pressure to an area of lower hydrostatic pressure

3. Which problem results from the genetic defect associated with phenylketonuria?
   a. Excessive levels of tyrosine and deficient levels of phenylalanine
   b. Excessive levels of tyrosine and normal levels of phenylalanine
   c. Excessive levels of phenylalanine and deficient levels of tyrosine
   d. Excessive levels of phenylalanine and normal levels of tyrosine

4. If a man with Gaucher type 1 has children with a woman who is a carrier for the disorder, what is the expected risk pattern?
   a. All sons will be unaffected; all daughters will be carriers.
   b. All sons will be carriers; all daughters will be affected.
   c. Each child of either gender has a 50% risk of having the disease.
   d. Each child of either gender has a 50% risk of being a carrier, a 25% risk of having the disease, and a 25% risk of neither being a carrier nor having the disease.

5. Why does a person with Hurler syndrome have an enlarged abdomen?
   a. The excess mucopolysaccharides accumulate inside the lysosomes within the liver cells.
   b. The excess mucopolysaccharides accumulate inside the macrophages located in the spleen.
   c. The excess glycosaminoglycans weaken the muscles of the abdomen and all contents move forward.
   d. The excess glycosaminoglycans cause the person to develop type 2 diabetes, with greatly increased abdominal fat.

6. How does intravenous enzyme replacement therapy for Gaucher disease reduce the organ storage of glucosylceramide?
   a. The enzyme increases the destruction of glucosamide-filled macrophages.
   b. The drug acts as a cofactor, increasing the activity of the mutated enzyme.
   c. The drug increases production of all blood cells in the bone marrow, including white blood cells, which have not stored glucosylceramide.
   d. The enzyme is absorbed through the plasma membranes of affected cells and converts the stored glucosylceramide into its constituent molecules.

7. Which health problem could be expected as a result of a gene mutation that affects the correct production and function of type 1 collagen?
   a. Failure of blood to clot after minor trauma
   b. Increased incidence of arterial and venous aneurysms
   c. Increased incidence of hearing loss among children and adults
   d. Restrictive lung disease from excessive stiffening of alveolar walls

8. The mother of a teenager recently diagnosed with osteogenesis imperfecta type I asks if the problem is related to the fact that she adhered to a vegetarian diet during pregnancy. What is the most appropriate response?
   a. Your diet is not related to this disease because it is an inherited disorder.
   b. Although this problem can be inherited, low calcium levels are a major cause.
   c. That is one possibility, especially because collagen requires proteins to form.
   d. More likely, it is related to the fact that you were older than 35 years of age when you became pregnant.

Continued

9. A 12-year-old boy with Marfan syndrome complains to his nurse-practitioner, "My mother won't let me play football or do anything else. Isn't there something I can do besides sitting and playing video games?" Which activities listed below may be considered less risky for this child to perform? Circle all that apply.

   a. Soccer (not the goalie position)
   b. Riding his bike with his friends
   c. Playing table tennis
   d. Competitive swimming
   e. Archery
   f. Recreational ice-skating
   g. Hiking moderate to steep trails
   h. Hiking low to moderate trails
   i. Basketball

CASE STUDY

A 30-year-old woman has just been diagnosed with Fabry disease. The health problems that caused her health-care providers to consider this disorder include renal insufficiency, high blood pressure, and poor circulation to her hands and feet that causes her considerable pain. At first, her care providers considered that she must have hypercholesterolemia; however, her lipid panel showed levels of the usual types of cholesterol to be within normal limits. In addition, her blood glucose levels are normal. Now that the diagnosis is made, she is very concerned that she may have passed the disorder to her two children, a son aged 2 and a daughter aged 6. In reviewing her family history, she tells you that her mother is living and has no identified health problems at age 62. The patient has two older brothers, 32 and 36 years old, who also have no identified health problems. She tells you that her father's family is a different story. Her father died of a heart attack at age 35. His sister died at 40 from a stroke, and another brother died at 40 from kidney failure. When you ask about her father's parents, she tells you that she never met her grandmother because she died at age 41 from heart failure and that her paternal grandfather was killed in the Korean conflict.

   1. Draw the pedigree and identify possible affected individuals.

   2. What, if any, pattern of inheritance is evident?

   3. Is her concern for her children realistic?

   4. Would genetic counseling be of any benefit to her and her family? Explain why or why not.

References

Bijarnia, S., Shaw, P., Vimpani, A., et al. (2009). Combined enzyme replacement and hematopoietic stem cell transplantation in Hurler syndrome. *Journal of Paediatrics and Child Health, 45*(7–8), 469–472.

Chen, M., and Wang, J. (2008). Gaucher disease: Review of the literature. *Archives of Pathology and Laboratory Medicine, 132*(5), 851–853.

DeRoche, K., and Welsh, M. (2008). Twenty-five years of research on neurocognitive outcomes in early-treated phenylketonuria: Intelligence and executive function. *Developmental Neuropsychology, 33*(4), 474–504.

Ehlers-Danlos National Foundation. (2008). Retrieved January 2011 from www.ednf.org/.

Gonzales, E. (2009). Marfan syndrome. *Journal of the American Academy of Nurse Practitioners, 21*(12), 663–670.

Iams, H. (2010). Diagnosis and management of Marfan syndrome. *Current Sports Medicine Reports, 9*(2), 93–98.

Little, C., Gould, R., and Hendriksz, C. (2009). The management of children with Hunter syndrome: A case study. *British Journal of Nursing, 18*(5), 321–322.

McCance, K., Huether, S., Brashers, V., and Rote, N. *Pathophysiology: The biologic basis for disease in adults and children,* 6th ed. St. Louis: Elsevier/Mosby, 2010.

MD Consult (2010). Retrieved January 2011 from www.mdconsult.com/das/pharm/body/231608677-3/0/full/3578 (must have a membership to access).

National Institutes of Health (NIH). (2010). Genetics Home Reference. Retrieved January 2011 from http://ghr.nlm.nih.gov/gene/

Online Mendelian Inheritance in Man (OMIM). (2010). Retrieved January 2011 from www.ncbi.nlm.nih.gov/omim/.

Osteogenesis Imperfecta Foundation. (2007). Retrieved January 2011 from www.oif.org/.

Schaefer, R., Tylki-Szymariska, A., and Hilz, M. (2009). Enzyme replacement therapy for Fabry disease: A systematic review of available evidence. *Drugs, 69*(16), 2179–2205.

Weinreb, N., Charrow, J., Andersson, H., et al. (2002). Effectiveness of enzyme replacement therapy in 1028 patients with type I Gaucher disease after 2 to 5 years of treatment: A report from the Gaucher Registry. *American Journal of Medicine, 113*(2), 112–119.

Workman, M., LaCharity, L., and Kruchko, S. Understanding pharmacology: Essentials for medication Safety. St. Louis: Elsevier/Saunders, 2011.

Wright, K., and Roberts, G. (2007). Phenylketonuria. *Journal of Continuing Education Topics & Issues, 9*(1), 8–12.

Self-Assessment Answers

1. c **2.** a **3.** c **4.** c **5.** a **6.** d **7.** b **8.** a **9.** b, c e, f, h

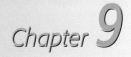

Chapter 9

Common Childhood-Onset Genetic Disorders

Learning Outcomes

1. Use the genetic terminology associated with common childhood-onset genetic disorders.
2. Describe the genetic/genomic contributions to sickle cell disease (SCD), inheritance patterns, and other factors that may influence disease expression.
3. Describe the genetic/genomic contributions to cystic fibrosis (CF), inheritance patterns, and other factors that may influence disease severity.
4. Describe the genetic/genomic contributions to Duchenne muscular dystrophy (DMD), inheritance patterns, and other factors that may influence disease severity.
5. Describe the genetic/genomic contributions to classic hemophilia (hemophilia A), inheritance patterns, and other factors that may influence disease severity.
6. Describe the genetic/genomic contributions to von Willebrand disease, inheritance patterns, and other factors that may influence disease severity.
7. Describe the genetic/genomic contributions to achondroplasia, inheritance patterns, and other factors that may influence disease severity.
8. Explain the gene-environment interactions involved in development of type 1 diabetes.
9. Explain the gene-environment interactions involved in development of atopic asthma.

KEY TERMS

Achondroplasia

Asthma

Autoimmune disease

Classic hemophilia

Cystic fibrosis (CF)

Duchenne muscular dystrophy (DMD)

Dystrophin

Hyperglycemia

Insulitis

Sickle cell crisis

Sickle cell disease (SCD)

Sickle cell trait

Diabetes mellitus type 1

Von Willebrand disease (VWD)

Introduction

A variety of disorders that have a major genetic cause manifest during infancy and childhood. Some of these disorders, such as asthma and diabetes mellitus type 1, require an environmental contribution for the disorder to develop fully. For other disorders, such as sickle cell disease and cystic fibrosis, the basic underlying pathology is a genetic mutation; however, the severity of the disease and when it is first diagnosed may be related to environmental factors. Some of these disorders can be managed and their consequences delayed or altered. For others, few management techniques slow the consequences of the disease, and life expectancy and physiological function are profoundly affected. This chapter focuses on the most common genetic disorders that manifest in childhood.

Monogenic Disorders

As discussed in Chapters 1 and 4, a monogenic or single gene trait or condition is one in which one gene controls the expression of a specific structure, protein, or function. Monogenic disorders can be transmitted in an autosomal dominant, autosomal recessive, or sex-linked pattern.

Sickle Cell Disease

Sickle cell disease (SCD) is a genetic disorder caused by a single nucleotide polymorphism (point mutation) in both alleles of a single gene that results in the abnormal formation of the beta chain of hemoglobin (beta globin). The disorder is transmitted in an autosomal recessive pattern and is most common among people with African or other equatorial ancestry (from geographic regions near the equator). The incidence of SCD in the United States among African Americans is about 1 in 400 live births. Carrier status, in which a person has only one mutated beta globin gene allele is estimated at 1 in 15 African Americans (Sickle Cell Disease Association of America, 2005). Both SCD and sickle cell trait have a far greater incidence in East Africa and other equatorial countries.

Genetic Contribution to the Disorder

As discussed in Chapter 2, transcription and translation of the wild-type beta globin gene *(HBB)* produce a 146 amino acid protein with glutamic acid (GLU) as the sixth amino acid (the DNA triplet is CTC). In the classic form of sickle cell disease, both beta globin alleles have a mutation in which the DNA triplet coding for glutamic acid has adenine substituted for thymine (instead of CTC, the triplet now reads CAC). This mutation results in valine as the sixth amino acid in the protein sequence.

Usually, two beta globin molecules associate with two alpha globin molecules and four "heme" molecules to form normal adult hemoglobin (HbA) in red blood cells (RBCs). The function of hemoglobin is to reversibly bind with up to four molecules of oxygen in arterial blood and unload the oxygen in various body tissues. (There are hundreds of thousands of hemoglobin molecules in a single RBC.)

When both alleles of the beta globin gene are mutated, RBCs have a high percentage of hemoglobin S (HbS) rather than HbA. It can bind with four molecules of oxygen in the same way that HbA does. However, HbS is very sensitive to low tissue levels of oxygen, and the shape of the four associated globin molecules (two alpha and two beta) folds differently as tissue oxygen levels decrease. This change in folding pulls the cell membranes inward, causing the RBC to form a sickle shape that does not flow smoothly through blood vessels (Fig. 9–1). Instead, the sickled RBCs clump together and block blood flow, causing tissues distal to the blockage to be poorly perfused and poorly oxygenated, which then leads to more sickling of RBCs and ischemia in the affected tissues. The membranes of the sickled RBCs also become abnormal and tend to stick together, making the clumping worse. In addition, the RBCs

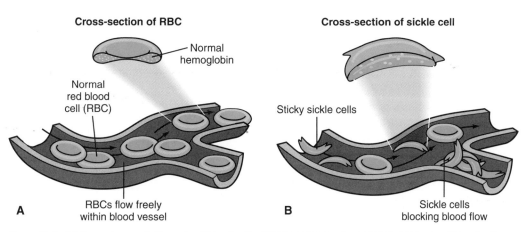

Cross-section of RBC

Normal hemoglobin

Normal red blood cell (RBC)

A RBCs flow freely within blood vessel

Cross-section of sickle cell

Sticky sickle cells

B Sickle cells blocking blood flow

Figure 9–1. (A) Normal, smooth flow of red blood cells. (B) Clumping together of sickle-shaped red blood cells, reducing or blocking blood flow.

containing largely HbS have a much shorter life span than normal, only about 16 to 20 days instead of 120 days.

When only one beta globin allele has the mutation, the person has **sickle cell trait.** In this disorder, the percentage of HbS in RBCs is usually less than 40%. Although cells with just this much HbS can assume a sickle shape, the degree of tissue hypoxia required for this change is far greater than that needed for RBCs with 90% or more HbS to form sickled cells.

Inheritance Patterns

The specific gene mutation causing SCD or sickle cell trait has a low incidence of developing spontaneously. The most common transmission is from parent to child in an autosomal recessive pattern. Figure 9–2 shows Punnett square transmission inheritance probability for people without a mutated beta globin allele, those with one mutated beta globin allele, and those with two mutated beta globin alleles.

Genetic testing is not used to diagnose SCD. It is diagnosed based on the large percentage of hemoglobin S (HbS) seen on electrophoresis. A person who has SCD usually has 80% to 90% HbS, and a person with sickle cell trait usually has less than 40% HbS. The number of RBCs with permanent sickling also is an indicator of SCD. Those without the disease have less than 1% sickled cells, those with sickle cell trait have less than 40%, and those with SCD may have as high as 90% permanently sickled cells at any one time.

Physical Manifestations

The poor perfusion and oxygenation of body tissues in the person with SCD results in pain, disability, organ damage, increased infections, and early death. The short life span of the RBCs results in chronic anemia, although these patients are not iron deficient. Conditions that trigger hypoxia or poor blood flow and lead to episodes of sickling include dehydration, infection, venous stasis, alcohol consumption, high altitude, low environmental or body temperature, acidosis, strenuous exercise, pregnancy, and anesthesia. Acute sickling periods are known as **sickle cell crises.** During these periods, extensive sickling occurs and disrupts blood flow to an entire organ(s) or body area. Severe pain in the affected area is the most common symptom during crises.

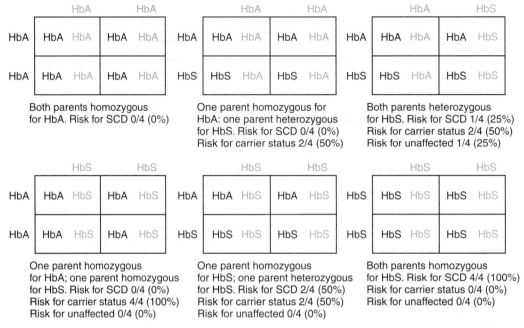

Figure 9–2. Comparison of risks to inherit HbA, HbS, sickle cell disease, and sickle cell trait.

Although some sickled RBCs resume a normal shape when tissue oxygen levels increase and the crisis is over, some cells remain sickled and all are more fragile. This fragility increases the risk for repeated sickling, even when tissue oxygen levels fall only slightly below normal.

Over time, the repeated blood vessel blockage leads to hypoxic damage of most tissues and organs, especially those that are highly dependent on oxygen, such as the liver, heart, brain, spleen, kidney, bones, and retinas. Hypoxic tissues become anoxic and ischemic, followed by necrosis (cell death). Small infarcts and necrotic tissue areas first appear. These areas become fibrotic and no longer function. The tissue or organ has progressively larger areas of fibrosis and scarring with fewer areas of functional cells. Eventually, too few functional cells remain and the tissue or organ is permanently nonfunctional. Table 9–1 lists the health problems caused by SCD. There is great variation among patients with SCD for disease severity and the onset of serious complications. Most children who receive supportive and preventive care for SCD live into adulthood; however, the complications of the disease can only be delayed, not eliminated. The only cure for SCD is a stem cell transplant. However, the many serious complications of this serious procedure, including death, and its cost limit the use of this treatment strategy.

Disease Variability

As noted above, disease expression varies. This is unusual for a genetic disorder in which the actual mutation is so specific and so stable. Unlike other genetic disorders, such as cystic fibrosis, in which the base or bases substituted or deleted can vary from family to family, all people who have the main form of SCD have the exact same amino acid change of valine for glutamic acid in the sixth position of beta globin. So, what accounts for the variability—*nature* (genetic influences) or *nurture* (environmental influences)? The answer is both, although the exact genetic mechanisms have not all been identified.

TABLE 9-1

Progressive Complications of Sickle Cell Disease

Pain	Increased susceptibility to infections, especially pneumonia
Priapism	Liver and spleen destruction and failure
Jaundice	Chronic kidney disease and kidney failure
Heart failure	Foot and leg ulceration
Fatigue	Brain infarcts, strokes, seizures
Weakness	
Joint damage	

Environmentally, those individuals who are able to avoid triggers for extreme sickling and crises have a slower onset of permanent complications. Those individuals whose crisis episodes are managed promptly and correctly also have better long-term physical function. However, there are many people who manage their disease appropriately and diligently who still have an early onset of serious complications, disability, and death.

One of the best predictors for which patients who have SCD will have delayed complications is the percentage of fetal hemoglobin (HbF) that remains in circulation. HbF is a type of hemoglobin normally expressed at high levels only during fetal life, where all oxygen is derived secondhand from the maternal circulation. It tolerates low oxygen conditions well without sickling. After a baby is born, RBCs begin to synthesize the adult form of hemoglobin (HbA) and the amount of HbF usually drops dramatically during the first months. Most people express less than 2% HbF and about 98% HbA by early childhood. Some patients with SCD continue to express as much as 20% HbF throughout childhood and adulthood. This percentage dilutes the percentage of HbS and results in better tolerance of conditions that could cause sickling. It is most likely that continued production of HbF is a genetically controlled function, although the gene or genes responsible have not yet been identified.

The drug hydroxyurea can increase the percentage of HbF in anyone who receives it, including a person with SCD. It is often used as long-term therapy to maintain higher levels of HbF and delay the complications of SCD.

Another interesting variation in the expression of SCD occurs when the person also has a disorder of the alpha chains of hemoglobin, alpha-thalassemia. In this genetically inherited condition, the actual loss of any one of the four gene alleles that code for alpha globin chains (two each on chromosome 16) causes alpha-thalassemia. It is not a case of "two wrongs making a right," but the anemia caused by alpha-thalassemia has long been known to reduce the effects of SCD in several possible ways (Embry et al., 1984). First, people with alpha-thalassemia are anemic, which reduces the amount of RBCs and the RBC concentration of HbS. In addition, these RBCs are less dense than SCD RBCs, resulting in less cell sickling and breakage. In addition, the alpha-thalassemia increases the amount of RBC cell membrane, which then protects against cell breakage. One final difference that may explain how alpha-thalassemia moderates the effects of SCD is that RBCs with both alpha-thalassemia and SDC do not dehydrate and lyse as easily as SCD RBCs alone. Regardless of the specific mechanism, the condition of alpha-thalassemia does modify the effects of SCD in a positive way.

Potential Disease Advantage

You may be asking yourself how can a disease such as SCD ever be an advantage? It does actually have one and that may be the reason that SCD developed in the first place! In equatorial regions of the world, the infectious disease malaria is common and deadly. The hemoglobin change caused by the genetic mutation of SCD reduces the susceptibility to severe malaria on exposure or infection with the organism. This benefit occurs in both those who are homozygous for the gene mutation and in those who are heterozygous. Clearly, the benefit to people who have SCD, even in areas where malarial infection is prevalent, is limited. However, the benefit to those who have the trait in areas in which malarial infection is prevalent is enormous. There really is no advantage for people who live in areas in which malarial infection is uncommon.

Cystic Fibrosis

Cystic fibrosis (CF) is a monogenic disorder in which both alleles of a gene have one or more mutations that result in problems with the transmembrane transport of chloride. The disorder is inherited as an autosomal recessive single gene trait and is most common among whites of Northern and Western European heritage, although it can be found among people of all races and ethnicities. The incidence of CF in the United States among Caucasians is about 1 in 3000 live births. Carrier status, in which a person has only one mutated gene allele, is estimated at 1 in 20 to 30 Caucasian Americans. About 30,000 children and adults in the United States have been diagnosed with CF (Cystic Fibrosis Foundation, 2011).

Genetic Contribution to the Disorder

CF is caused by inheriting a gene mutation in both alleles of the cystic fibrosis transmembrane conductance regulator *CFTR* gene, which is located at chromosome 7q31. This gene produces a protein that serves as a chloride channel and regulates both chloride and bicarbonate transport. Additionally, the *CFTR* gene product controls or influences other transport pathways.

The *CFTR* gene is very large and complex, containing different coding regions. Different parts of the protein it produces have varying roles in development and physiological function. At present, more than 1400 different mutations in this gene have been identified (Cystic Fibrosis Foundation, 2011). Mutation differences are believed to account for much of the variance in the severity, the age of symptom onset, and differences in organ involvement. Even with so many mutations, some are more common than others. The $\triangle$F508 is the most common mutation (among Caucasians) and produces the most severe disease. Interestingly, *CFTR* mutations do not prevent production of the protein but instead change the protein sequence so that it still functions but with varying degrees of activity and efficiency. As a result, the mutation genotype does correlate with the specific manifestations (phenotype) expressed by the person with CF (Kulczycki, Kostuch, and Bellanti, 2003).

Inheritance Patterns

Transmission of CF is autosomal recessive from parent to child. This pattern follows the same probability for the unaffected state, the affected state, and the carrier state demonstrated in Figure 9–2 for sickle cell disease.

Genetic testing is not used to diagnose the homozygous expression of CF. It is diagnosed on the basis of physical manifestations and the results of the sweat chloride test. Positive results are those indicating a high concentration of sodium chloride in the person's sweat (60 to 200 mEq/L or mmol/L) compared with the normal value (5 to 35 mEq/L). However, the heterozygous carrier cannot be identified with the sweat chloride test and has no distinctive disease manifestations. Genetic testing by direct sequencing of the *CFTR* gene is useful for establishing carrier status, identifying affected children prenatally, and, to some degree, predicting disease severity.

Physical Manifestations

The two main organ systems affected that involve epithelial cells are the lungs and the pancreas. The epithelial cells in these tissues produce a thick, sticky mucus as a result of poor chloride transport that, over time, plugs up the glands in these organs, causing glandular atrophy and organ dysfunction or failure. Other organs that are affected to a lesser degree include the liver, salivary glands, and testes.

The most serious complications of CF occur in the lungs from the constant presence of thick, sticky mucus. The mucus narrows airways, reducing airflow, and permits chronic lower respiratory bacterial infections. Due to the infections, chronic bronchitis, bronchiectasis, and increased alveolar compliance result, and lung abscesses form. Common lung complications of CF include pneumothorax, arterial erosion and hemorrhage, antibiotic-resistant infection, and respiratory failure.

The thick mucus also plugs the ducts of the pancreas, causing glandular atrophy and progressive fibrotic cyst formation. These changes first reduce and then halt production of the digestive enzymes needed for fat and protein digestion. This enzyme loss leads to malnutrition, smaller stature, fatty diarrhea (steatorrhea), and a deficiency of fat-soluble vitamins. Although the endocrine function of the CF pancreas also is affected, this occurs much later in the disease process and causes diabetes.

The liver and gall bladder also are damaged by mucus deposits, and the liver eventually fails. In many people with CF, the salivary gland ducts dilate and produce abnormal saliva.

Male infertility is associated with CF, usually as a result of failure of the vas deferens to develop (agenesis of the vas deferens). The vas deferens is a tubular structure that transports sperm from testicular storage sites to the urethra. Without a vas deferens, the man does not have sperm in the seminal fluid, even though he produces sperm in the testes.

Disease Variability

CF is extremely variable in disease severity and in organ involvement, although expression of the clinical course is less variable within a given affected family. Greater variation in severity is seen in different families, with pancreatic problems more extreme in some families and lung problems more extreme in others. For example, in some families, affected children are diagnosed in early infancy and often progress quickly to severe lung or pancreatic disease before the teenage years. In other families, manifestations may not be apparent until later childhood or adolescence. More recently, some adults have been identified as being homozygous for *CFTR* mutations but have minimal or no obvious manifestations.

There is no cure for CF, although aggressive management of lung infections and therapies, such as lung transplantation, can extend life. Gene therapy has been tried but is not a currently approved therapy for CF. For those who have obvious manifestations of lung involvement, life expectancy is considerably reduced, although it has increased from childhood to adulthood to an average of 37.5 years as a result of improvements in medical therapy (Cystic Fibrosis Foundation, 2011).

Potential Disease Advantage

The high frequency of the heterozygous carrier state for CF among Caucasians from Northern and Western Europe suggests that being a CF carrier might have a potential advantage. Scientists now believe people who are heterozygous for specific common *CFTR* mutations have greater resistance to typhoid and to cholera toxin when exposed to these disease-causing microorganisms (Pier et al., 1998).

Duchenne Muscular Dystrophy

Duchenne muscular dystrophy (DMD) is a genetic disorder of progressive muscle weakness caused by any one of a variety of mutations in an allele of the *DMD* gene, which codes for the protein dystrophin. It is the most common inherited *myopathy* (muscle degrading disease). The disorder is inherited in an X-linked transmission pattern and is most common among males. The incidence of DMD worldwide is about 1 in 3300 to 3500 live births of males. It occurs at about the same rate in all races (Muscular Dystrophy Association, 2010). Becker muscular dystrophy (BMD), a milder form of the disease, results from a less-damaging mutation of the same gene and follows the same inheritance patterns.

Female carriers, who have one normal X chromosome and one with an abnormal dystrophin allele, can express some manifestations of the disorder but to a much lesser degree than affected males. The actual incidence of female carriers is not known.

Genetic Contribution to the Disorder

The gene for dystrophin is located on the X chromosome (locus is Xp21). It is the largest gene in the human genome, and its product, dystrophin, also is large. Muscular dystrophies of several types are associated with mutations in this gene. Mutation types include large deletions, small deletions, large duplications, insertions, and base changes. The most common mutation consists of large deletions, and the disorder is exclusively genetic in origin.

Dystrophin is a structural protein that functions to maintain muscle integrity. It is found inside skeletal, cardiac, and smooth muscle cells. A variant of dystrophin also is found in brain cells. In muscle cells, dystrophin surrounds muscle fiber membranes and secures the contractile protein strands, especially actin, so they remain anchored in place and are stable. With too little dystrophin (BMD) or completely nonfunctional dystrophin (DMD), each muscle contraction loosens actin, gradually breaking down the muscle fibers and destroying the integrity of individual muscle cells. Because muscles are not mitotically active after birth, damaged and dead cells are not replaced. The muscles lose muscle fibers and become filled with connective tissue and fat.

Inheritance Patterns

The *DMD* gene is located on the X chromosome (Xp21). Because males have only one X chromosome, which is inherited exclusively from their mothers, DMD has a sex-linked (X-linked) transmission pattern. Figure 9–3 shows Punnett square inheritance probability for people without a mutated dystrophin allele, those with one mutated dystrophin allele, and those with two mutated dystrophin alleles (rare). Additionally, in about 30% to 35% of males who have DMD, the mother is not a carrier. Thus, the spontaneous mutation rate for this gene is very high. This rate is thought to be related to the large size of the gene, making it a very large target for mutational events during DNA replication, protein synthesis, and gametogenesis (the formation of mature sperm and ova).

The diagnosis of DMD is first suggested by a history of progressing muscle weakness in a male child along with hugely elevated blood levels of the enzyme creatine kinase (CK) and the protein myoglobin. Both are normally present inside intact muscle cells. When the cells are damaged or die, they are released into the blood. These levels decrease as the child ages because there is a limit to how much muscle is available to be destroyed. Additional testing can include a muscle biopsy to determine whether muscle weakness results from muscle cell degeneration or from inflammation. Genetic testing with the polymerase chain reaction (PCR) on blood or skin cells can determine specific areas of mutations on the *DMD* gene. This is useful in identifying carrier status and the DMD status of a fetus.

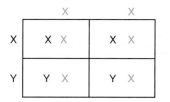

Mother homozygous for normal dystrophin.
Father hemizygous for normal dystrophin.
Risk for Inherited DMD is 0/4 (0%).
Risk for spontaneous mutation leading
to DMD is not known.

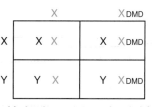

Mother heterozygous (carrier) for DMD.
Father hemizygous for normal dystrophin.
Risk for DMD is 1/4 (25%)
Risk for carrier status 1/4 (25%)

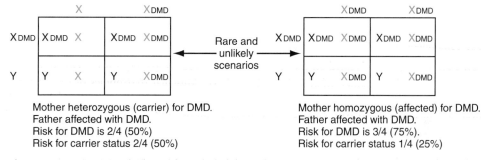

Rare and
← unlikely →
scenarios

Mother heterozygous (carrier) for DMD.
Father affected with DMD.
Risk for DMD is 2/4 (50%)
Risk for carrier status 2/4 (50%)

Mother homozygous (affected) for DMD.
Father affected with DMD.
Risk for DMD is 3/4 (75%).
Risk for carrier status 1/4 (25%)

Figure 9–3. Comparison of risks to inherit normal dystrophin, DMD carrier status, or DMD.

For DMD, female carriers also may be identified on the basis of elevated CK levels and the presence of slightly weaker than expected skeletal muscle strength. However, whether these tests are conclusive depends on the percentage of skeletal muscles in which the affected X chromosome (the maternal derived X or the paternal derived X) is the one that remains active. (Remember from Chapter 4, in females one X is inactivated in most cells, and which X is inactivated is a random process.)

Physical Manifestations

Muscle weakness in DMD is first seen in the neck and hip girdle muscles. Young boys who have learned to sit up and to walk usually start to show difficulty in walking and remaining upright between 2 and 5 years of age. The child has difficulty directly standing from a sitting position or when getting up from the floor. The arms are used to push himself into an upright position rather than depending on the legs to raise the body. The gait becomes clumsy and falling occurs frequently. The calf muscles start to appear large in relation to the rest of the child's muscles. This size increase represents replacement of muscle fibers with fat and connective tissue rather than a strengthening of the muscle itself. Usually, the child is unable to walk by the teenage years.

Most boys with DMD develop cardiac muscle problems because these cells also rely on dystrophin to maintain their integrity. The most common problems are dilated cardiomyopathy and chronic heart failure. Although dystrophin is needed in smooth muscle, DMD has fewer effects on smooth muscles. However, some children with DMD do develop bladder paralysis or gastric dilation.

Most children with DMD demonstrate cognitive impairment. The actual cause is not known but is thought to be related to the fact that some dystrophin is required in the brain.

Disease Variability

There is little variability in the manifestations and severity of DMD, but those that exist are believed to be related to the type of mutation in the DMD gene. For BMD, there is greater variability, depending on how much functional dystrophin is produced. Some men have few manifestations and are not diagnosed with the disorder until they are 30 years of age or older.

Female carriers may express considerable manifestations if the healthy X chromosome is the one that is inactivated more frequently in muscle cells. Generally, women have more difficulty with cardiac issues than with skeletal muscle. The theoretical basis for this common problem is that, while skeletal muscle strength is adequate when only 50% of the cells are fully functional, adequate heart activity, especially left ventricular function, needs at least 80% of the cardiac muscle cells to be fully functional. These women often develop dilated cardiomyopathy and left ventricular failure at earlier than expected ages.

Currently, there is no cure for DMD. Management focuses on corticosteroid therapy, which slows the rate of muscle cell degeneration. Weight management is used to allow weaker muscles to maintain mobility for as long as possible. Although moderate exercise is recommended, too much exercise causes faster muscle breakdown. Cardiac and respiratory support are also needed as the disease progresses. The major causes of death are respiratory failure, pneumonia, and heart failure in the late teenage years or early adulthood. No therapy prevents these outcomes; however, appropriate support can delay functional organ failure.

Classic Hemophilia

Classic hemophilia or hemophilia A is a monogenic disorder in which the production of blood-clotting factor VIII is either absent or well below normal levels. The disorder is inherited as an X-linked single gene trait and is most common among males. The incidence of classic hemophilia worldwide is about 1 in 5000 live births of males. It occurs at about the same rate in all races and ethnicities. A less common form of hemophilia is hemophilia B, formerly known as *Christmas disease* (the first child identified with this form of hemophilia had "Christmas" as his last name). The clotting factor affected by this disease is factor IX, the gene for which is also located on the X chromosome.

Genetic Contribution to the Disorder

The gene for factor VIII is located on the X chromosome and is known as *F8*. This clotting factor (also known as *antihemophilic factor* [AHF] A and *antihemophilic globulin* [AHG]) is one of many synthesized in the liver that are required to be activated and work in a cascade-like series to form a stable blood clot after blood vessel injury (Fig. 9–4). When factor VIII is activated, its purpose is to work with other activated clotting factors and von Willebrand factor to form a complex of several activated factors, platelets, and calcium. This complex is known as *prothrombin activator,* and its purpose is to activate prothrombin to thrombin. Thrombin is an active enzyme that converts fibrinogen to fibrin molecules. Once fibrin molecules are present, they then rapidly self-assemble into long strands that form a network or scaffold that serves as the basic frame upon which platelets, proteins, and blood cells collect to create a stable clot (Fig. 9–5). When little or no factor VIII is present, the cascade stops before it generates the complex needed to activate prothrombin. As a result, fibrinogen is not converted to fibrin, the scaffold does not form, and blood does not clot.

The *F8* gene is fairly large, and a variety of mutations can impair its function. Often, a unique, specific mutation is responsible for the expression of classic hemophilia within a kindred. Mutation types include point mutations, deletions, errors in mRNA splicing, and a problem in which the area of

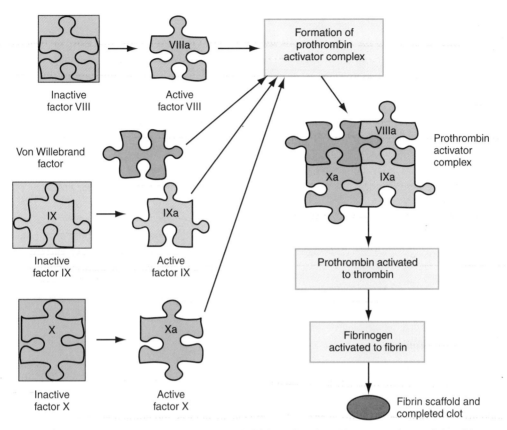

Figure 9–4. Basic parts of the blood-clotting cascade, highlighting the roles of factor VIII and von Willebrand factor.

the X chromosome where *F8* is located is inverted (Kumar et al., 2010). This essentially results in "backward" gene encodement that cannot be transcribed or translated.

Inheritance Patterns

The *F8* gene is located on the X chromosome (Xq28). Because males have only one X chromosome, which is inherited exclusively from their mothers, hemophilia has a sex-linked (X-linked) recessive transmission pattern. This pattern follows the same probability for the unaffected state, the affected state, and the carrier state, demonstrated in Figure 9–3 for Duchenne muscular dystrophy. Additionally, in about 25% to 30% of males who have classic hemophilia, the mother is not a carrier (Kumar et al., 2010). Thus, the spontaneous new mutation rate for this gene is relatively high.

Physical Manifestations

Babies born with classic hemophilia usually have no clinical manifestations of excessive bleeding at birth, and many may have only minimal bleeding in the immediate neonatal period, even when circumcised. Bruising and excessive bleeding begin to occur in response to any trauma during infancy. The episodes of bleeding increase when the infant begins to crawl and walk (because the child is not as protected from small environmental traumas as he was when he was less mobile). Interestingly, petechiae do not form in areas of trauma and bruising.

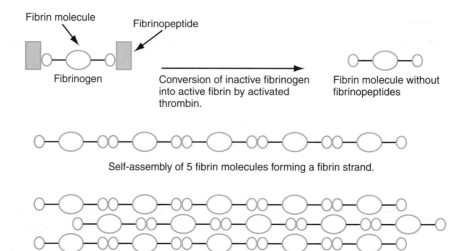

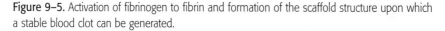

Figure 9–5. Activation of fibrinogen to fibrin and formation of the scaffold structure upon which a stable blood clot can be generated.

In addition to hemorrhage, the most common problem associated with hemophilia is the extensive joint damage that occurs in weight-bearing joints (hips, knees, and ankles), with spontaneous bleeding into the joint as a result of normal walking. With clotting factor replacement therapy, it is hoped that younger people with hemophilia will no longer suffer this debilitating and activity-limiting damage.

The diagnosis of classic hemophilia is made first on the basis of a history of excessive bruising and bleeding. Clotting studies demonstrate a normal prothrombin time (PT) coupled with an abnormally prolonged partial thromboplastin time (PTT). Blood levels of factor VIII are low to absent. Carriers can be identified by the presence of lower than normal levels of factor VIII, longer than average PTT, and *F8* gene sequencing to determine the presence of the specific mutation identified within the family.

Female carriers often have excessive bruising and bleeding from lower than normal F8 levels. The amount of F8 produced by carriers varies, depending on the percentage of liver cells that have the normal *F8* gene inactivated. Many have significantly less than 50% of normal factor VIII levels, but the amount usually is more than enough to prevent spontaneous bleeding, major hemorrhage from trauma, and damage from joint bleeding.

Disease Variability

The degree of excessive bruising and bleeding correlates with the abnormal levels of factor VIII. Patients who have 1% to 2% of normal factor VIII levels have very severe disease and excessive bleeding. Those with 5% to 10% of normal factor VIII levels have moderate disease and bleeding. Those with 15% or higher of normal factor VIII levels have only mild disease and episodic bleeding.

The only cure for classic hemophilia or hemophilia B is a liver transplant. The scarcity of this organ for transplantation, the expense, and the dangers inherent in the procedure make this an uncommon form of treatment. Synthetic forms of both factor VIII and factor IX are now available through the process of recombinant DNA technology. This process virtually eliminates the danger of blood-borne disease transmission that existed when the factors were obtained from pooled human serum (cryopre-cipitate). Regularly scheduled infusions of recombinant factor VIII have increased the life expectancy of a person with classic hemophilia from less than 5 years (in the early 20th century) to about 65 years (National Hemophilia Foundation, 2010).

Von Willebrand Disease

Von Willebrand disease (VWD) is a monogenic disorder in which the affected person produces less than normal amounts of von Willebrand factor (vWf). The disorder is inherited as an autosomal dominant trait and is the most common inherited blood-clotting disorder worldwide, with an incidence of 1 to 3 out of 100 live births (Kumar et al., 2010; Mittal, James, and Valentino, 2009).

Genetic Contribution to the Disorder

The gene for von Willebrand factor is *VWF* and is located on chromosome 12p13.3. This factor is produced by blood vessel endothelial cells and works with factor VIII as a "glue" that holds various blood-clotting factors together to form the prothrombin activator complex needed to convert prothrombin to thrombin in the blood-clotting cascade (see Fig. 9–4).

   VWF also activates platelets. Although extensive blood vessel damage can change the production of vWf in a body area, deficiency is really a genetic-based problem.

Inheritance Patterns

The *VWF* gene is located on an autosome—chromosome 12. The most common forms of the disorder are from mutations inherited in an autosomal dominant pattern. However, because of reduced penetrance, a family pedigree can sometimes give the appearance of an autosomal recessive pattern, although there is not a true carrier status. However, with reduced penetrance, a person who does not manifest the disorder can transmit the affected gene to his or her children who then may express the disorder. In addition, the rarest form of the disorder, which is also the most severe, is autosomal recessive.

Physical Manifestations and Disease Variability

There are three main types or categories of VWD, depending on the degree of von Willebrand factor produced. In addition, there are many more subtypes within each main type.

   Type 1 VWD is the most common, and people with this type have lower than normal circulating levels of vWf. The person has frequent nosebleeds, occurring without trauma, that bleed for prolonged periods (more than 30 minutes). Excessive mouth bleeding with tooth eruption, tongue biting, and after tooth extractions or aggressive dental work is common and may require medical intervention to stop. Skin lacerations cause bleeding for 30 minutes or longer. Large bruises form with minimal trauma. In girls who are menstruating, menstrual flow is heavy and the girl may be anemic. Many children and adults in this category remain undiagnosed.

   Type 2 VWD, the second most common form, also is inherited in an autosomal dominant pattern. This type is associated with abnormal or defective vWf, even though the amount produced is normal. Manifestations range from mild to moderate, depending on the type of defect in vWf. It is often the most difficult to diagnose because the vWf levels are normal, and further testing is required to determine the specific subtype. In addition, among the different subtypes, levels of vWf may not correlate to disease severity.

   For both types 1 and 2, affected individuals may not be diagnosed during childhood because symptoms are not viewed as serious, others in the family have the same problems and have learned how to manage them, or too few serious bleeding episodes have occurred in the younger years. Heavy menstruation and postpartum bleeding are often the triggers for investigating a genetic cause in young adulthood.

Type 3 VWD is the rarest and has the most serious bleeding problems. The levels of vWf are extremely low, and bleeding is so excessive that the person may first be thought to have hemophilia. This form of the disorder demonstrates an autosomal recessive pattern of inheritance.

Mild to moderate manifestations of VWD are managed with desmopressin injections or nasal spray. This synthetic analog of vasopressin increases both vWf levels and, to some extent, factor VIII levels. It is believed to do this by releasing preformed factors from cellular storage sites. The effect is rapid but temporary. When bleeding is severe, caused by type 3 VWD, or fails to respond to desmopressin therapy, the patient may need infusions of plasma with concentrated levels of vWf; however, this therapy has a risk for transmission of blood-borne viral disease.

Achondroplasia

Achondroplasia is a monogenic disorder of human short-limbed dwarfism that occurs as a result of a mutation in the gene that codes for the fibroblast growth factor receptor 3 (*FGFR3*). It is the most common disorder of dwarfism and occurs in all races and ethnicities at an incidence rate of about 1 in 15,000 to 40,000 live births (National Institutes of Health, 2010). The word **achondroplasia** literally means "without cartilage." This designation is not accurate because people with achondroplasia do have normal cartilage in appropriate locations. However, bone formation starts with cartilage in the embryonic stage, which then hardens (ossifies) to become bone. Problems in the formation and growth of the long bones result from mutations in the *FGFR3* gene.

Genetic Contribution to the Disorder

Although short stature and disordered bone growth can have environmental causes, achondroplasia is directly caused by a mutation in the *FGFR3* gene. Normally, the product of this gene is a protein that is involved in the development and maintenance of bone (and brain) tissue. It is a receptor that limits the formation of bone from cartilage, especially in the long bones. Two specific point mutations are responsible for 99% of all cases of achondroplasia. Either of these mutations results in the substitution of the amino acid arginine for glycine in position 380 of the protein (National Institutes of Health, 2010). The protein produced by this mutation is an excessively active receptor for fibroblast growth factor, which results in shortened long bone growth during embryonic and fetal life. Other bones, including those that compose the trunk and face, are less affected.

Inheritance Patterns

The *FGFR3* gene is located on chromosome 4p16.3 and, in about 10% to 15% of cases, is inherited in an autosomal dominant pattern of transmission. However, this large gene has a high rate of spontaneous new mutations, and close to 80% of affected children do not have a parent with achondroplasia. The spontaneous new mutations arise most often as a result of advanced paternal age. The disorder is highly penetrant. The homozygous condition is associated with excessive pregnancy loss and mortality in the neonatal period (Kumar et al., 2010).

Physical Manifestations

The initial appearance of achondroplasia in a newborn is striking. The infant's head and torso appear generally normal, but the extremities are disproportionately short. These proportions are maintained throughout life although the head is large (Fig. 9–6). The humerus and femur are more disproportionately short than the lower arms or legs. The skin and soft tissues on the arms and legs form extra creases (as if the skin and soft tissue are longer than the bones). The neck is very short with an abnormal junction between the posterior head and neck. This abnormality can compress the cervical spinal cord and is

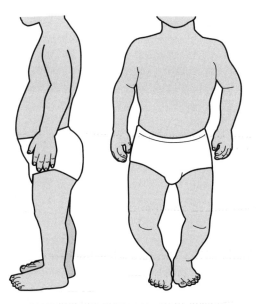

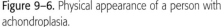

Figure 9–6. Physical appearance of a person with achondroplasia.

believed to be a factor in the common occurrence of sleep apnea in these individuals. In addition, infants with achondroplasia have a higher incidence of sudden infant death syndrome (SIDS) than children without achondroplasia, which may be attributable to the abnormal head and neck junction or to stenosis of the opening in the skull through which the spinal cord exits (foramen magnum). The face has a large and prominent forehead (bossing). The midline of the face is somewhat less developed than the upper segments. Intelligence and cognitive function have the same ranges as seen in the general population.

Most children with achondroplasia have delayed motor development. As they grow, the teeth are crowded and poor bite often occurs. Otitis media is a frequent occurrence because of the position of the eustachian tubes within the less developed facial midline. When the child starts to walk, an exaggerated lordosis spinal curvature develops (Richette et al., 2008).

Achondroplasia cannot be cured. Reconstructive surgery can alter the physical appearance. Bone-lengthening surgery can increase overall height, making the everyday activities of adults with achondroplasia a little easier, although this practice is controversial (Shirley, 2009). Injections with growth hormone are minimally effective (or not at all) at increasing height, as these individuals are not growth hormone deficient. Weight control is advised to reduce stress on hip and leg joints and to prevent obstructive sleep apnea.

Disease Variability

Most of the physical features of achondroplasia are present in all individuals who have the disorder. One variable feature is hydrocephaly. This occurs in some but not all children with the disorder. If it is not corrected, brain damage results.

Complex Disorders

Complex disorders are those that require both genetic and environmental input to develop. The genetic input increases the individual's susceptibility to developing the health problem, but unless one or more specific environmental triggers occur at the right time, the problem may never develop.

In many cases, the genetic component of complex disorders involves more than one gene, and these are often not identified. Two common complex disorders that manifest in childhood are type 1 diabetes mellitus and asthma.

Type 1 Diabetes Mellitus

Human cells require glucose to generate the chemical energy needed to perform all cellular work. Glucose comes from the carbohydrates we eat and from liver production of glucose. In order to be used as cellular fuel, glucose must enter cells even though many cells have membranes that are impermeable to glucose. This is where insulin is needed. In addition to the digestive portion of the pancreas, the endocrine portion contains about 1 million small glands, known as the *islets of Langerhans,* scattered through the organ. Within these islets are beta cells that produce and release insulin when blood glucose levels are elevated (**hyperglycemia**). Insulin enters circulation and binds to insulin receptors on cells' plasma membranes. The result of insulin binding to an insulin receptor is a change in the membrane structure so that glucose can cross the membrane and enter the cell for metabolic purposes.

Insulin's main function is related to carbohydrate metabolism by preventing hyperglycemia. Other functions of insulin are related to the regulation of fat and protein metabolism. Table 9–2 lists the body's positive responses and actions to the presence of insulin.

Diabetes mellitus type 1 is an autoimmune, metabolic, endocrine disorder in which insulin-producing cells in the pancreas have been destroyed and the person no longer synthesizes insulin to prevent hyperglycemia. An **autoimmune disease** is one of inflammation and immune action excess in which components of a person's immune system no longer recognize the person's own cells, tissues, and organs as "self" and attack them as if they were invading organisms. The predisposition to developing an autoimmune response leading to type 1 diabetes is inherited; however, expression of the autoimmune disorder requires additional input from the environment. In addition, although the incidence of such disorders is higher in some families than in the general population, it does not follow any specific pattern for single gene inheritance. Usually, type 1 diabetes as an autoimmune disease manifests in childhood, sometimes as early as age 4 to 6 weeks.

Genetic Contribution to the Disease

Susceptibility to the development of type 1 diabetes as an autoimmune problem is partially determined by the inheritance of certain human leukocyte antigen (HLA) genes coding for a specific tissue type located on chromosome 6. The tissue types most closely associated with an increased risk for type 1

TABLE 9–2

Positive Physiological Responses to the Presence of Adequate Insulin Levels

Prevention of hyperglycemia

Increased amino acid uptake by cells

Increased production of cellular proteins

Decreased muscle cell breakdown

Increased cell division

Increased liver storage of excess glucose as glycogen

Movement of fats, especially triglycerides and cholesterol, out of the blood and into fat cells (reduced blood lipid levels)

diabetes are the HLA-DR and HLA-DQ tissue types (remember that the tissue type is expressed on all of your cell membranes and serves as a unique universal "product code" for you; Kumar et al., 2010). However, even though inheritance of these particular tissue types increases the risk for autoimmune responses, most people with these tissue types do not develop type 1 diabetes or any other autoimmune disease.

The overall risk for developing any autoimmune disease in the general population is about 1%. In examining 100 people who have any autoimmune disease, especially whites, at least 90 of them also will have the HLA-DR and HLA-DQ tissue types. However, if we checked 100 people who have the HLA-DR or HLA-DQ tissue type, only about 2% of them also have an autoimmune disease. So, having an HLA-DR or HLA-DQ tissue type doubles the risk for developing an autoimmune disease (from 1% to 2%), but the risk is still low.

So why doesn't everyone or even most of the people who have that tissue type develop an autoimmune disease? The risk is present for all of them, but unless at least one environmental event occurs at a particular time, the risk doesn't lead to disease expression. Actual expression or development of the disease requires that an environmental factor interact with the genetic predisposition (increased susceptibility). The risk for type 1 diabetes in the general population ranges from 1 in 400 to 1 in 1000. This risk increases to 1 in 20 for those people who have one parent with type 1 diabetes or another autoimmune disorder.

In addition to specific tissue types increasing the risk for the development of autoimmune disease, other genetic variations may also increase this risk. Results from genome-wide association studies (GWAS) that examined the DNA sequences from large numbers of people who have specific health problems (in this case autoimmune diseases) and consistent single nucleotide polymorphisms, particularly on chromosomes 6 and 18, have been found to associate with type 1 diabetes, Crohn disease, and inflammation (Hindorff et al., 2009). Although these associations are not strong, and some occur in regions where no genes have yet been identified, their potential common role in autoimmune disease development needs to be explored.

Environmental Contribution to the Disease

Unlike type 2 diabetes, obesity and a sedentary lifestyle do not increase the risk for type 1 diabetes. The most common cause appears to be related to certain viral infections, such as mumps, rubella, and Coxsackie virus infection, which trigger autoimmune destruction of pancreatic beta cells (Kumar et al., 2010). The typical course is the child becomes ill with a viral infection, such as Coxsackie B4 (Dotta et al., 2007). Symptoms of this viral infection include fever, headache, sore throat, gastrointestinal distress, and muscle aches. The child is sick for 3 to 5 days and then recovers seemingly good health. However, about 6 weeks later, the child appears thinner and is constantly hungry and thirsty. He or she is tired and does not engage in his or her normal activities. The child also remarks about needing to urinate frequently. The parents notice a change in behavior and decide to consult their health-care provider. A random check of blood glucose level reveals a value of 340 mg/dL (normal is less than 140 mg/dL). Other tests are made, and the child is diagnosed with type 1 diabetes. The mother tells the health-care provider that her twin sister has had diabetes since age 5.

How does the viral infection lead to diabetes? First, when a virus infects the body, it invades many individual cells. The virus uses the cell's internal mechanisms to make more viruses, including breaking and entering the cell's DNA. As a result, the infected cell expresses some viral proteins on its surface. White blood cells, especially natural killer cells (NK cells or CD16 cells), recognize the viral signal on the infected cell's surface and exert cytotoxic actions against the infected cell. The plan is to destroy the infected cell and all of its viral contents to prevent the infection from spreading throughout the body. When the Coxsackie B4 viruses infect the body, they also infect the beta cells of the pancreas, where insulin is produced. The viruses do not directly kill or even really damage these cells. It is the person's own white blood cells (natural killer cells) that take out the infected body cells. Unfortunately, when most or all of the beta cells of the pancreas are infected, they are all attacked and can be destroyed by the immune system cells. Biopsy of the pancreatic tissue at that time will show **insulitis,** which is infiltration of the islet cells by white blood cells, resulting in inflammation of these cells. In addition, other immune system cells make antibodies against the islet cells (islet cell autoantibodies). The islet cells, including the beta cells, die and the islets become fibrotic and nonfunctional over time. The pancreas actually weighs less as a result of fibrosis replacing glandular tissue.

When enough of the islet beta cells have been destroyed by inflammatory and immune responses, the pancreas no longer produces insulin. The person has symptoms of hyperglycemia, and islet cell autoantibodies can be detected in the blood, along with other markers of inflammation.

Although infection with the Coxsackie B4 virus is known to lead to islet cell autoimmune destruction and beta cell loss, it is not the only infectious organism that can stimulate this reaction. Only a small percentage of people who become infected with the virus go on to develop islet cell destruction and diabetes. Most recover without islet cell damage. Only those people who have a genetic predisposition or susceptibility respond to the infection this way. Proposed mechanisms include that their immune systems overreact and respond inappropriately by attacking and destroying self cells, even though they are virally infected. Another proposed mechanism is that the islet cells of some people are less resistant to infection and more easily express proteins of the infecting virus, making these cells better "targets" for immune system attack.

Interestingly, even among people with increased genetic susceptibility to islet cell damage as a result of a viral infection, the timing of the environmental event that can trigger the self-cell destruction also affects the outcome. Apparently, some periods of life are a window of increased susceptibility to a gene-environment interaction leading to autoimmune disease, such as early childhood for type 1 diabetes. If the environmental exposure occurs much later than this age window, the disease does not result. It is speculated that the "window of susceptibility" is different for specific diseases and may, in fact, be different among individuals. In addition to the timing of exposure to a triggering event, there is also a gender difference for susceptibility. Females are affected by autoimmune disease about four times more often than males. The basis of this gender difference is not known.

Other evidence for a gene-environment interaction that stimulates an autoimmune response against islet cells includes the fact that type 1 diabetes is associated with allergy to cow's milk. (This is a true allergy to the milk proteins, not lactose intolerance. The person with a milk allergy has actual circulating antibodies directed against cow's milk proteins.) In addition, many people who have type 1 diabetes also have another autoimmune disease or have other first-degree relatives who have an autoimmune disease. Table 9–3 lists examples of diseases that have an autoimmune component.

Physical Manifestations

The person who has type 1 diabetes has a serious lack or absence of insulin and must inject insulin from other sources for the rest of his or her life. The initial manifestations of type 1 diabetes are related to the lack of insulin and the resulting hyperglycemia. The high blood glucose levels increase blood osmolarity, stimulating thirst. The person starts to drink much more than normal *(polydipsia),* and, most often, the person craves water. The increased water intake coupled with the increased osmolarity of the blood drawing interstitial fluid into the vascular space leads to excessive urination *(polyuria).* Although the blood glucose levels are high, little glucose enters cells, making the person feel hungry and tired. In

TABLE 9–3

Examples of Disorders With an Autoimmune Basis

Addison disease (chronic adrenal insufficiency)

Alopecia areata

Autoimmune thrombocytopenia purpura

Celiac disease

Crohn disease

Dermatomyositis

Diabetes mellitus (type 1)

Hashimoto thyroiditis (hypothyroidism)

Goodpasture syndrome

Graves disease (hyperthyroidism)

Guillain-Barré syndrome

Multiple sclerosis

Myasthenia gravis

Pernicious anemia

Psoriasis

Rheumatoid arthritis

Scleroderma

Sjögren syndrome

Systemic lupus erythematosus

Ulcerative colitis

response, he or she eats more *(polyphagia)* but does not gain weight (in fact, loses weight). The fatigue leads to increased sleepiness and a loss of interest in usual activities. If the conditions continue, the person starts using fats for cellular fuel. A by-product of fat breakdown is the formation of ketone bodies, which are acidic. When these products become excessive in the blood, the person experiences diabetic ketoacidosis, a life-threatening condition that requires careful insulin therapy to resolve.

When a person uses insulin from other sources rather than from his or her own pancreas, blood glucose levels can fluctuate widely and chronic hyperglycemia is common. The effects of long-term hyperglycemia dramatically change blood vessels, generally thickening their basement membranes and making vessel walls more fragile, so the exchange of nutrients and waste products at the tissue level is reduced. Over time, cells in many organs are damaged from chronic hypoxia and the buildup of waste products. Complications result from poor tissue circulation and cell death. When enough cells in any organ are damaged beyond repair, the organ fails to function. The long-term results of hyperglycemia are the same whether the hyperglycemia is caused by type 1 or type 2 diabetes (see Chapter 10). For most people with diabetes, the cause of death is from the organ complications of the disease rather than from the diabetes itself. Table 9–4 lists the many long-term consequences and complications of chronic hyperglycemia. Maintaining good control over blood glucose levels, which means keeping the level within the individual target range through drug therapy, diet, and exercise, can delay or even prevent these serious complications.

TABLE 9–4

Long-Term Consequences and Complications of Diabetes

Atherosclerosis

Bladder atony

Cataract formation

Cerebrovascular accidents

Charcot foot

Coronary artery disease

Dysphagia

Erectile dysfunction

Gastroparesis

Hyperlipidemia

Hypertension

Increased risk for infection

Increased risk for lower limb gangrene with progressive amputation

Myocardial infarction

Nephropathy and kidney failure

Orthostatic hypotension

Peripheral neuropathy

Poor intestinal peristalsis

Poor wound healing, stasis ulcers

Retinopathy leading to blindness

Asthma

Breathing to inhale oxygen is a vital function. Actual entrance of oxygen into the blood occurs deep within the lungs at the alveolar-capillary membrane. The tubular structures (airways) of the upper aerodigestive tract and lungs are critical to moving air into and out of the alveoli (ventilation) so that oxygen can enter the body and carbon dioxide, a waste gas formed during metabolism, can exit. For ventilation to be effective, the airways must be patent and of a sufficient internal diameter to allow free airflow.

Asthma is a chronic inflammatory disease of the airways that is usually characterized by intermittent periods of reversible airflow obstruction. (For some people, some degree of airway obstruction is always present, but this is not common.) The intermittent episodes are commonly called *asthma attacks*. Asthma can occur as a result of three actions: (1) constriction of the smooth muscles surrounding the smaller airways, (2) swelling of the mucous membranes lining the airways, or (3) excessive mucus collecting in and plugging the airways. The most common type of asthma is atopic asthma, which is a hypersensitivity reaction (allergic response) involving the release of immunoglobulin E (IgE). This type of asthma can have any one or even all three actions occurring at the same time. It usually begins in childhood and is often present in more than one family member. Because of this familial connection, asthma was once thought to be a learned, attention-getting behavior. This misconception has been pretty well debunked for all asthma, especially atopic asthma, in which specific chemical and laboratory changes can be identified.

Most people have mild to moderate asthma that can be controlled easily with proper drug therapy and the avoidance of environmental triggers. A severe attack, however, can greatly impair gas exchange. About 3400 deaths from asthma occur yearly in the United States alone (Centers for Disease Control and Prevention, 2010).

Genetic Contribution to the Disease

The fact that asthma appears to "run in families" has been noted for years and suggests a possible genetic influence in its development. Studies conducted more than 20 years ago provided evidence to support this suggestion, although opinions differed on the degree of heritability. Townley et al. (1986) proposed a polygenic influence for the induction of asthma symptoms among large numbers of people exposed experimentally to an inhaled drug that often causes bronchial responses. Longo et al. (1987) proposed a Mendelian dominant influence for bronchial hyperreactivity in a very large epidemiological study of families with asthma. As early as 1997, scientists proposed possible candidate genes as ones in which mutations were most likely to result in increased expression of asthma (Holgate et al., 1997). So, who was right, and which genes are involved in atopic asthma?

Between 50 and 100 genomic variations are known to be consistently associated with development of atopic asthma (Kumar et al., 2010; OMIM, 2010; Weiss et al., 2009). Some have greater influence than others, especially within certain racial or ethnic groups, and may act alone in causing asthma. Others, although consistent, appear to have lesser influence and may require a "group effort" for atopic asthma expression. Common areas of identified genomic variation associated with atopic asthma include 1q31 (especially among African Americans and Euro-Americans); 1p32 (especially among Hispanic Americans); 5q31, 6p21 (especially among Euro-Americans); 8p23, 11q21 (especially among African Americans); and 12q22, 15q13, and 17q21 (especially among Euro-Americans; OMIM, 2010; Sleiman et al., 2010). Many of these areas are those in which genes coding for proteins that are important in regulating inflammatory reactions and immune responses are located.

One of the strongest associations currently identified with susceptibility to asthma involves 8 to 12 different single nucleotide polymorphisms at the 1q31 locus (Sleiman et al., 2010). This area encodes the gene *DENND1B*, which produces a protein strongly active in the work of two cells of the immune system—the macrophage and the mast cell. Both of these cell types are involved in nonspecific inflammatory responses and in acquired (adaptive) immune responses that develop individually in susceptible people when they are exposed to an allergen. Some of these acquired responses are mediated by the antibody IgE along with various intracellular inflammatory biochemicals (e.g., histamine, bradykinin, tumor necrosis factor, interleukin13 [IL13]). Thus, the major genetic/genomic issues of asthma are, as suspected decades ago, an increased responsiveness of airway tissues when contacted with an environmental irritant (hyperresponsiveness) and an increased amount of the mediators of inflammation, especially immunoglobulin E (IgE).

Environmental Contribution to the Disease

All people have airways that respond with bronchoconstriction and inflammation to contact with major irritants in the air we breathe, such as heavy smoke or chemical particles. The presence of these irritants stimulates nerve fibers in airway tissues, causing constriction of bronchial smooth muscle. However, children with hyperresponsive airways have these reactions even when only a small amount of irritant is present. Common environmental irritants that make airways respond with constriction of bronchial smooth muscle include cold air, dry air, or fine airborne particles; microorganisms; aspirin; and exercise that increases the respiratory rate.

For the allergic (hypersensitivity) responses of swelling of the mucous membranes and producing excessive amounts of mucus, the immune system must adapt and learn how to release mediators of inflammation and IgE rapidly in response to the presence of a specific environmental allergen. Immune system "learning" is a complex process that starts with exposure to a particular substance (which substances a person becomes allergic to can be unique to the person, although there are many common allergens). This ability to produce IgE as a response to exposure to an allergen and the degree of response is genetically controlled and related to genomic variations; however, the exposure needed to start the process is environmental.

Physical Manifestations

The tissue changes that lead to narrowing of the airways start at the cellular level in the person who has genetic variation and result in airway hyperresponsiveness. Environmental triggers come into contact with the airway tissues, and they respond by constricting the bronchial smooth muscle.

The inflammatory and immune responses to the presence of an allergen involve different airway tissue changes. The allergen, which is most commonly inhaled but can enter the body in other ways, binds to specific antibody molecules, especially IgE. These molecules are attached to mast cells and basophils. These cells are filled with granules containing biochemicals such as histamine, which start an immediate inflammatory response that dilates blood vessels, increases capillary leak, and causes the mucous membranes to swell and produce large amounts of mucus. These cells also secrete other biochemicals that prolong the inflammatory responses. In addition to stimulating tissue inflammation, these substances attract more eosinophils, macrophages, and basophils to the area, causing the release of even more inflammatory-inducing mediators. When the tissue swelling and/or mucus production are extreme, the airways can be blocked internally. Usually, these tissue responses also stimulate nerve endings in the airways and result in constriction of the bronchial smooth muscle, causing external airway obstruction in addition to internal airway obstruction.

Most children with atopic asthma have no manifestations between asthma attacks but often have other allergic-type problems, including rhinitis, skin rash, or itching. During an actual asthma attack, the child has some difficulty breathing along with chest tightness, coughing, wheezing, and increased mucus production. Audible wheezing is the most common recognizable symptom. At first, the wheeze is louder on exhalation but as the attack worsens, loud wheezing also is heard on inhalation. The respiratory cycle (one inhalation followed by one exhalation) is longer and requires more effort, especially exhalation. Usually, when the attack is severe and the work of breathing increases, the child uses the accessory muscles. This response shows as muscle retractions at the sternum, the suprasternal notch, and between the ribs. Shortness of breath may become so intense that the child can speak only a few words between breaths. The lips and nail beds may show cyanosis.

Pulse oximetry shows hypoxia with oxygen saturation below 90%. A peak flow meter reading shows a decrease in peak flow below the child's usual value. The arterial oxygen level (PaO_2) decreases during a severe asthma attack, and the arterial carbon dioxide level ($PaCO_2$) rises. Other laboratory tests obtained during an atopic asthma attack often show an elevated serum eosinophil count and IgE levels.

Summary

Common monogenic disorders that usually manifest in childhood include sickle cell disease, cystic fibrosis, Duchenne muscular dystrophy, hemophilia, von Willebrand disease, and achondroplasia. Those that have obvious anatomic manifestations, such as achondroplasia, or those that show other problems early, such as sickle cell disease, cystic fibrosis, and hemophilia, may be diagnosed within the first few weeks or months of life. Patterns of inheritance are clear, although there may be considerable variation in disease expression. Some of these disorders have such severe associated problems that death in childhood was common. At present, even though most disorders cannot be cured, better supportive care has resulted in people with these disorders living into adulthood.

The complex disorders of type 1 diabetes and atopic asthma have less identifiable genetic origins and considerable variability in susceptibility. They both require an interaction with environmental factors for disease expression.

GENE GEMS

- Sickle cell disease (SCD) and sickle cell trait have a far greater incidence in East Africa and other equatorial countries.
- Sickle cell disease results in most of a person's hemoglobin to be HbS instead of normal adult hemoglobin (HbA).
- HbS does bind oxygen in the same way that HbA does; however, HbS is very sensitive to low tissue levels of oxygen and makes the red blood cell pull inward, forming a sickle shape when tissue oxygen levels decrease.
- A person with sickle cell trait can form sickled red blood cells, but the degree of hypoxia has to be severe and prolonged for this to occur.
- The genetic mutation that causes sickle cell disease is the same for every person who has the disease, does not arise spontaneously, and is the most stable of the disease-causing mutations.
- Genetic testing is not needed for the diagnosis of sickle cell disease.
- Pain is the most common symptom associated with sickle cell disease.
- Two additional genetic factors that moderate SCD effects are a higher percentage of fetal hemoglobin (HbF) and the coexisting presence of alpha-thalassemia, another genetic disease.
- Carriers for SCD have inherent reduced susceptibility to death from malarial infection.
- Cystic fibrosis (CF) is most common among Caucasians from Northern and Western Europe, although it can be found in any race or ethnicity.
- More than 1400 mutations in the cystic fibrosis gene *(CFTR)* have been identified and are thought to be responsible for the extreme variation in expression of disease severity.
- The most common clinical test used to diagnose cystic fibrosis is the sweat chloride test. Genetic testing is used to identify carrier status, specific mutations, and an affected fetus.
- Carriers of CF appear to have an inherent reduced susceptibility to death from typhoid and cholera.
- Duchenne muscular dystrophy (DMD) is the most common inherited muscle-degrading disease; a more mild form is Becker muscular dystrophy (BMD).
- DMD is an X-linked recessive disorder that affects males more severely and more frequently than females.
- The DMD gene is the largest gene in the human genome and is very susceptible to mutation, including a high percentage of spontaneous mutations.
- The spontaneous mutation rate for the large gene responsible for classic hemophilia (the *F8* gene) is high.
- Many different mutations of *F8* can cause hemophilia, and these may vary from family to family, making genetic testing for hemophilia more difficult.

Continued

- von Willebrand disease (VWD) is inherited as an autosomal dominant trait and is the most common inherited blood-clotting disorder worldwide.
- The majority of people who have VWD have the mildest form and often have never been diagnosed with the disorder.
- Two specific point mutations in the *FGFR3* gene are responsible for 99% of all cases of achondroplasia.
- The *FGFR3* gene is very large, and at least 80% of achondroplasia is a result of spontaneous new mutations associated with advanced paternal age.
- Most children with achondroplasia have delayed motor development and normal intellectual development.
- Obstructive sleep apnea is a potential lethal complication of achondroplasia.
- Type 1 diabetes is an autoimmune disease that results from an increased genetic susceptibility coupled with an environmental trigger, most commonly a viral infection.
- The tissue types most associated with type 1 diabetes and other autoimmune diseases are the HLA-DR and HLA-DQ tissue types.
- People who have the HLA-DR and HLA-DQ tissue types are twice as likely to develop an autoimmune disease than the general population, but the risk is still low (2%).
- A person with type 1 diabetes has a loss of pancreatic islet cells and produces no insulin.
- Unlike type 2 diabetes, obesity and a sedentary lifestyle have no role in the development of type 1 diabetes.
- The chronic hyperglycemia and hyperlipidemia associated with any type of diabetes are responsible for pathological changes starting at the blood vessel level in almost all tissues and organs.
- Asthma is an airway disease problem and does not cause changes in the alveoli.
- Genome-wide association studies link variations in 50 to 100 genes for increased risk to develop atopic asthma.
- Gene variations most strongly associated with asthma differ among races and ethnicities.
- The major genetic/genomic issues of asthma are an increased responsiveness of airway tissues when contacted with an environmental irritant (hyperresponsiveness) and an increased amount of the mediators of inflammation, especially immunoglobulin E (IgE).

Self-Assessment Questions

1. For which genetic problem does the heterozygous state confer an advantage?
   a. Achondroplasia
   b. Type 1 diabetes
   c. Classic hemophilia
   d. Sickle cell trait

2. Which feature or factor is the best predictor for delay of complications in a person who has sickle cell disease (SCD)?
   a. Male gender
   b. 20% or greater of HbF
   c. Having survived malaria
   d. Living in a geographic area that has cold winters

3. A 16-year-old girl whose younger sister was just diagnosed with cystic fibrosis is pregnant with a male fetus. Her boyfriend (the baby's father) has no relatives with the disorder. She asks what the chances are that her son could be affected. What is your best response?
   a. "Because it is likely that you are a carrier and your boyfriend does not have any affected relatives, only your daughters can develop the disease."
   b. "Because you may be a carrier and your boyfriend does not have any affected relatives, your son will not have the disease but could also be a carrier."
   c. "Because your sister actually has cystic fibrosis, the risk for your children having the disorder is 50% with each pregnancy."
   d. "Because you are a woman, your daughters will each have a 50% risk for having the disease, and all of your sons will be carriers."

4. Which statement regarding Duchenne muscular dystrophy (DMD) is true?
   a. Females are not affected.
   b. Because DMD is X-linked recessive, females are affected and males are carriers.
   c. Because DMD is X-linked recessive, males are affected and females are carriers.
   d. The sons of women who are older than age 40 when pregnant are at an increased risk for DMD.

5. A son with classic hemophilia is born to parents with no family history of the disease. Genetic testing reveals that the mother does not have the mutation on either of her X chromosomes. What is the most likely explanation for the son's disorder?
   a. The son is not biologically related to the mother.
   b. One of the mother's ova had a spontaneous mutation of the X chromosome.
   c. One of the father's sperm had a spontaneous mutation of the X chromosome.
   d. The son's DNA underwent a spontaneous mutation during the second trimester of pregnancy.

6. A 12-year-old girl is diagnosed with von Willebrand disease (VWD) when she developed profound anemia from very heavy menstrual periods. Her levels of von Willebrand factor are normal. What specific type of von Willebrand disease is she most likely to have?
   a. Type 1 VWD
   b. Type 2 VWD
   c. Type 3 VWD
   d. Type 4 VWD

7. Which health problem occurs at a higher rate among children with achondroplasia than among the general population?
   a. Mental retardation
   b. Hearing impairment
   c. Color blindness
   d. Sudden infant death syndrome

8. For individuals who have increased genetic susceptibility for type 1 diabetes, what is the most common environmental trigger for disease expression?
   a. Obesity and a sedentary lifestyle
   b. Exposure to radiation
   c. Premature birth
   d. Viral infection

Continued

9. Which gene-environment interaction is most likely for the development of atopic asthma in childhood?
   a. Equal gene and environmental contribution
   b. Greater environmental contribution than gene contribution
   c. Greater gene contribution than environmental contribution
   d. Minimal gene or environmental contribution, greater psychosocial contribution

CASE STUDY

Daniel, a 35-year-old man who has mild type 1 von Willebrand disease, has a 4-month-old daughter. He and his wife express concern to the pediatrician that their daughter may have inherited the disorder. Daniel explains that his mother also has it and that although neither of her parents was affected, his maternal grandfather had two out of five siblings (all females) express the disease. Daniel's three cousins from his mother's only sibling do not have the disease.

1. Draw the pedigree and indicate any obvious pattern of inheritance.

2. What are the possible explanations for Daniel's mother having the disorder but neither of her parents expressing it?

3. Is the concern that Daniel's daughter may have the disorder valid?

4. What questions should you ask Daniel and his wife?

References

Centers for Disease Control and Prevention. (2010). FastStats. National Center for Health Statistics. Retrieved January 2011, from www.cdc.gov/nchs/fastats/.

Cystic Fibrosis Foundation. (2011). Frequently asked questions. Retrieved February 2011, from www.cff.org.

Dotta, F., Censini, S., van Halteren, A., et al. (2007). Coxsackie B4 virus infection of beta cells and natural killer cell insulitis in recent onset type 1 diabetic patients. *Proceedings of the National Academy of Science, 104*(12), 5115–5120.

Embry, S., Clark, M., Monroy, G., and Mohandas, N. (1984). Concurrent sickle cell anemia and alpha-thalassemia. Effect on pathological properties of sickle erythrocytes. *Journal of Clinical Investigation, 73*(1), 116–123.

Hindorff, L., Sethupathy, P., Junkins, H., et al. (2009). Potential etiologic and functional implications of genome-wide association loci for human diseases and traits. *Proceedings of the National Academy of Sciences, 106*(23), 9362–9367.

Holgate, S. (1997). Asthma genetics: Waiting to exhale. *Nature Genetics, 15*(3), 227–229.

Kulczycki, L., Kostuch, M., and Bellanti, J. (2003). A clinical perspective of cystic fibrosis and new genetic findings: Relationship of CFTR mutations to genotype-phenotype manifestations. *American Journal of Medical Genetics, 116A*(3), 262–267.

Kumar, V., Abbas, A., Fausto, N., and Aster, J. Robbins and Cotran: Pathologic basis of disease, 8th ed. Philadelphia: Saunders, 2010.

Longo, G., Strinati, R., Poli, F., and Fumi, F. (1987). Genetic factors in nonspecific bronchial hyperreactivity: An epidemiological study. *American Journal of Diseases of Children, 141*(3), 331–334.

Mittal, N., James, P., and Valentino, L. (2009). Diagnosis of von Willebrand disease in children. *Current Pediatric Reviews, 5*(3), 169–175.

Muscular Dystrophy Association. (2010). *Facts about Duchenne and Becker muscular dystrophies: (DMD and (BMD)*. Retrieved December 2010 from www.mdsusa.org.

National Heart Lung and Blood Institute. (2009). Von Willebrand Disease. Retrieved December 2010 from www.nhlbi.nih.gov/health/dci/Diseases/vWD/vWD.

National Hemophilia Foundation. (2010) MASAC recommendations concerning products licensed for the treatment of hemophilia and other bleeding disorders. Retrieved December 2010 from http://hemophilia.org.

National Institutes of Health. (2010). Genetics Home Reference: Achondroplasia. Retrieved December 2010 from http://ghr.nlm.nih.gov/condition/achondroplasia.

OMIM (Online Mendelian Inheritance in Man). (2010). Asthma, susceptibility to. Retrieved December 2010 from www.ncbi.nlm.nih.gov/omim.

Pack-Mabien, A., and Haynes, J. (2009). A primary care provider's guide to preventive and acute care management of adults and children with sickle cell disease. *Journal of the American Academy of Nurse Practitioners, 21*(5), 250–257.

Pier, G., Grout, M., Zaidi, T., et al. (1998). Salmonella typhi uses CFTR to enter intestinal epithelial cells. *Nature, 393*(6680), 79–82.

Richette, P., Bardin, T., and Stheneur, C. (2008). Achondroplasia: From genotype to phenotype. *Joint Bone Spine, 75*(2), 125–130.

Shirley, E. (2009). Achondroplasia: Manifestations and treatment. *Journal of the American Academy of Orthopedic Surgeons, 17*(4), 231–241.

Sickle Cell Disease Association of America. (2005). About sickle cell disease. Retrieved December 2010 from www.sicklecelldisease.org.

Sleiman, P., Flory, J., Imielinski, M., et al. (2010). Variants of *DENND1B* associated with asthma in children. *New England Journal of Medicine, 362*(1), 36–44.

Townley, R., Bewtra, A., Wilson, A., et al. (1986). Segregation analysis of bronchial response to methacholine inhalation challenge in families with and without asthma. *Journal of Allergy and Clinical Immunology, 77*(1, Part 1), 101–107.

Weiss, S., Raby, B., and Rogers, A. (2009). Asthma genetics and genomics 2009. *Current Opinion in Genetics & Development, 19*(3), 279–282.

Self-Assessment Answers

1. d **2.** b **3.** b **4.** c **5.** b **6.** b **7.** d **8.** d **9.** c

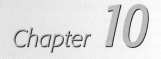
Common Adult-Onset Genetic Disorders

Learning Outcomes

1. Use genetic terminology associated with common adult-onset disorders.
2. Describe the implications of incomplete penetrance in hereditary hemochromatosis.
3. Distinguish between genetic causes of diabetes mellitus type 2 and maturity-onset diabetes of the young (MODY).
4. Discuss the genetic and environmental contributions to complex autoimmune disorders.
5. Compare the genetic risk for family members of patients with early-onset Alzheimer disease and those with late-onset Alzheimer disease.
6. Compare genetic contributions to age-related vision and hearing impairment.

KEY TERMS

Alzheimer Disease (AD)

Gestational diabetes mellitus (GDM)

Hereditary hemochromatosis (*HFE*-HHC)

Human leukocyte antigens (HLA)

Maturity-onset diabetes of the young (MODY)

Multiple sclerosis (MS)

Presbycusis

Rheumatoid arthritis (RA)

Self-tolerance

Systemic lupus erythematosus (SLE)

Introduction

Many single-gene disorders are first evident during childhood. Most complex or multifactorial disorders are first seen during adulthood. However, this is not always the case. This chapter will discuss disorders that have their onset during adulthood. Some are due to problems in a single gene, such as hemochromatosis. Others are due to a combination of several gene variants working together along with the environment, such as diabetes mellitus type 2.

As people get older, they are more likely to have been exposed to environmental factors that can trigger the onset of disease in someone who has a genetic susceptibility. Finding out what genes increase a person's susceptibility to a complex (multifactorial) disease that clearly runs in the family is a continuing challenge. Knowing who is most likely to get a particular disease based on their genome variations allows the targeting of interventions to those people who are at highest risk.

Adult-onset genetic diseases carry with them a unique set of problems. These include when and if a person should have genetic testing to determine their risk, when and if prophylactic treatment or monitoring should begin, and when and if genetic counseling is appropriate. For example, in 2001, the American Academy of Pediatrics (and several other organizations) recommended against predictive genetic testing of children at risk for adult-onset disorders, unless there is a clear benefit to the child (Nelson, 2001). Therefore, testing children for the gene variant that causes Huntington disease would not be supported, while testing a 6-year-old for hereditary nonpolyposis colon cancer may be useful because guidelines for monitoring by colonoscopy can be altered based on genetic risk. This policy statement was reaffirmed in 2005 and in 2009. You can read more about genetic testing of minors in Chapter 14. This chapter will discuss disorders that more commonly appear during adulthood and will consider the genetic contributions to each of them. A number of adult-onset disorders, such as cardiovascular diseases and many cancers, are described in later chapters.

Monogenic Disorders

A few disorders with symptoms that appear during adulthood are caused by single-gene problems. For some, it is clear why we do not see any obvious signs and symptoms until adulthood, but for others, it is a bit puzzling. Three relatively common adult-onset single-gene problems are hemochromatosis, maturity-onset diabetes of the young (MODY), and alpha-1 antitrypsin (AAT) emphysema.

Hereditary Hemochromatosis

Hereditary hemochromatosis (*HFE*-HHC) is associated with excessive absorption of dietary iron by the gastric mucosa. This excess iron accumulates in the liver, pancreas, heart, joints, and testes. It also accumulates in the skin, causing the affected person to have a bronzelike skin discoloration. An older name for this disorder was "bronze diabetes." Even though an affected person has had the genotype since birth, clinical symptoms usually do not begin until age 40 to 60 years. It takes some time for the buildup of iron to damage the organs and cause clinical evidence. The first symptoms patients notice are weakness, abdominal pain, and weight loss. Unless the disease is identified early and treatment is begun, affected people will develop liver cirrhosis, diabetes mellitus, cardiomyopathy, arrhythmias, arthritis, and hypogonadism.

Affected people carry mutations in the *HFE* gene. About 11% of the general population of Caucasians is heterozygous for one of the mutations that cause *HFE*-HHC. The percentage of carriers is much lower in other populations. For example, only 2.3% of African Americans are heterozygous for mutations in this gene (Kowdley, 2006). *HFE*-HHC is an autosomal recessive trait; people who are either *homozygous* or *compound heterozygous* are at risk. Fortunately, the penetrance for *HFE*-HHC is quite low, so not everyone who carries the genotype will show the phenotype. This makes the biochemical rather than the genetic testing of people who are at risk most useful. What matters most is whether the person is clinically affected.

The transferrin saturation test is the biochemical test that is used clinically to exclude the presence of *HFE*-HHC or to support the need for further evaluation, such as genetic testing or liver biopsy. Several different types of genetic testing can be useful in families that are at risk for *HFE*-HHC. For example, *diagnostic testing* can be used to confirm that a person who shows the phenotype has this disease and not something else that causes similar symptoms. *Carrier testing* can identify heterozygotes who are at risk of passing on the trait to their offspring. *Predictive testing* can be used to identify people who are homozygous or compound heterozygous for the genotype and therefore at risk of developing symptoms over time. These people can be monitored periodically for iron overload, so if symptoms do occur, they can be treated promptly.

Therapeutic phlebotomy is a simple, effective, and inexpensive treatment that can bring iron levels close to normal. Each unit of whole blood (400 to 500 ml) normally contains between 160 to 200 mg of iron. Many people affected with HHC have regularly scheduled phlebotomies. Women with *HFE*-HHC often do not show signs of iron overload until well after menopause, because the menstrual cycle provides natural and regular blood iron loss every month (Kowdley, 2006). Without treatment, excess iron accumulates in the organs and tissues, causing fatigue, joint pain, and abdominal pain. Over the long term, iron overload leads to arthritis, liver cirrhosis, diabetes, cardiomyopathy, heart failure, and hypopituitarism.

Maturity-Onset Diabetes of the Young

Maturity-onset diabetes of the young (MODY) is a single-gene problem that causes hyperglycemia, usually before the age of 25. This disorder is transmitted in an autosomal dominant pattern, and mutations in six different genes cause the six major types of MODY. Recent work has identified three additional genes in small populations, so there is now MODY 7, 8, and 9. However, approximately 85% of people with MODY have types 1, 2, or 3.

Clinical genetic testing is available for the six major genes that cause MODY. Sometimes people with MODY have been misdiagnosed as having diabetes mellitus type 1 or type 2 (DMT1 or DM type 2). Genetic testing can confirm or refute whether a person has MODY. Even though the name implies that MODY affects the young, some people with MODY 1 do not have symptoms until they are older, suggesting either a gene-environment interaction or variability in expression. One study of people with MODY 1 found that diabetes developed by age 25 in only 65% of those who carried the gene mutation. MODY was found in 100% of study subjects by age 50 (Klupa, 2002).

Each of the genes involved in MODY plays a role in glucose metabolism, insulin action, or insulin release from the pancreas. The six major types of MODY and the genes that have been identified as causing them are listed in Table 10–1. Mutations in hepatocyte nuclear factor 1 alpha gene (*HNF-1α*), located on chromosome 12, cause MODY 3, which accounts for approximately 65% of cases. *HNF-1α* is involved in the metabolism of glucose, cholesterol, and fatty acids. Defects in the glucokinase gene (*GCK*) on chromosome 7 (*GCK*) cause MODY 2. Sometimes children who carry *GCK* mutations will have mild hyperglycemia, and some cases of gestational diabetes are also caused by mutations in this gene. Glucokinase regulates the release of insulin from the beta cells of the pancreas in response to the presence of glucose in the blood. People with MODY 2 tend to have a less severe form of the disease, but they need higher levels of glucose in the blood to trigger the release of insulin than people with glucokinase that is working properly. MODY 1 is caused by mutations in hepatocyte nuclear factor 4 alpha (*HNF-4α*), which is located on chromosome 20. Variations in this gene result in problems with insulin secretion.

Because MODY is transmitted as an autosomal dominant trait, only one copy of the defective gene is needed for a person to have the disease. Rarely, people are homozygous (or compound heterozygous) for mutations in one of these genes and tend to have more severe forms of the disease. Those who are homozygous for defects in the gene that codes for glucokinase can have severe DM as a newborn (severe neonatal DM). Those who are homozygous for mutations in the *IPF1* gene, which causes MODY 4, may not grow a pancreas at all (pancreatic agenesis).

TABLE 10–1

Genetic Defects of β-Cell Function

	Chromosome	Gene	Incidence
MODY 1	20	*HNF-4α*	∼ 5%
MODY 2	7	*GCK*	∼ 15%
MODY 3	12	*HNF-1α*	∼ 65%
MODY 4	13	*IPF 1*	
MODY 5	17	*HNF-1β*	< 3%
MODY 6	2	*NeuroD1*	
Mitochondrial DNA			

Data for this table from: Diabetes Care. (2010). Diagnosis and classification of diabetes mellitus. *Diabetes Care, 33 Suppl 1*, S62–69.

Alpha-1 Antitrypsin (AAT) Deficiency

Alpha-1 antitrypsin deficiency (AATD) was first described as a risk factor for chronic obstructive pulmonary disease (COPD) in 1963. AATD is caused by mutations in the *SERPINA1* gene, which codes for alpha-1 antitrypsin. Adults who are homozygous for one of these mutations have a high risk of chronic lung disease (COPD), specifically emphysema. AATD also causes liver disease in some children as well as in adults.

Trypsin is a proteolytic enzyme (or proteinase) that breaks down proteins into their peptides and amino acids during digestion. Trypsin is produced in its inactive form by the pancreas. Alpha-1 antitrypsin (AAT) is an antiproteinase enzyme that is produced by the liver. It protects lung tissue and bile ducts from damage by destructive proteins such as trypsin. Not having enough AAT leads to inflammation in the lungs, emphysema, liver cirrhosis, and liver fibrosis. Too much trypsin (or not enough antitrypsin) can be very damaging to tissue.

The air we breathe often contains microscopic particulate matter that can irritate and damage the lungs. Thus, the lungs have proteolytic enzymes to break down these particulates and protect the lungs. However, these "protective" enzymes must be controlled so that their effects are directed only against particulate matter and not the lung tissues. Alpha-1 antitrypsin limits the activity of these enzymes and prevents them from auto-digesting a person's lung tissues. So when a person does not produce enough active AAT, the normally protective enzymes go beyond degrading inhaled particulate matter and begin degrading the lung's elastic tissue. Over time, the loss of elastic tissue leads to early-onset emphysema.

The severity of AAT depends on which forms of the gene are inherited. People who are homozygous for the allele associated with the most severe deficiency (the Z allele) have very little alpha-1 antitrypsin in their serum; therefore, their lungs and livers are most vulnerable to destruction by excess trypsin. This genotype is described as PI-ZZ, and it is passed through families as an autosomal recessive trait. People with two ZZ alleles account for 95% of all people with AATD (Schlade-Bartusiak, 2008). The other alleles are M and S, and they confer varying degrees of risk (Table 10–2). Severe AATD is found in only 1% to 2% of all people who have emphysema. Other forms of COPD are more complex and clearly involve the actions of several susceptibility genes working together with the environment.

TABLE 10–2

Alpha-1 Antitrypsin Genotypes

Genotype	Level of AAT and/or Risk for Disease
MM	Results in normal concentrations of AAT
MZ	Heterozygotes have a slightly increased risk of poor lung function.
SZ	A higher risk of lung problems among smokers, but not usually associated with increased risk in nonsmokers
ZZ	Often associated with clinical disease and a plasma concentration of AAT that is less than 20% of normal

Adapted from: Schlade-Bartusiak, K., and Cox, D. W. (2008). Alpha-1 antitrypsin deficiency. Retrieved October 16, 2010, from www.ncbi.nlm.nih.gov/bookshelf/br.fcgi?book=gene&part=alpha1-a.

While AATD is considered a single-gene disorder, there are still environmental factors that can affect the clinical progression of the disease. For example, tobacco smoking greatly increases the risk of COPD in a person who carries the AATD genotype. For smokers who are at genetic risk, respiratory disease begins between the ages of 40 and 50 years, or even younger. In nonsmokers, lung disease may not appear until they are well into their 60s. People at genetic risk are counseled to avoid not only active and passive smoking, but also exposure to environmental pollutants such as mineral dust, gas, or other fumes.

Complex Disorders

There are many more complex (multifactorial) disorders that have adult onset than there are single-gene disorders with adult onset. However, finding the genes that contribute to the risk of complex diseases is always difficult. Multifactorial disease is often due to a large number of genes, each exerting a small effect, combined with environment. Advances in genetic testing technologies, such as genome-wide association studies (GWAS), have added greatly to our ability to find genes associated with adult-onset complex diseases. These are often among our top causes of morbidity and mortality, so finding who is genetically susceptible before they develop symptoms could have a powerful impact on public health. When people find out they are at genetic risk for a particular disease, they tend to follow recommendations for monitoring their health better than when they just know that a disease runs in their family. In this section, we will discuss diabetes mellitus type 2, obesity, and autoimmune disorders.

Diabetes Mellitus Type 2

There are many different types of diabetes mellitus (DM), and together they affect approximately 220 million people worldwide (WHO, 2009). Chapter 9 discusses type 1 diabetes mellitus. MODY was described earlier in this chapter with other monogenic disorders of adult onset. This section will focus on DM type 2 and gestational diabetes. The fasting blood glucose levels that are diagnostic for impaired glucose tolerance and actual DM are listed in Table 10–3. When people have random blood glucose levels of 200 mg/dL or higher, plus clinical signs such as increased urination and increased thirst, fatigue, blurred vision, and poor wound healing, they should have further testing to determine whether they have DM (NIDDK, 2008).

TABLE 10–3

Fasting Glucose Values and the Diagnosis of Diabetes Mellitus

Plasma Glucose Result (mg/dL)	Diagnosis
99 or below	Normal
100 to 125	Impaired Fasting Glucose
126 or above*	Diabetes

*This value must be confirmed by repeating the test on another day.
Data for this table from: ADA. (2010). Diagnosis and classification of diabetes mellitus. *Diabetes Care*, *33 Suppl 1*, S62–69.

What all forms of DM share in common is persistent hyperglycemia and the profound impact that this has on the health of people who are affected. When the body's organs are exposed to high blood sugar levels for long periods of time, severe damage or failure of organ systems can occur. The most commonly affected organs are the heart and blood vessels, the eyes, the kidneys, and the nerves. We also see the accompanying loss of lipid control. The result is the macrovascular and microvascular complications we see in patients with DM.

DM type 2 is the most common form of DM, accounting for about 90% to 95% of all people with DM (Diabetes, 2010). DM type 2 is caused by a relative (rather than an absolute) problem with the secretion of insulin or, more commonly, a severe decrease in insulin sensitivity (insulin resistance). This means that even when insulin is produced in normal amounts, it fails to bind well to the insulin receptor. It is the correct binding of insulin to its receptor that changes a cell's permeability to glucose (see Chapter 9). There is also excessive liver glucose production and a decrease in the cellular uptake of glucose. That means that even though people with DM type 2 can make insulin, they cannot make enough to compensate for the difficulty they have in using insulin. Many older people with DM type 2 are not diagnosed early, because symptoms tend to appear gradually over time, so they may not identify the classical signs of DM, such as polyuria or polydipsia.

Sometimes people do not find out they have DM type 2 until they start experiencing complications such as retinopathy or neuropathy. Often, DM type 2 is found during laboratory testing for an unrelated problem. The National Institute of Diabetes, Digestive, and Kidney Disease suggests that nearly 6 million people in the United States have DM type 2 and have not been diagnosed (NIDDK, 2008). This is surprising because we know that DM type 2 clearly runs in families. As health-care providers, we would hope that when a person has a first-degree relative with DM type 2, they would be on the lookout for signs and symptoms in themselves. We can help alert patients to their increased risk of DM type 2 and suggest periodic monitoring in accordance with guidelines (AHRQ, 2010).

The contribution of genetics to the onset of DM type 2 has been demonstrated in a large number of studies, but because this disease does not follow simple rules of Mendelian inheritance, it can be very difficult to tease out the specific genetic factors that contribute to its onset. About 7% of people in the general population will get DM type 2 at some point in their lives, but 30% to 40% of people who have one affected parent will become affected. The risk is 70% for people who have two affected parents (Vimaleswaran, 2010). With DM type 2 becoming more and more prevalent, having two affected parents is not uncommon.

Another way of determining how big a part genetics plays in the risk of having a complex or multifactorial disease is to look at twin concordance studies. You may remember from Chapter 4 that *twin concordance* refers to the percentage of second twins who are affected with a disease that affected the first twin. In DM type 2, the monozygotic (identical) twin concordance rate has been estimated at being between 60% and 90%. That means that if one twin is affected, the other twin will be affected 60% to 90% of the time. That is very strong evidence for a genetic contribution because monozygotic twins share their genotypes in common. The twin concordance rate for dizygotic (fraternal) twins is usually estimated at about 30%. Remember that dizygotic twins share only about 50% of their DNA in common, just like regular siblings.

Even though most people who have DM type 2 are diagnosed in middle to late adulthood, there is a disturbing rise in the diagnosis of younger people. Children and adolescents are being diagnosed with DM type 2 (not MODY, but actually DM type 2). According to the World Health Organization, at highest risk are females from minority groups whose mothers are also affected (WHO, 2009). The incidence of DM type 2 is increasing dramatically worldwide, and it is most often associated with obesity, which is also increasing at an alarming rate.

One theory that attempts to explain why DM type 2 has become so common describes what was called the "thrifty genotype" (Neel, 1962). Historically, when populations experienced periods of plenty followed by times of famine, those people who were better at storing fat survived to pass on their genes to their offspring. People who were not metabolically "thrifty" would be less able to store fat, and they would not survive during times when there was little food. Now, when many people have access to lots of calorie-dense food, the ability to get the most energy from every calorie and easily store fat is not such a great advantage! People with thrifty genotypes are so good at storing fat that they carry around lots of excess body weight. This leads to the increasing prevalence of obesity and DM type 2. The most important risk factors for DM type 2 are obesity and its usual partner, a sedentary lifestyle. Obesity, which will be discussed in the next section, causes some degree of insulin resistance all by itself (ADA, 2010). Even if the thrifty genotype explains why obesity and DM type 2 are on the rise, lots of work must be done to identify the specific genetic factors that make someone's genotype thrifty in the first place!

Candidate Genes Associated With Diabetes Mellitus Type 2

Candidate gene and genome-wide association studies (GWAS) have identified a number of genes that increase susceptibility to DM type 2, and these vary somewhat from population to population. For example, calpain 10 *(CAPN10)* is a gene that appears to be very important in the onset of DM type 2 in about 40% of Mexican-American family clusters, while it has much less importance for people of British descent (Malecki, 2005). It is still unclear exactly how *CAPN10* increases the risk for DM type 2. We do know that it has a role in breaking down proteins (it is a protease), and it affects the action of other enzymes. How that connects to impaired glucose metabolism remains to be seen.

Genes are considered candidates for study if the proteins they encode have an important role in pathways of insulin secretion or insulin action. One example of a great candidate gene for DM type 2 is peroxisome proliferator-activated receptor-γ *(PPARγ)*. *PPARγ* encodes a protein involved in both lipid and adipocyte (fat cell) metabolism. One form of this gene decreases insulin sensitivity significantly. This gene variant is also really common among Caucasians. About 98% of Europeans are at least heterozygous for this allele, so having one copy apparently does not cause DM type 2 all by itself; otherwise, 98% of people with European descent would have DM type 2. Even though the number of affected people is growing, it is not quite that high!

ATP binding cassette, subfamily C, member 8 *(ABCC8)* is a gene that encodes a sulfonylurea receptor, and it is joined with a potassium channel encoded by the gene *KCNJ1*. These genes are important in controlling the release of hormones such as insulin and glucagon from the beta cells of the pancreas. It seems likely that they would have a good chance of being associated with DM type 2 when one or both of them was not working properly. This makes them good candidates for study. The other reason why they are of particular interest is that these genes, along with *PPARγ*, are important targets for drugs that are used to treat DM type 2. Variations in these genes may affect how patients respond to their oral antidiabetic drugs in addition to placing them at higher risk of having DM type 2. There is much to learn about the genes that make someone susceptible to DM type 2.

Gestational Diabetes Mellitus

Although numbers vary from study to study, up to 7% of pregnancies are complicated by gestational diabetes mellitus (GDM). For some time, GDM has been defined as any amount of glucose intolerance that is first identified during pregnancy. Sometimes women with GDM need insulin therapy, and sometimes diet alone is sufficient to normalize their blood sugars. Typically, the elevations in blood sugar are first noticed around 28 weeks of gestation, and they resolve after delivery. It is thought that a genetic predisposition is triggered by insulin resistance that occurs during pregnancy. However, GDM does seem to run in families. Also, mutations in some of the genes that can cause MODY have been found in women with GDM (Lambrinoudaki, 2010).

If the hyperglycemia is discovered early in pregnancy or on the first prenatal visit, it will be unclear whether the glucose intolerance started with the pregnancy or if it existed before the pregnancy and was just undiagnosed. Although the elevated blood sugar levels usually go down after delivery, for some women, the hyperglycemia persists, and if it persists for 6 weeks after delivery, they are reclassified as having actual DM type 2. The American Diabetes Association suggests that women who have high blood sugar levels at their first prenatal visit should be diagnosed as having DM and not just GDM (ADA, 2010). About 90% of women who develop GDM go on to develop DM type 2 later in life.

Genetic Syndromes Associated With Diabetes Mellitus

Some genetic syndromes include an increased risk of DM. These include chromosomal problems such as Down syndrome, Turner syndrome, and Klinefelter syndrome. Single-gene disorders can also result in increased incidence of DM. Wolfram syndrome is transmitted in an autosomal recessive manner and causes DM type 1, usually beginning between the ages of 5 and 15. People with Wolfram syndrome also have a collection of other problems, including hearing loss and visual impairment.

Obesity

Obesity is a problem that affects growing numbers of people worldwide. Having a body mass index (BMI) greater than 25 defines overweight, and a BMI greater than 30 is considered obese. According to the World Health Organization, 1.6 billion adults were overweight and 400 million were obese in 2005 (Fawcett, 2010). Approximately 70% of people in the United States are currently either obese or overweight. People who are obese are at high risk for many concerning health problems, including DM type 2, cancer, and heart disease. Finding genetic links to obesity could be key in developing therapies that work to alleviate the burden of this major health problem. Obesity runs in families. Genetics accounts for between 40% and 90% of the variation in BMI. However, finding the genes responsible is an enormous challenge.

Many interesting locations on the genome have been found using candidate gene or linkage studies, but very few of these have been supported by additional studies. Since 1996, people searching for genes associated with obesity have been able to catalogue their findings in the Human Obesity Gene Map. This map lists 127 genes that have been associated with obesity in at least one study (Loos, 2009). These are simply associations, and no one is saying that they have found the genes that "cause" obesity.

Candidate Genes Associated With Obesity

The melanocortin 4 receptor *(MC4R)* seems like an important candidate gene. It plays a critical role in both the regulation of food intake and the regulation of energy balance. Recently, one variation in this gene has been found to be protective against obesity. People who carry this variant have a 50% lower risk of being obese than people who do not carry this variation. Unfortunately, this variant is found in only 1% to 2% of the population!

Prohormone convertase 1/3 *(PCSK1)* looks like another promising choice. The gene encodes an enzyme that is important in the regulation of energy metabolism, and people with rare mutations in this gene suffer from an extreme form of childhood obesity. Large studies have suggested that this gene has little influence on obesity in the general population.

Brain-derived neurotrophic factor *(BDNF)* is thought to play a role in development and in the stress response. It has been shown to be involved in eating behaviors, controlling body weight, and hyperactivity. As with *PCSK1,* there are rare variations in this gene that result in severe obesity and an uncontrolled appetite. Several studies have found that other variations in this gene are associated with a lower BMI.

The adrenergic β3 receptor gene *(ADRB3)* is involved in the regulation of lipid breakdown and in thermogenesis. Diet-induced thermogenesis refers to the increase in the metabolic rate above baseline that happens following the ingestion of food. It is of major importance in determining daily energy expenditure. There have been several inconclusive studies, but one variation of this gene was associated with a higher BMI in East Asians but not in other populations (Vimaleswaran, 2010).

While GWAS have identified interesting loci that may be useful in determining risk for obesity in the future, the results of association studies are not clinically useful in the short term. In 2007, a study found an association between common variations *(single nucleotide polymorphisms* or *SNPs)* in the fat mass and obesity-associated *(FTO)* gene and BMI. This gene encodes a protein that plays an important role in controlling both feeding behavior and energy expenditure (Fawcett, 2010). It is important to remember that even if there is an association between a gene or locus and a disease process (such as obesity), this does not mean that one causes the other. There is still much work to be done before we can say that we have found the genes that cause an increased risk of obesity.

Autoimmune Disorders

The immune system is very complex. The work it does is challenging. It has to identify foreign invaders and destroy them, but it also has to be able to identify self-cells and keep them safe. This ability to distinguish self- from nonself cells is tricky. It usually works amazingly well, but sometimes it breaks down. When immune factors start to attack self-cells, we have autoimmune disease, which can have devastating symptoms and be very difficult to treat. We do not completely understand the mechanism for **self-tolerance**, the ability of immune system cells to recognize and not attack the cells of the body in which they reside. This chapter will discuss multiple sclerosis (MS), systemic lupus erythematosus (SLE), and rheumatoid arthritis (RA).

Most autoimmune diseases are complex, and the genetic contribution is not that easy to tease out, although many autoimmune problems do seem to run in families. While the twin concordance is higher in monozygotic twins than in dizygotic twins, it is still not 100%, so there are factors other than genotype that make someone more likely to get an autoimmune disease. These factors are most likely from the environment.

Some investigators have suggested that environmental factors that change DNA methylation (*epigenetic* changes) may be the key to environment-gene interaction in autoimmune disease. This is an important area of ongoing research. For example, we know that women are much more vulnerable to autoimmune diseases than men, but we do not really understand why this is. SLE is eight times more common among women than among men. Some have suggested that the inactive X chromosome that all women carry could be the culprit.

Remember that in each cell of a woman's body, one X is inactivated, so she does not make twice as much protein as men do from the genes on her two X chromosomes. This is an epigenetic effect on gene expression in the genome. It is just one place that researchers are looking, because it is a clear difference between the genetics of men and women (Hewagama and Richardson, 2009). You can read more about epigenetics and X inactivation in Chapter 4.

Even though it is difficult, finding genetic contributions to common autoimmune disorders can provide a valuable contribution to understanding the mechanisms and pathophysiology of the disorders. Therefore, there is great interest in locating susceptibility genes. As we have seen with DM type 2 and obesity, genome-wide scans have helped to move the science forward.

Systemic Lupus Erythematosus

Systemic lupus erythematosus (SLE) is a classic autoimmune disorder caused by immune cells attacking self-cells all over the body. Symptoms appear in the skin, heart, lungs, kidneys, joints, and the nervous system. Affected people often have a "butterfly" rash over the cheeks of the face, a patchy skin rash, light sensitivity, arthritis, ulcers of the mucous membranes, pericarditis, pleuritis, or seizures. It certainly seems that the body is attacking itself. SLE usually begins between 20 and 45 years of age, and women are affected much more often than men. Some women with SLE experience worsening of their symptoms around the time of menstruation. This might indicate that the hormones women produce at this time could be involved in SLE onset.

The genetic contributions to SLE susceptibility are significant. If we look at twin studies, we can see that the twin concordance rate for monozygotic twins is between 25% and 75%. For dizygotic twins, the concordance rate is only between 2% and 9% (Hewagama and Richardson, 2009). Remember that monozygotic twins share close to 100% of their genotype, while dizygotic twins share only about 50% of their genotype. It is not surprising that several areas of the genome have been associated with SLE, but because monozygotic twin concordance is not 100%, there must be environmental factors as well. Suggested environmental triggers for the onset of SLE in genetically susceptible people include viruses, drugs, and exposure to sunlight.

One region of the genome that is implicated in many problems with immunity and autoimmunity is the **human leukocyte antigens (HLAs)** coded for by the major histocompatibility complex (MHC) genes located on chromosome 6 (Fig. 10–1). Remember that the HLAs function as unique identifiers on the surface of almost all cells in the body. When an immune system cell recognizes an invader, the immune cell "examines" the HLA proteins on the invader's surface to determine if it is a self-cell or a nonself cell. If the proteins do not perfectly match the body's HLAs, then the cell is identified as foreign and the attack begins. There are about 40 different major HLAs and an unknown number of minor HLAs.

Genes encoding proteins in the complement pathway are also found in this region. The complement system includes several different plasma proteins that are activated in a cascade to destroy pathogens. These proteins either destroy invaders directly or they "complement" the action of antibodies. Because both HLAs and the complement system are important for effective immune functioning, it is not surprising that genes in this region are associated with autoimmune disease.

Some locations on chromosome 1 contain genes that are important in clearing immune complexes from the circulation after they have done their work. People with SLE have been found to have lower levels of the enzyme DNase1. This enzyme's job is to take cellular debris and chop it into small pieces

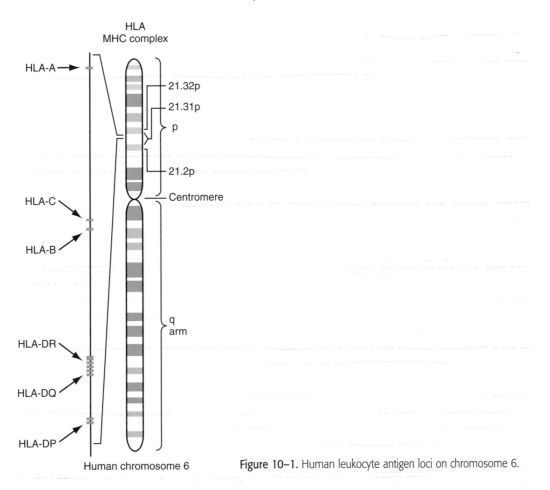

Figure 10–1. Human leukocyte antigen loci on chromosome 6.

so that it can be disposed of more easily. When researchers turned off this gene in mice, they found that even though the mice appeared to be healthy when they were born, they developed signs of SLE after several weeks. It seems possible that a mutation in the gene that codes for this enzyme could interfere with the body's ability to dispose of cellular waste and trigger an autoimmune reaction, causing SLE.

Multiple Sclerosis

Multiple sclerosis (MS) is the most common autoimmune disorder that involves the nervous system. In this disorder, the myelin coating of neurons is destroyed by inflammation (demyelination). Scattered regions of plaque found in the white matter of the central nervous system damage the myelin sheath until it becomes too thin to allow the transmission of neural impulses from the brain to the spinal cord and periphery. The disease is characterized by episodes of exacerbation and remission and is the most common cause of neurological disability in young people.

As with SLE, it has been clear for some time that MS runs in families. Having an affected first-degree relative (parent, child, or sibling) raises your risk of getting MS from 1 in 750 to 1 in 100; some studies even found the risk to be 1 in 40 (Hoppenbrouwers and Hintzen, 2010). We also know that the risk of getting MS differs among ethnic populations. MS is most common among people whose ancestors came from Northern Europe. While people whose ancestors came from other regions can still get MS, it is much less likely. Just as we saw with other autoimmune disorders, most people believe that there is an environmental trigger that sets off disease in a person who is genetically susceptible.

MS is clearly complex and is probably due to a combination of variations in many genes, each exerting a small, increased risk, added to environmental contributions. Some of the genes that have been implicated are those you will probably recognize as the "usual suspects." The first gene variants associated with MS were located on chromosome 6. They are the HLA genes that also seem to be important in the onset of SLE, as well as many other autoimmune problems. Much work is in process looking for associations between variants in the HLA genes and MS. For example, one gene in the HLA region (*DRB5*) seems to be protective against MS. There are a significant number of people of African descent who do not have this allele, and this may help to explain why MS can be very severe in some African Americans but not in others. Additional genes important to effective immune function have been associated with MS. These include interleukin-7 (IL-7) and interleukin-2 (IL-2). Interleukins are cytokines, or chemical messengers, within the immune system.

The geographical distribution of MS risk has led some to wonder if limited exposure to sunlight might be an environmental risk factor because it reduces the body's ability to make vitamin D. Some studies have demonstrated that having an adequate dietary intake of the vitamin D reduces the risk of MS in people with the *HLA-DRB1* risk allele. This is biologically plausible, because vitamin D has an important role in the development and function of both the central nervous and the immune systems. There is also evidence that when people who have *HLA-DRB1* risk allele get mononucleosis, their risk of getting MS goes up (Hoppenbrouwers, 2010).

Rheumatoid Arthritis

Rheumatoid arthritis (RA) is a chronic and progressive autoimmune disorder that most frequently affects women and the elderly. It is considered the most common connective tissue disease, affecting more than 2 million people. RA is characterized by synovitis (inflammation of the membrane that lines the joints) and production of autoantibodies. Rheumatoid factors, consisting mainly of IgA and IgM, attack tissue in the joints and cause inflammation.

Approximately 50% of the risk for RA is genetic. The most powerful environmental risk factor is smoking. Some investigators believe that RA is best understood as a collection of different subsets of inflammatory diseases that share a pathway leading to synovial inflammation. The genetic factors involved seem to be different, depending on whether a patient has antibodies directed against citrullinated peptides (ACPA). Being positive for these antibodies means that a person is more likely to have progressive joint destruction and a generally poor prognosis. There are some differences in the particular HLA alleles associated with RA in ACPA-positive and ACPA-negative patients.

Thirty different regions of the genome have been associated with RA. One of the problems is that alleles that have been found in RA patients are very common in the general population, so they really do not help determine who is at greatest genetic risk. Genes that have long been associated with RA include protein tyrosine phosphatase (*PTPN22*). *PTPN22* is involved in many autoimmune diseases, including type 1 diabetes, autoimmune thyroid disease, and SLE.

Autoimmune Summary

As you can see, there are many regions of the genome that are associated with autoimmune diseases in general. This leads us to believe that immune system dysfunction shares many common mechanisms of pathogenesis. It is somewhat puzzling that we do not always see many different kinds of autoimmune diseases in every family that is affected with one kind. Studies on whether this happens commonly have reported conflicted results. We know it certainly appears to happen in some families. Autoimmune disorders share much, but not everything, in common. If we were to construct a diagram of all the genes associated with autoimmune disorders, we would have overlapping circles, with some genes involved in the risk of each of these diseases (such as the HLAs), some involved in two, and some involved in only one. It is most likely the unique combinations of susceptibility alleles combined with environmental risk factors, such as smoking or lack of exposure to sunlight, that makes for the variations in autoimmune dysfunction. There is still much to learn about the genetic contribution to autoimmune diseases.

Diseases Affecting Older Adults

Our bodies go through many changes as we age. Some of these changes make us more vulnerable to disease. Certainly, aging means that our bodies have had more time to be exposed to environmental factors that could interact with genetic susceptibilities, resulting in illness. This section will review age-related changes in vision and hearing as well as genetic contributions to Alzheimer disease and cognitive decline.

Alzheimer Disease and Cognitive Decline

Some cellular changes that occur with aging can have profound effects on the way our brains function. However, age-related cognitive decline does not happen to everyone in the same way, and genetic variations probably play an important role in how aging affects our ability to solve problems and process new information. For example, we know that *telomeres*, those repetitive sequences of DNA at the tips of the chromosomes, shorten as cells age. The enzyme *telomerase* protects the telomeres from shortening in stem cells and many cancer cells. The ability to preserve telomere length is partly inherited, but estimates of just how heritable it is vary widely, from between 4% heritability to 80% heritability! Recent studies have suggested that the length of a person's telomeres can provide an estimate of not only their physical aging, but also their mental aging and the likely onset of dementia. It is unclear how useful this will be, but the authors suggest that measuring telomere length could be a relatively simple way to biologically assess the aging brain (Yaffe, 2008).

Alzheimer disease (AD), which affects about 24 million people worldwide, is the most common age-related cause of dementia. It is an irreversible disease that progresses from mild memory loss to complete incapacitation. Neurons lose their ability to connect, and eventually there is brain cell death. Approximately 50% of cases of dementia are caused by Alzheimer disease, and the number of affected people is expected to grow as our population ages. AD appears to run in families, and people have suspected for some time that there must be a genetic contribution to disease susceptibility.

There are two types of AD—early and late onset. A small number of AD cases (between 1% and 6%) occur in people between the ages of 30 and 60 years. This is considered early-onset AD. The vast majority of cases are considered late-onset AD. This occurs in people older than 60 years. Between 25% and 45% of people older than 85 years have some kind of dementia. It is difficult to distinguish AD from other forms of dementia without completing a postmortem examination of the brain that looks for the characteristic signs of dense amyloid plaques and neurofibrillary tangles (Bekris, 2010).

Early-Onset Alzheimer Disease

Genetic contributions are fairly clear with early-onset AD. About 60% of families with one case of early-onset AD report that there are other cases among their close family members. There is even an autosomal dominant form of early-onset AD that affects about 13% of these families. The genes that have been identified with autosomal dominant forms of AD are located on chromosomes 21 (amyloid precursor protein, or APP), 14 (presenilin 1), and 1 (presenilin 2). Because the APP gene is located on chromosome 21, people with Down syndrome (trisomy 21) who carry an APP gene variant get an extra dose of the dysfunctional protein (Bekris, 2010). Mutations in any of these genes result in increased beta-amyloid protein, which forms a large part of the plaques that are associated with AD.

Genetic testing is available for family members of people with disease-causing mutations in one of these genes. Deciding whether to have predictive genetic testing for a devastating disease with limited treatment is very difficult. Family members are encouraged to seek counseling from genetics professionals prior to agreeing to any genetic testing, particularly when no effective treatment is available.

Late-Onset Alzheimer Disease

Most cases of AD occur after age 60 and are not caused by problems in single genes alone. They are complex (multifactorial) and involve a combination of many gene variations that contribute a small increase in susceptibility along with environmental factors. We do know that even in families in which one person is affected with late-onset AD, his or her first-degree relatives (parents, children, siblings) are twice as likely to get AD than someone from the general population.

The only gene that has been associated with the complex form of AD is apolipoprotein E *(APOE)*, which is found on chromosome 19. APOE has four different alleles, or forms of the gene, but only three occur commonly (E2, E3, and E4). We each get one allele from our mothers and one from our fathers, so there are lots of possible combinations of these three alleles. The E2 allele is less common and seems to offer some protection from AD. The E3 allele is most common and does not appear to alter the risk for AD one way or the other. The E4 allele is found in about 40% of people who develop late-onset AD. However, the E4 allele is also carried by people who live well into old age without any signs of dementia, so there must be other major factors that put a person at risk for significant cognitive decline. Having two copies of the E4 allele does seem to be associated with a higher risk of getting AD than having only one copy, and people with two copies tend to get late-onset AD earlier than those who carry one copy. In addition, people who carry the E4 allele tend to have poorer outcomes following head injury or stroke. Even so, we do not completely understand how the *APOE* gene variants affect brain tissue. However, people with the E4 variant do seem to have more plaque and tangles. Women with two copies of E4 have a 45% risk of getting AD by age 73, and men with two copies have a 25% risk, so there is some unknown factor that accounts for this difference between the sexes.

To make things even more complicated, approximately 42% of people who get AD do not have even one copy of the E4 risk allele. Individual studies have suggested that five to seven additional genes are associated with AD, but these studies have not been replicated, so it is difficult to determine whether the genes they found are really involved in causing dementia. It is clear that there are other genetic risk factors out there that have not been identified, and much work is ongoing (Bekris, 2010).

Age-Related Macular Degeneration

Age-related macular degeneration (AMD) is the most common cause of central vision loss among older people in affluent countries. Approximately 1.8 million Americans over the age of 50 have vision loss due to AMD, and that number is expected to increase to 2.9 million by 2020. Losing central vision can be devastating, because it means that what you are looking at directly will be the hardest to see. AMD is caused by deterioration in the retina that occurs with the accumulation of extracellular deposits of a protein called *drusen*. The macula, which is located in the center of the retina, controls our ability to clearly see what is central in our visual fields. That means that daily functions such as reading, recognizing familiar faces, and driving can be challenging if not impossible because images in the area we are trying to focus on will appear blurred.

There are two types of AMD. **Atrophic** or **non-neovascular AMD**, also called *dry AMD*, is caused by the breakdown of light-sensitive cells in the macula. While dry AMD accounts for about 85% of cases, it usually progresses slowly. **Exudative** or **neovascular AMD** is called *wet AMD*, and it occurs when abnormal blood vessels grow underneath the macula and leak protein and blood. While wet AMD accounts for only 10% of overall cases, those affected tend to have a rapid progression of the disease. About two-thirds of people with advanced AMD have the wet type. As with many of the adult-onset diseases we have discussed, AMD is complex. It is caused by a combination of variations in susceptibility genes and environmental factors.

Genome-wide association studies suggest that genes in the complement pathway, which is important in inflammation and immunity, are probably involved. Genes that have a role in cholesterol management may be involved as well. However, we do not clearly understand how gene variants in these systems increase risk. Inflammation seems to be particularly important in the development of wet AMD, so the involvement of complement and/or cholesterol makes some sense, because they each have been connected with inflammation. Drusen deposits are "highly enriched" with cholesterol, although having high blood cholesterol levels does not predict AMD, so the cholesterol pathways in the eye and the cholesterol pathways in the blood must be different (Hampton, 2010).

The most powerful environmental risk factor for AMD is smoking, but all of those other risk factors that we commonly associate with coronary artery disease also seem to increase the risk of AMD. To decrease the risk of getting AMD, people should maintain a healthy weight, exercise regularly, and not smoke! Does that all sound familiar? Diet also seems to play a part in protecting people from AMD. Risk goes down when the diet includes high levels of vitamins C, D, and E; omega-3 fatty acids; beta carotene; zinc; lutein; and zeaxanthin (Hampton, 2010). Identifying the people who are at genetic risk and helping them to make lifestyle modifications can be important in reducing the prevalence of AMD.

Age-Related Hearing Loss

Hearing is a very complicated process, and there are lots of genetic causes of both syndromic and non-syndromic hearing loss. There are more than 400 different syndromes that include hearing loss as a feature. These include Alport syndrome, Jervell and Lange-Nielson syndrome, neurofibromatosis, Stickler syndrome, and Treacher Collins syndrome (all of these are typically diagnosed in childhood). There are also causes of hearing loss that are not directly genetic, including exposure to teratogens, infections, and trauma.

Age-related hearing loss, which is also called **presbycusis**, is a complex disorder with both genetic and environmental contributions. Hearing impairment due to aging affects about 50% of people who are over age 60, and men are more commonly affected than women (Van Eyken, 2007). Everyone experiences some hearing loss with aging. However, for some people, the age of onset is younger and the hearing impairment is more severe. The genetic contributions to presbycusis have been supported by studies of hearing loss in monozygotic and dizygotic twins. The environmental contributions to age-related hearing impairment include ototoxic drugs (such as aminoglycosides and loop diuretics), alcohol, tobacco intake, and exposure to chemicals. Medical conditions, such as diabetes mellitus, renal disease, or cardiovascular disease, can also contribute.

Exposure to loud noises can cause both metabolic and mechanical damage to the cochlea. Most of the studies of the impact of noise exposure on hearing have focused on occupational or military exposures. Now people are investigating exposures to loud noises coming from digital media players and the use of earbuds, as well as from loud music from concerts. Of course, all people who are exposed to the same noise levels over time will not experience the same impact on their hearing. Studies are now being done to identify those people who are most susceptible to noise-induced hearing loss using candidate gene studies and GWAS. The genes involved in handling oxidative stress have been studied, as have the genes involved in potassium recycling. While we do not have clear indications about how to determine who is at risk for noise-induced hearing impairment, one thing is certain—reducing environmental exposure to loud noises will reduce the risk for virtually anyone (Konings, 2009).

Hearing is a very complicated process with lots of opportunities for things to go wrong. Age-related changes can alter gene function in many of the molecular pathways associated with processing sound. For example, the hairlike fibers in the ear, which convert sound waves into the nerve signals, are partly maintained by the proteins β- and γ-actin. Studies in mice have indicated that variations in the genes that encode these proteins may be involved in age-related hearing loss. Researchers are very close to finding gene variants that make some people more likely to have progressive age-related hearing loss. However, there is much work yet to do.

Summary

Common adult-onset diseases are usually complex, involving contributions from both genes and the environment. It makes sense that environmental exposures increase over time, making the environmental contributions a much bigger factor in disease onset as we age. The good news is that, for many of these diseases, particularly those associated with aging, making lifestyle changes can have an impact on age at disease onset and overall disease severity. Maintaining a healthy weight, exercising, and eating well seem to have a significant impact on risk for many of the complex adult-onset disorders, including DM and age-related vision and hearing impairment. For others, such as the autoimmune disorders, making lifestyle changes has a less clear impact. For the rare, single-gene disorders, early diagnosis can lead to protective therapies, such as phlebotomy for people with hemochromatosis. As genetic/genomic knowledge progresses, options for both protective and therapeutic interventions will also increase.

GENE GEMS

- As people get older, they are more likely to have been exposed to environmental factors that can trigger the onset of disease in someone who has a genetic susceptibility.
- Hereditary hemochromatosis is an autosomal recessive trait with incomplete penetrance.
- Maturity-onset diabetes of the young (MODY) is a single-gene disorder that causes hyperglycemia in people younger than age 25.
- People who are homozygous for the allele associated with the most severe deficiency (the Z allele) have very little alpha-1 antitrypsin in their serum.
- DM type 2 is a complex disorder with a very large genetic contribution.
- Several candidate genes for DM type 2 are currently being studied.
- GWAS have identified interesting loci that may be useful in determining the risk for obesity; however, the results may not be clinically useful in the short term.
- Human leukocyte antigens (HLA), located on chromosome 6, function as unique identifiers on the surface of almost all cells in the body.
- Some early-onset Alzheimer disease is transmitted in an autosomal dominant manner.
- Some late-onset Alzheimer disease has been associated with the E4 allele of apolipoprotein E.
- Age-related macular degeneration has been associated with the genes involved in complement and cholesterol management.
- Smoking increases the risk of both age-related macular degeneration and age-related hearing loss.
- Both genetic and environmental factors contribute to age-related hearing loss.

Self-Assessment Questions

1. Your patient's family comes from Ireland. Both her parents are carriers of gene mutations causing hereditary hemochromatosis (*HFE*-HHC). What is your patient's risk of having the clinical signs of this disorder?
   a. HHC is an autosomal recessive condition; the risk is 25%.
   b. HHC has incomplete penetrance; we cannot accurately predict the clinical risk.
   c. HHC is a complex trait; we cannot accurately predict the clinical risk.
   d. HHC is an autosomal dominant trait; the risk is 50%.

2. A fasting urine sample indicates that your 24-year-old male patient has new onset hyperglycemia. What is the most likely cause of this?
   a. Type 1 diabetes mellitus
   b. Type 2 diabetes mellitus
   c. Maturity-onset diabetes of the young (MODY)
   d. Gestational diabetes mellitus.

3. Which autoimmune disorder has the greatest environmental contribution?
   a. Stickler syndrome
   b. Rheumatoid arthritis
   c. Multiple sclerosis
   d. Systemic lupus erythematosus

4. What is the risk of a person becoming affected with Alzheimer disease if his father developed AD during his 40s?
   a. Early-onset AD is usually transmitted in an autosomal dominant manner, so the risk is 50%.
   b. Before his risk can be determined, he should be screened for the E4 allele in APOE.
   c. To accurately determine his risk, we must find out if his mother is a carrier.
   d. Because early-onset AD is a complex problem, we cannot determine his risk.

5. Which statement is true regarding age-related macular degeneration (AMD)?
   a. It is the most common cause of peripheral vision impairment among the elderly.
   b. It is transmitted in an autosomal recessive manner.
   c. Smoking increases the risk in those who are genetically susceptible.
   d. Predictive genetic testing can identify the genes that cause AMD.

6. Multiple sclerosis is more common in people from what geographic area?
   a. Western Africa
   b. Southeast Asia
   c. Mediterranean region
   d. Northern Europe

7. Which of these are potential causes of age-related hearing loss?
   a. Consistent exposure to loud noises
   b. Genetic variants
   c. Alcohol and tobacco intake
   d. Any and all of these

CASE STUDY

Bonnie Tribble is 84 years old and has been a cigarette smoker for most of her life. She lives independently and drives herself around town on short errands to the grocery store and to church. Her 82-year-old brother, Dustin, has just been diagnosed with age-related macular degeneration (AMD). His doctor has told the family that he should no longer be allowed to drive. Bonnie is very quiet when her niece tells her that Dustin will no longer be driving. Being able to get around town independently is extremely important to Bonnie's sense of self. Bonnie comes in for a routine physical and blood work and reluctantly reports that she has not had her scheduled regular eye examination.

1. Because her brother is affected, what is Bonnie's risk of having age-related macular degeneration?

2. What is the risk to Bonnie's children if she is affected? Could they do anything to reduce their risk?

3. What clinical signs might she be experiencing?

4. What environmental factor(s) might play a role in Bonnie's risk of AMD?

5. If Bonnie is diagnosed with AMD, what factors would you expect to be particularly important in planning her ongoing care?

References

ADA. (2010). Diagnosis and classification of diabetes mellitus. *Diabetes Care, 33 Suppl 1*, S62–69.

AHRQ. (November 8, 2010). Diagnosis and management of type 2 diabetes mellitus in adults. Retrieved November 10, 2010, from www.guideline.gov/content.aspx?id=14856

Bekris, L. M., Yu, C. E., Bird, T. D., et al. (2010). Review article: Genetics of Alzheimer disease. *Journal of Geriatric Psychiatry and Neurology 23*(4), 213–227.

Fawcett, K. A., and Barroso, I. (2010). The genetics of obesity: FTO leads the way. *Trends Genet, 26*(6), 266–274.

Hampton, T. (2010). Genetic research provides insights into age-related macular degeneration. *Journal of the American Medical Association 304*(14), 1541–1543.

Hewagama, A., and Richardson, B. (2009). The genetics and epigenetics of autoimmune diseases. *Journal of Autoimmunity 33*(1), 3–11.

Hoppenbrouwers, I. A., and Hintzen, R. Q. (2010). Genetics of multiple sclerosis. *Biochimica et Biophysica Acta*.

Klupa, T., Warram, J. H., Antonellis, A., et al. (2002). Determinants of the development of diabetes (maturity-onset diabetes of the young-3) in carriers of HNF-1alpha mutations: Evidence for parent-of-origin effect. *Diabetes Care, 25*(12), 2292–2301.

Konings, A., Van Laer, L., and Van Camp, G. (2009). Genetic studies on noise-induced hearing loss: A review. *Ear Hear, 30*(2), 151–159.

Kowdley, K. V., Tait, J. F., Bennett, R. L., et al. (2006). *HFE*-associated hereditary hemochromatosis. Retrieved October 15, 2010, from www.ncbi.nlm.nih.gov/bookshelf/br.fcgi?book=gene&part=hemochromatosis

Lambrinoudaki, I., Vlachou, S. A., and Creatsas, G. (2010). Genetics in gestational diabetes mellitus: Association with incidence, severity, pregnancy outcome and response to treatment. *Curr Diabetes Rev, 6* (6), 393-399

Loos, R. J. (2009). Recent progress in the genetics of common obesity. *Br J Clin Pharmacol, 68*(6), 811–829.

Malecki, M. T. (2005). Genetics of type 2 diabetes mellitus. *Diabetes Research and Clinical Practice 68 Suppl*, S10–21.

Neel, J. (1962). Diabetes mellitus: A thrifty genotype rendered detrimental by "progress"? *American Journal of Human Genetics, 14*, 353–362.

Nelson, R. M., Botkjin, J. R., Kodish, E. D., et al. (2001). Ethical issues with genetic testing in pediatrics. _Pediatrics, 107_(6), 1451–1455.

NIDDK. (November 2008). Am I at risk for type 2 diabetes? Retrieved November 11, 2010, from http://diabetes.niddk.nih.gov/dm/pubs/riskfortype2/

Schlade-Bartusiak, K., and Cox, D. W. (2008). Alpha1-antitrypsin deficiency. Retrieved October 16, 2010, from www.ncbi.nlm.nih.gov/bookshelf/br.fcgi?book=gene&part=alpha1-a

Van Eyken, E., Van Camp, G., and Van Laer, L. (2007). The complexity of age-related hearing impairment: Contributing environmental and genetic factors. _Audiology & Neuro-otology 12_(6), 345–358.

Vimaleswaran, K. S., and Loos, R. J. (2010). Progress in the genetics of common obesity and type 2 diabetes. _Expert Reviews in Molecular Medicine 12_, e7.

WHO. (November, 2009). Diabetes. Retrieved October 8, 2010, from www.who.int/mediacentre/factsheets/fs312/en/print.html

Yaffe, K., Lindquist, K., Kluse, M., et al. (2008). Telomere length and cognitive function in community-dwelling elders: Findings from the Health ABC Study. _Neurobiology of Aging 4_(4), T708.

Self-Assessment Answers

1. b **2.** c **3.** c **4.** d **5.** c **6.** d **7.** d

Genomic Influences on Selected Complex Health Problems

Chapter 11

Cardiovascular Disorders

Learning Outcomes

1. Use the genetic terminology associated with cardiovascular disorders.
2. Describe the genetic/genomic contributions to common cardiovascular disorders.
3. Explain how genetics and the environment interact in the development and severity of coronary artery disease.
4. Compare the monogenic and multifactorial causes of stroke.
5. Explain how factor V Leiden contributes to an increased risk of blood clots.
6. Explain why finding the genetic causes of hypertension is so difficult.
7. Describe the genetic contributions to selected heart rhythm problems.
8. Discuss the genetic contributions to the different types of cardiomyopathy.

KEY TERMS

Acquired disease

Arrhythmogenic right ventricular dysplasia/cardiomyopathy (ARVD/C)

Cardiomyopathy

Channelopathy

De novo mutation

Epistasis

Factor V Leiden

Familial dilated cardiomyopathy (DCM)

Familial hypercholesterolemia (FH)

Familial hypertrophic cardiomyopathy (HCM)

Genetic heterogeneity

Jervell and Lange-Nielsen syndrome

Knockout mice

Long QT syndrome (LQTS)

Private mutations

Romano-Ward syndrome

Thrombophilia

Introduction

Clinicians have known for some time that cardiovascular (CV) disease "runs in families." Primary health-care providers ask patients about their family histories and nod knowingly when patients report that their parents or siblings also have heart problems. But clinicians also know that environment has an important role in increasing or decreasing risk for many CV problems. For example, high-fat diets can increase CV risk, and regular exercise can lower it. So how can we figure out how important a role genetics plays in determining someone's risk for CV disease? Well, that really depends on the disease in question.

In the United States alone, more than 81,100,000 adults have CV disease; some have more than one type, which means that more than one in three Americans are affected (AHA, 2010). Coronary artery disease (CAD) and hypertension (HTN) are common complex (multifactorial) disorders. That means that many different gene mutations work together; some probably increase risk while others protect against disease. In addition, environment and lifestyle factors modify the severity of disease and whether a person will get sick at all. Additionally, there are rarer CV disorders, such as long QT syndrome and dilated cardiomyopathy, that are caused by mutations in single genes and generally follow mendelian inheritance patterns (with some variations, such as incomplete penetrance and/or variable expressivity). In this chapter, we will discuss coronary artery disease, hypertension, arrhythmias, cardiomyopathies, and stroke. This introduction provides only a brief overview of the genetics involved in these serious cardiovascular conditions but should help you understand the importance of knowing the family history.

Atherosclerosis and CAD

CAD is the most common cause of both mortality and morbidity worldwide. Large-scale studies indicate that a person's lifetime risk of experiencing a cardiovascular event is greater than 60%. "Cardiovascular events" include myocardial infarction and serious arrhythmias that can lead to sudden cardiac death. While we have known for some time that both genetics and environment play major roles in the onset of CAD, we are just beginning to tease out the specific genes involved in increasing a person's susceptibility to this life-threatening problem.

Genes Associated With Multifactorial Atherosclerosis

The major cause of CAD is *atherosclerosis,* the fatty buildup of plaque in and on the arterial walls. When plaque ruptures, a blood clot forms more easily and limits blood flow. We can see problems due to ischemia in major organs like the heart, brain, peripheral arteries, and kidneys. About 50% of the risk for atherosclerosis has been attributed to genetics. That takes into consideration gene variations associated with diseases that increase risk for atherosclerosis, such as hypertension and diabetes mellitus.

The process of atherosclerosis involves a series of events occurring at the level of the endothelium, the innermost lining of arteries. These events include endothelial dysfunction, a buildup of lipids, the production of reactive oxygen species, the oxidation of LDL, and inflammation. Imagine all the proteins involved in those processes and you can see what a complicated job finding all the genetic contributions can be. For example, if we just look at the genes that have been found to be associated with inflammation in atherosclerosis, we have the genes that code for the interleukins (IL-1, IL-Ra, IL-6, IL-10), cytokines and cytokine receptors (TNF-χ, TNF-receptor, LTA), adhesion molecules (ICAM-I, VCAM-I, PECAM), chemokines and chemokine receptors (CS3CR1, CCR5, CCR2, CXCL12, RANTES, MCP-1), eicosanoids (ALOX5, ALOX5AP, LTA4H, LTC4S, PTGS1, PTGS2, L-PGDS), and many others (connexin 37, TLR-4, CRP, RNFS4)! Add to those the genes that code for proteins involved in lipid and cholesterol metabolism, endothelial dysfunction, oxidative stress, vascular remodeling, arterial thrombosis, and cell cycle regulation (Roy et al., 2009). There are so many places to look for genetic contributions.

Apolipoprotein E (ApoE) is a component of very-low-density lipoproteins (VDRL). When people carry the ApoE4 allele, they tend to have higher levels of LDL than people who carry other alleles. In one study, men with either the ApoE4 or the ApoE2 alleles had higher risk of CAD; however, another study showed that people who are heterozygous for ApoE2 and ApoE3 actually have lower LDL levels. There has not been clear evidence of exactly how much having these alleles increases or decreases overall risk, because atherosclerosis is usually a complex multifactorial problem (Roy et al., 2009).

Studies of large numbers of affected and unaffected people have shown that, in most cases, atherosclerosis is caused by many different genes working together, with each single gene having only a small effect. Studying areas of interest in the genome requires the use of thousands of DNA markers (usually SNPs) and multiple studies of different large populations. Currently, the effect of the interactions of some SNPs appears to vary by ethnicity. For example, the genes involved appear to be different for Caucasian populations than they are for the Han Chinese. When genome-wide association studies (GWAS) are done, they must be redone in many different ethnic groups before we can say that these genes or loci are truly important for people whose ancestors came from a particular geographic area.

A number of GWASs have identified an association between a region of chromosome 9 (9p21) and the onset of CAD. Of particular interest is the fact that this area of the genome does not code for protein. The locus 9p21 is in a noncoding region on the short arm (p arm) of chromosome 9 (Consortium, 2007). This region used to be considered part of "junk DNA." Recall from Chapters 1 and 2 that 98% of the genome does not code for proteins, so there is much more DNA in noncoding regions than in regions that do code for protein. Scientists have often wondered why we have so much noncoding DNA, but now we are starting to find out.

Scientists used genetic engineering to breed **knockout mice** without the 9p21 region of chromosome 9. Knockout mice are those that are bred, using genetic engineering, with one or several genes "turned off" or "knocked out." The results of these studies indicated that not having this region affected the expression of two genes that were located more than 100,000 base pairs away! These genes were important in controlling cell growth in the heart (and other places) by controlling the cell cycle. Mice without this region often died prematurely, and some developed tumors (Helgadottir et al., 2007). More recent studies suggest that mutations in the 9p21 region predict the onset of CAD in about 25 different populations (Horne et al., 2008). Studies have differed in reporting whether variations in this region increase the risk of early myocardial infarction (MI). When CAD is diagnosed in a person younger than age 50, the genetic contribution is probably much greater than environmental factors, compared with people who develop CAD at a later age.

Environmental Contributions to Atherosclerosis

The influence of environmental risk factors makes it very difficult to determine which genes are involved in the development of atherosclerosis (Roberts et al., 2009). In a laboratory setting, we can carefully control the environment of the mice in our experiment. When we are studying people, who are out in the community living their lives, it is very difficult to accurately monitor lifestyle choices. Is there really any way to be certain that a participant stuck to his low-fat diet and exercised every day? That means that comparing the impact of a low-carbohydrate diet with the impact of a low-fat diet in people with certain genetic variants can be really challenging.

In addition, some risk factors that are considered modifiable lifestyle choices have strong genetic components. For example, let's look at tobacco use and nicotine dependence. Smokers have a risk of atherosclerosis that is directly related to the number of cigarettes they smoke a day. Men who smoke 20 or more cigarettes per day have three times the risk of having an MI than nonsmokers. For women the risk is six times higher. Smoking directly damages the arterial wall by increasing the amount of carbon monoxide in the blood; it also decreases HDL cholesterol (good cholesterol) and increases LDL cholesterol (bad cholesterol). Using tobacco products makes the arteries more likely to constrict and increases the likelihood of blood clot formation.

Studies of the genetic contributions to nicotine dependence are in progress. For some people, a mutation in the gene that codes for the nicotine receptor greatly increases the risk of nicotine dependence.

However, just like atherosclerosis itself, it now appears that nicotine dependence is a problem that involves the effects of many genes working together *(polygenic)*. Genetic studies are continuing and will need to include thousands of people, but the early work supports that idea that being drawn to smoking and having great difficulty quitting has a biological basis (Bierut, 2009).

Single-Gene Causes of Atherosclerosis

A number of monogenic disorders of lipid metabolism have been identified as causes of atherosclerosis. While the most common is familial hypercholesterolemia, which is discussed shortly, there are other single-gene disorders as well. Some examples include Tangier disease, which is an autosomal codominant disorder that results in very low levels of HDL or no HDL at all. Familial hyperlipidemia is transmitted in an autosomal recessive manner and results in both high LDL and high triglyceride levels. Familial apolipoprotein A-1 deficiency is an autosomal recessive disease with very low levels of HDL, even though patients have normal levels of VDRL and LDL levels (Roy et al., 2009). While most of these disorders are rare, familial hypercholesterolemia is relatively common.

Familial Hypercholesterolemia

Familial hypercholesterolemia (FH) is a single-gene disease that is primarily transmitted in an autosomal dominant manner. About 1 in 500 persons is heterozygous for a mutation in genes associated with familial hypercholesterolemia. Individuals who are heterozygous tend to have plasma cholesterol levels between 300 mg/dL and 400 mg/dL and have a rate of CAD much higher than the general population. About 50% of men who are heterozygous die from a myocardial infarction (MI) before the age of 60. Only about 15% of women will have a fatal MI before the age of 60 because heart disease is less common in premenopausal women (Marks et al., 2003).

For people who are homozygous (about 1 in 1 million), the effects of FH are much more severe. Cholesterol levels can be between 600 mg/dL and 1200 mg/dL. If they are not treated, most homozygotes will die before they reach age 30, and there is even a report of a child having an MI at 18 months of age (Marks et al., 2003). Affected people sometimes have other signs of high blood lipid levels, like yellowish cholesterol deposits in the eyelids *(xanthelasmas)* or the skin *(xanthomas)*. Xanthomas are particularly common on the Achilles tendons, elbows, and knees.

Cholesterol can be taken in from the environment (eaten) and is synthesized in the liver, and it is a necessary component of the plasma membrane. Wherever it comes from, cholesterol is not water soluble, and it must be carried in the blood by a complex that is water soluble. Low-density lipoprotein (LDL), or "bad cholesterol," is one of the carriers of cholesterol in the blood. The LDL receptor is a cell surface protein that binds LDL and takes it into the cell by the process of endocytosis. FH is caused by having too few working LDL receptors. When there are not enough working LDL receptors, cholesterol accumulates in the blood and can contribute to *atherosclerotic plaques* that form on the blood vessel walls.

The LDL receptor protein is coded for by the gene *LDLR*. More than 1000 different mutations have been identified, and they have been grouped into four different classes (Hobbs et al., 1990):

- Class I: A defective protein is produced
- Class II: The protein cannot move from the endoplasmic reticulum to the Golgi apparatus.
- Class III: The receptor is unable to bind with LDL properly.
- Class IV: The protein can get where it is supposed to go on the cell's surface, and it can bind with LDL, but it is not able to complete the process of endocytosis.

Another autosomal dominant form of hypercholesterolemia is familial defective apolipoprotein B-100 (ApoB). This disorder looks clinically similar to FH. ApoB is a glycoprotein that serves as a ligand (a molecule that binds to another chemical and forms a larger complex) for the LDL receptor. When LDL binds properly to its receptor, two mechanisms control its blood levels: reduced liver LDL production and enhanced enzymatic breakdown and removal of LDL. The result of defective ApoB is reduced blood clearance of LDL, causing plasma levels that are two to three times normal.

Dietary management has been the recommended initial treatment of people with FH, but dietary modification alone can reduce LDL levels by only about 10%, so medications are often begun early. Bile-acid-absorbing resins (e.g., cholestyramine) can be used to decrease cholesterol reabsorption into the gut and recycling through the liver. When there is a reduction in circulating cholesterol, the liver makes more LDL receptors and cholesterol levels are lowered, but only by about 15% to 20%, so combination therapies are more common.

High doses of HMG-CoA reductase inhibitors (the "statin" drugs such as atorvastatin, rosuvastatin, and simvastain) are usually part of the initial treatment of FH. Children who are homozygous are treated aggressively and may also require a cholesterol absorption inhibitor (e.g., ezetimibe) and LDL apheresis for better control. LDL apheresis physically removes LDL from the blood in a process that is similar to dialysis.

Stroke

Whatever the cause, the heart is not the only organ affected when lipids build up in the arteries and when there is inflammation and artery constriction. The brain (and really any other organ that is highly dependent on good circulation of oxygenated blood) can also experience ischemia and even infarction because of the reduced delivery of oxygen to the tissues.

Stroke is defined as a sudden-onset problem in the brain that is most likely due to a problem in the blood vessels. It is a major cause of both morbidity and mortality and often leaves patients with significant permanent disability. Stroke comes on suddenly and lasts for at least 24 hours (Ikram et al., 2009).

It is clear that genetic risk factors are important in the development of all vascular diseases, including stroke. A person with a family history of stroke has two to three times the risk of having a stroke than a person without a family history. It is less clear exactly what genetic changes make a person likely to have a stroke. Strokes certainly "run in families," and several SNPs have been associated with the risk of stroke. There are also some rare single-gene disorders that can increase the risk of stroke, but, overall, the genes involved in the development of stroke in the general population have not yet been found.

Strokes are heterogeneous, meaning that there are lots of variations, even within the general classifications (ischemic or hemorrhagic) of the disease. For example, hemorrhagic strokes can be classified according to whether they are caused by vascular malformations, saccular aneurysms, or as signs of small-vessel disease in the brain. They can also be classified according to where in the brain the problem lies. For example, is it in the thalamus, basal ganglia, brain stem, cerebral cortex, or cerebellum? Ischemic strokes can be classified as atherothrombotic (due to an atheroma in a major artery) or cardioembolic (due to debris, such as platelet aggregates or cholesterol from a cardiac source). There is also a catch-all category of "unknown" for strokes that do not conform to clinical or imaging standards for either ischemic or hemorrhagic stroke.

When the phenotype is not clearly defined, teasing out genetic causes can be really difficult. Stroke is usually a multifactorial (complex) problem involving many genes working together with the environment. Each gene may have only a small effect, but when their effects are combined, the risk for stroke is great. Whether a person has a stroke also is influenced by whether she or he has other complex disorders such as hypertension, hyperlipidemia, or diabetes mellitus. Add environmental risk factors (like smoking or chronic alcoholism) and it becomes even more difficult to sort out what genes are involved! Even so, investigators are applying new genetic research techniques to help us identify those people who are at an increased genetic risk of having a stroke. This is really important work because many strokes occur in people who have not reported any warning signs, so finding out who has a genetic predisposition can help identify those who need close monitoring.

There have been few genetic studies that separate ischemic stroke from hemorrhagic stroke, which is also called *intracerebral hemorrhage (ICH)*. Approximately 75% of strokes are ischemic, meaning they are caused by a decrease in blood flow to the brain usually due to a blood clot. Only 25% of strokes are hemorrhagic, meaning they are caused by a blood vessel in the brain breaking. For ICH, a family history increases a person's risk of having a stroke about two to six times that of a person without a family history. With subarachnoid hemorrhage, there appears to be an even greater gene-environment interaction with smoking compared to other causes of stroke.

Monogenic Causes of Stroke

Fewer than 1% of strokes are caused by single-gene variants. Monogenic strokes occur more often in children or young adults. Diseases such as Fabry disease, sickle cell disease, or some mitochondrial disorders can result in stroke. There is an adult-onset disease called CADASIL, an acronym for *cerebral autosomal dominant arteriopathy with subcortical infarcts and leukoencephalopathy*. People with this disorder begin experiencing strokes between the ages of 30 and 40 years. They may also develop migraine headaches and, eventually, dementia. Ehlers-Danlos type IV, Marfan syndrome, and fibromuscular dysplasia are single-gene, connective tissue disorders that increase the likelihood of artery dissections, aneurysms, and stroke. Neurofibromatosis type I increases the risk of aneurysms, carotid-cavernous fistulas, and vessel occlusions (Alberts, 2009).

Fabry disease is a lysosomal storage disease that is transmitted in an X-linked recessive manner. It is caused by the inability to make the enzyme alpha-galactosidase A, which is needed so that people can metabolize lipids. While enzyme replacement therapy is available, Fabry disease is probably underdiagnosed, meaning that many people who would benefit from treatment are not receiving it. One study found that 5% of young adults who experienced a stroke had mutations in the gene that codes for alpha-galactosidase A, even though they had not been diagnosed with Fabry disease (Alberts, 2009). You can read more about genetic disorders that affect metabolism, such as Fabry disease, in Chapter 8.

The mitochondrial disorder MELAS (mitochondrial encephalomyopathy, lactic acidosis, and stroke-like episodes) is another single-gene cause of stroke. Because it is a problem in mitochondrial DNA, it is maternally inherited (see Chapter 5). MELAS includes a collection of symptoms that may not appear to fit together at first. These include diabetes, lactic acidosis, myoclonus, hearing loss, headaches, dementia, and myopathy.

Mutations in several other genes can cause ICH. Familial cerebral amyloid angiopathy causes amyloid deposits and destruction of the capillary vessel walls. Recently, the gene that codes for type IV collagen has been identified as a cause of hemorrhagic stroke. It is transmitted as an autosomal dominant trait and can greatly increase a person's vulnerability to having a cerebral hemorrhage after even minor head trauma.

Factor V Leiden

Factor V Leiden is an example of a genetic **thrombophilia,** which means that it is a disease that increases the risk of blood clots. Most people who have factor V Leiden will not develop blood clots, but their risk of having blood clots is higher than that of the general population. Between 3% and 8% of people with European ancestry are heterozygous (they inherited a mutation from one parent) for factor V Leiden. About 1 in 5000 people are homozygous (they have inherited a mutant copy from each parent).

Factor V Leiden, which was identified in the city of Leiden in the Netherlands, creates problems by altering factor V of the clotting cascade. Proteins of the coagulation cascade are supposed to be degraded by activated protein C (APC) so that they do not become too large or stay around too long. The factor V Leiden variation *(F5)* results in a protein that cannot be degraded, so the person experiences a state of "hypercoagulation." One of the tests used to determine if a person has factor V Leiden is the activated protein C resistance test, but genetic testing is also available clinically.

Carrying one bad copy of the gene that codes for the factor V Leiden protein increases a person's risk of having a blood clot in a cerebral vein by eight times that of a person without this gene variant. The situation is even worse for women taking birth control pills (or any hormone-based contraceptive), which increase the risk of stroke, even in women without factor V Leiden (Baird, 2010). Remember that not everyone with factor V Leiden is going to have a stroke, and many will not even have excessive blood clot formation. Other examples of thrombophilias are caused by mutations in genes that code for prothrombin, antithrombin III, protein C, and protein S. Thrombophilias increase the risk of ischemic stroke, deep-vein thrombosis, and myocardial infarction.

Genes Associated With Multifactorial Causes of Stroke

Because the pathophysiology of ischemic stroke is similar to that of coronary artery disease, it is no surprise that many of the genes associated with atherosclerosis are considered candidates for genes involved in the development of stroke. Association studies have found several regions of the genome that appear to be related to stroke, but most have shown only small effects. If we consider only ischemic stroke, we can include all that was said previously about the genetic risk for atherosclerosis, but hemorrhagic stroke is a very different animal.

One finding that has been supported by several studies indicates that a person who has the E4 allele of the apolipoprotein E (ApoE) gene is likely to have a poorer prognosis after hemorrhagic stroke (this allele does not seem to affect the outcome after ischemic stroke) (Alberts, 2009). Novel experimental procedures will probably uncover many more genetic variants that can lead to the development of vascular diseases such as stroke.

One major cause of secondary stroke is hypertension. People with hypertension are four to six times more likely to have a stroke than people without hypertension. Hypertension contributes to atherosclerosis and directly weakens blood vessel walls, increasing the likelihood of both ischemic and hemorrhagic stroke.

Hypertension

Hypertension (HTN) is a major cause of morbidity and mortality worldwide. In the United States, one in three people have hypertension. Worldwide, there are more than 1 billion affected people (Arnett, 2009). The American Heart Association provides several criteria for determining if a person has hypertension (AHA, 2009). A person must meet one or more of the following:

1. Have a systolic pressure greater than or equal to 140 mm Hg, without taking any medication.
2. Have a diastolic pressure greater than or equal to 90 mm Hg, without taking any medication.
3. Take medication used to treat hypertension.
4. Be told on two or more occasions by a health-care professional that she or he has high blood pressure.

Hypertension can be either "primary (essential)" or "secondary." About 90% to 95% of all people with HTN have primary HTN, which means that there is no clear single cause of the disease. It most likely results from a combination of many genes working together, each contributing a small amount, in association with lifestyle and environmental influences. Does that sound like a familiar story? Blood pressure (BP) in general is controlled by many genes that interact with each other.

A gene-to-gene interaction is called **epistasis.** One gene will modify the effects of another; one gene will increase the expression of another gene, while another gene suppresses its expression.

Secondary hypertension is a consequence of another disease; for example, a person with sleep apnea may have an increased blood pressure that will go back down once the apnea is treated and the person is sleeping well (Arnett, 2009). People with hormonal imbalances such as hyperaldosteronism or hyperthyroidism can also have secondary hypertension. In addition, many drugs can cause secondary hypertension. For example, people who take corticosteroids daily retain more sodium and water, which leads to hypertension. There are fewer than 12 single-gene disorders (monogenic) that can result in hypertension. Of course, more may be found in the future.

Most of these monogenic disorders affect the way the kidneys control salt. When salt is retained, excess fluid is not excreted, which can cause hypertension. The genes involved are usually part of complex pathways, such as the renin, angiotensin, aldosterone (RAAS) pathway, although other hormonal imbalances may also be involved. For example, glucocorticoid remedial aldosteronism (GRA) is caused by a "crossing over" mistake during meiosis I. The problem is on chromosome 8, and the trait is transmitted in an autosomal dominant manner.

We have known for a long time that hypertension runs in families, but teasing out how much is genetic and how much is environmental remains a challenge. Gene-environment interactions are suspected when two people with the same genotype have different phenotypes. For example, a person who eats a high-salt diet, is elderly, or is taking medication that affects the RAAS will probably have a different BP than a young person eating a low-salt diet and not taking any medication, even if he or she has the same genotype for all the genes involved.

Common gene variations, or polymorphisms, can also affect the way genes interact with the environment. For example, a common variation in the RAAS genes can affect whether hypertension responds to treatment with a low-salt diet. In one clinical trial, people with the polymorphism AGT-6-AA had a significant decrease in BP when they followed a low-sodium diet, but people with the AGT-6-GG genotype did not benefit from salt reduction. Having this information before a patient starts treatment for HTN could save time and result in better clinical outcomes. The way people respond to antihypertensive medications can also differ because of gene-environment interactions, as discussed in Chapter 15.

Even though the genetic basis of primary hypertension is complex and appears to involve a large number of genes in several pathways, in which each contributes a small amount, it is still clear that HTN runs in families. Identifying people at risk by collecting a thorough family history on those affected can improve the health of many people. In most people, simple prevention strategies, such as following diet and exercise recommendations, can reduce the risk of hypertension.

Arrhythmias

A number of arrhythmic diseases have genetic causes or contributions. Many are due to problems with genes coding for ion channels (sodium, potassium, and calcium) in the heart. These are sometimes referred to as **channelopathies.** Different mutations can result in different phenotypes. For example, mutations in the sodium channel gene *SCN5A* can cause long QT syndrome, Brugada syndrome, atrioventricular conduction defects, or congenital sick sinus syndrome. The physiological effect of the specific mutation probably causes the different phenotypes. Although there are many arrhythmias with genetic causes, we will focus on atrial fibrillation, because it is so common, and long QT syndrome, because it is a classic inherited channelopathy.

Atrial Fibrillation

Atrial fibrillation (AF) is the most common arrhythmia seen by clinicians and currently affects approximately 2% of the U.S. population (Darbar and MacRae, 2009). AF has been shown to run in families, but how much AF is genetic in origin has yet to be determined. Studies report that 5% of people with atrial fibrillation and 15% of people with isolated (lone) atrial fibrillation have a familial form of the disease (Darbar and MacRae, 2009); however, there are probably lots of different genes that can cause atrial fibrillation, which means that this arrhythmia has **genetic heterogeneity.** There are also many reasons why a person could have atrial fibrillation. AF is often secondary to several pulmonary or cardiac problems, and these may have genetic causes as well. In addition, AF is considered an underdiagnosed problem.

When AF is not present at birth, it is considered an **acquired disease.** Acquired disease can be indirectly caused by gene variants. Structural changes in the heart may lead to acquired AF, and the structural changes could have a genetic cause. For example, when there is a defect in a gene that codes for a cardiac sodium channel (*SCN5A*), the phenotype can include dilated cardiomyopathy along with atrial fibrillation.

Several single genes responsible for AF have been found, but they account for only a small number of cases. These genes code for potassium ion channels in the heart (*KCNQ1, KCNE1, KCNH2*), and they are involved in causing other heart rhythm problems as well as AF. We will discuss some of these genes when we talk about long QT syndrome.

Most cases of AF are probably multifactorial in origin. As we discussed with hypertension, it is very likely that AF is caused by small effects of many gene variants. A certain combination of gene variants might make a person more vulnerable to getting AF when conditions are right. The fact that AF occurs most commonly in older patients and does not always cause consistent symptoms makes studying the genetics of AF very difficult, but because it is so common, there is a lot of motivation to find the genes involved. New laboratory techniques are promising, but we are just scratching the surface of knowledge related to the genetics of AF.

Long QT Syndrome

Long QT syndrome (LQTS) is a group of disorders that involve a delay in repolarization during the cardiac cycle. This is seen on the electrocardiogram as a lengthening of the QT interval. Figure 11–1 shows a long QT interval. Approximately 1 in 2000 and 3000 people are affected by LQTS. The measured length of the QT interval must be corrected for heart rate, making the most accurate measurement the "QT corrected" or QTc. Most clinicians define "long" as a QTc greater than 440 msec in men and 460 msec in women. This repolarization delay makes the heart vulnerable to developing a potentially lethal polymorphic ventricular tachycardia called *torsade de pointes* (twisting around a point; Fig. 11–1). Triggers for developing this serious arrhythmia include electrolyte imbalances, activities like swimming, loud sudden sounds, or bradycardia.

A number of different gene mutations can cause LQTS. Most of the genes involved code for cardiac ion channels. For example, LQT1 is caused by mutations in the potassium channel gene *KCNQ1* (*KVLQT1*). Approximately 42% of cases of LQTS are caused by mutations in this gene. Another 45% of cases are designated as LQT2, which is caused by mutations in another potassium channel gene *KCNH2* (*HERG*). Other types of LQTS involve sodium or calcium channels or their subunits. Many mutations causing LQTS are considered **private mutations,** meaning that they appear unique to only one person or one kindred and are not found consistently in the general population.

The vulnerability to a specific trigger varies with the gene involved. For example, it is more likely that a person will experience a cardiac event, such as torsade de pointes, before age 10 if he or she has

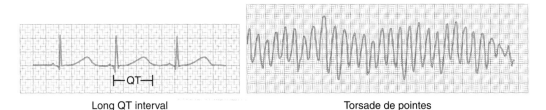

| Long QT interval | Torsade de pointes |

Figure 11–1. A long QT interval, which can lead to torsade de pointes.

LQT1. Events in LQT1 are often triggered by exercise, particularly swimming, while events for people with LQT2 are often triggered by auditory stimuli, such as an alarm clock ringing (so a ringing alarm clock can be harmful as well as obnoxious). People with LQT3, a sodium channel problem, often have their events during periods of rest or while they are asleep.

Although LQTS often does not appear until adolescence or later, sometimes evidence of LQTS can be seen prenatally. This is considered *congenital LQTS*. There are two types (phenotypes) seen in congenital LQTS. **Romano-Ward syndrome** usually follows autosomal dominant transmission and includes QT prolongation and tachyarrhythmias. **Jervell and Lange-Nielsen syndrome** has an autosomal recessive transmission pattern, and the QT prolongation and tachyarrhythmias are accompanied by deafness.

The effectiveness of standard treatments also varies by type of LQTS. Beta-blockers work best for people with LQT1, while mexiletine is often able to shorten the QT interval in people who have LQT3 but not in people with mutations in other genes that cause LQTS.

For another subset of patients, LQTS appears only when they take certain medications. These people have *acquired LQTS*. There is a growing list of drugs that can lengthen the QT interval and/or trigger torsade de pointes. The list includes antibiotics, antihistamines, antipsychotics, antidepressants, and bronchodilators. The Arizona Center for Education and Research on Therapeutics (AzCERT) keeps an updated list of drugs that have been shown to prolong the QT interval or trigger torsade de pointes (www.qtdrugs.org).

Cardiomyopathy

There are several types of **cardiomyopathy,** and they all involve a weakened or diseased heart muscle, which results in an inefficient pumping of blood. Cardiomyopathy often has a genetic cause, although there are a number of other causes as well. These include alcohol or cocaine abuse, viral infection, malnutrition, pregnancy, and end-stage kidney disease. Cardiomyopathy can be caused by a number of genetic diseases that affect multiple systems. See Table 11–1 for a list of some of these diseases. We will be discussing hypertrophic cardiomyopathy, dilated cardiomyopathy, restrictive cardiomyopathy, and arrhythmogenic right ventricular cardiomyopathy. See Figure 11–2 for illustrations of the major types of cardiomyopathy.

While clinical genetic testing is available for most forms of cardiomyopathy, it is important to remember that cardiomyopathy is diagnosed based primarily on clinical signs and symptoms. A clinician might recommend genetic testing for a person diagnosed with cardiomyopathy so that asymptomatic family members could be tested for a specific gene mutation, which is much more cost effective. Screening recommendations vary based on whether a family member carries the family mutation. When genetic testing is chosen, it is important for the person with the clearest phenotype (the most typical signs and symptoms) to be the one tested initially. This will make it much more likely that the family's mutation will be found.

TABLE 11–1

Genetic Diseases That Can Cause Cardiomyopathy

Hypertrophic cardiomyopathy	Beckwith-Wiedemann syndrome
	Down syndrome
	Friedreich ataxia
	Fabry disease
	Hunter syndrome
	Hurler syndrome
	Noonan syndrome
Dilated cardiomyopathy	Becker and Duchenne muscular dystrophy
	Emery-Dreifuss muscular dystrophy
	Fabry disease
	Fanconi anemia
	Mitochondrial myopathy
	Sickle cell disease
Arrhythmogenic right ventricular cardiomyopathy	Ventricular dysplasia
	Naxos disease
	Carvajal syndrome

Hershberger, et al., 2009.

Familial Hypertrophic Cardiomyopathy

Familial hypertrophic cardiomyopathy (HCM) affects approximately 1 in 500 adults, which makes it the most common genetic cardiac disorder worldwide. In HCM, the heart muscle becomes asymmetrically thick, and there are problems with ventricular filling and diastolic dysfunction. Left ventricular

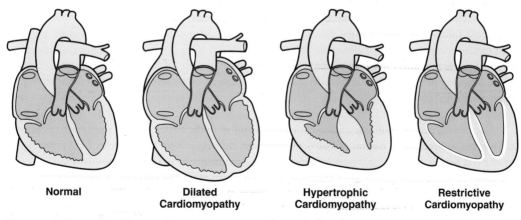

Normal **Dilated Cardiomyopathy** **Hypertrophic Cardiomyopathy** **Restrictive Cardiomyopathy**

Figure 11–2. Types of cardiomyopathy.

outflow tract obstruction happens in some patients because of hypertrophy of the septum and move-ment of the mitral valve. If you were to look at heart muscle tissue from a person affected with HCM under a light microscope, you would see disorganization (disarray) in the cardiac myocytes. This disor-ganization makes transmission of electrical impulses through the heart difficult, which can lead to cardiac rhythm problems.

HCM is diagnosed based on finding left ventricular hypertrophy, without any known cause, on the electrocardiogram or echocardiogram. This suggests that the problem is in the heart muscle itself and is not, for example, the result of muscle growth in order to pump larger quantities of blood against a high systemic pressure. HCM is transmitted as an autosomal dominant trait, but it can also be caused by **de novo mutations.** These are mutations that are not found in other family members and appear to be brand-new (de novo) in the person who is affected.

HCM, and several other forms of cardiomyopathy, are caused by mutations in genes that code for proteins of the sarcomere. The sarcomere is the contractile unit of the cardiac muscle cell (myocyte), and when there is a structural problem in the sarcomere, the heart loses its ability to contract effectively. More than 900 mutations in 12 genes have been found to cause HCM. These genes encode proteins such as β-myosin heavy chain, myosin-binding protein C, troponin T, troponin I, tropomyosin, and actin.

There is some disagreement about whether genetic diseases that include left ventricular hypertrophy (LVH) should be considered causes of HCM. The argument has to do with the way HCM is often defined, which currently is LVH that is not explained by another cardiac or systemic disease. Some genetic causes of ventricular hypertrophy are metabolic or infiltrative diseases, such as Pompe disease or Noonan syndrome. You can see these listed in Table 11–1, but some experts would say that these should not be considered HCM at all, because the hypertrophy is clearly caused by a known disease (Elliott and McKenna 2009; Maron et al., 2009).

While there are causes of HCM other than genetics, when more than one family member is affected, it is very likely that there is a genetic cause. It is very important that a complete three- or four-generation family history be recorded and updated frequently. HCM is often asymptomatic early on and has a varying age of onset and reduced penetrance. Many affected persons are identified as they reach adolescence or young adulthood; however, HCM has been diagnosed in infants and in 90-year-olds. Clinical genetic testing is available for people diagnosed with HCM. Recommendations for the care of family members of patients include obtaining an echocardiogram and electrocardiogram to screen all first-degree relatives. However, because the age of onset can vary, one normal echocardiogram does not mean that a person will never be affected. Some people do not develop symptoms until they reach mid-dle age, and they can have normal echocardiograms until that time. Screening guidelines are available from the American College of Cardiology, the American Heart Association, and other organizations.

One of the problems in identifying people who are affected with HCM is that they can be misdiag-nosed as having asthma, anxiety attacks, mitral valve prolapse, depression, or innocent murmurs. Some-times people are told that they have an "athletic heart" or exercise-induced asthma. The Hypertrophic Cardiomyopathy Association has collected data from more than 3000 patients who have HCM; 40% of these patients were initially diagnosed with something other than HCM, and some waited as long as 35 years before receiving a correct diagnosis (Maron and Salberg, 2006). That is one of the reasons why genetic testing can be so helpful in this population.

The most frequent cause of sudden cardiac death in young athletes is HCM. More than one-third of all athletes who die from sudden cardiac death before the age of 30 have HCM. Recommendations for activity restrictions for HCM patients are available. In general, affected people are told to avoid high intensity physical activities, particularly those that require a burst of effort, such as weight lifting or basketball, and to be moderate in all of their physical activities (Maron, 2003; Maron et al., 2003). The problem is that most people who die from HCM have not been diagnosed. That makes screening young athletes before they begin competition very important. The American Heart Association has developed guidelines for preparticipation sports physicals that are endorsed by the Hypertrophic Cardiomyopathy Association (Table 11–2).

Familial Dilated Cardiomyopathy

In **familial dilated cardiomyopathy (DCM),** there is left ventricular enlargement and poor pumping. DCM often results in heart failure and is a common cause for heart transplantation. The heart is distended (dilated), so that contraction of either ventricle is difficult (systolic dysfunction). DCM is most often the result of ischemic heart disease, but it can also be caused by exposure to toxins or infectious agents in susceptible people. Clinicians diagnose idiopathic DCM when the clinical signs are present and no cause can be found. Clinical signs include heart failure symptoms, such as those common to congestion (edema or dyspnea) or those associated with reduced cardiac output (fatigue). People can also present with arrhythmias or problems in the cardiac conduction system, or even with blood clots or stroke.

TABLE 11–2

Athletic Preparticipation Screening Guidelines

- Medical History*

Personal history	1. Exertional chest pain/discomfort
	2. Unexplained syncope/near-syncope
	3. Excessive exertional and unexplained dyspnea (shortness of breath)/fatigue associated with exercise
	4. Prior recognition of a heart murmur
	5. Elevated systemic blood pressure
Family history	6. Premature death (sudden and unexpected, or otherwise) before age 50 due to heart disease in one relative
	7. Disability from heart disease in a close relative younger than 50 years
	8. Specific knowledge of certain cardiac conditions in family members: hypertrophic or dilated cardiomyopathy, long QT syndrome or other ion channelopathies, Marfan syndrome, or clinically important arrhythmias
Physical examination	9. Heart murmur
	10. Femoral pulses to exclude aortic coarctation
	11. Physical stigmata of Marfan syndrome
	12. Brachial artery blood pressure (sitting position)

*Parental verification is recommended for high school and middle school athletes.
   Judged not to be neurocardiogenic (vasovagal), of particular concern when related to exertion.
   Auscultation should be performed in both supine and standing positions (or with Valsalva maneuver), specifically to identify murmurs of dynamic left ventricular outflow tract obstruction.
Preferably taken in both arms.
   At the discretion of the examiner, a positive response or finding in any 1 or more of the 12 items may be judged sufficient to trigger a referral for cardiovascular evaluation. Parental verification of the responses is regarded as essential for high school (and middle school) students.
**Cardiovascular screening should include ECG, echocardiogram, possible stress test, possible cardiac MRI, and follow-up plan as needed. In the opinion of the HCMA, these tests should be conducted by a cardiac professional, not a general practitioner or pediatrician.
Used with permission of the Hypertrophic Cardiomyopathy Association (www.4hcm.org/hcm/diagnosis/40255.html).

DCM is considered familial when two or more close family members are also affected. Studies have found that between 20% and 50% of DCM cases are inherited, but because DCM also shows reduced penetrance in some families, finding no history in family members does not necessarily mean the disease was not inherited. There are more than 20 genes that can cause DCM, which is usually transmitted in an autosomal dominant manner with a variable age of onset. DCM can also be transmitted as an X-linked or autosomal recessive trait. Just as in HCM, most of the genes causing DCM code for proteins in the sarcomere.

In 2009, the Heart Failure Society of America recommended that whenever a person is diagnosed with DCM, a family history must be taken, family members must be screened, and there should be genetic counseling with the offer of genetic testing. All first-degree relatives of people with DCM should have echocardiograms, electrocardiograms, physical examinations, and a thorough medical history, looking for symptoms such as arrhythmias and syncope. It is important that screenings are done at regular intervals because clinical manifestations may not appear until adulthood (Hershberger et al., 2009).

Familial Restrictive Cardiomyopathy

Restrictive cardiomyopathy is less common than the other types of cardiomyopathy, and some sources suggest that it is not a genetic disease. In this condition, there is a decrease in filling during diastole because of a rigid ventricle that does not expand as it should. There is usually normal systolic function. Some cases are idiopathic, and others are secondary to diseases such as scleroderma, sarcoidosis, amyloidosis, lymphoma, or hemachromatosis. While most cases of restrictive cardiomyopathy are probably not directly due to single-gene problems, families in which the trait shows autosomal dominant transmission have been documented. Mutations in the gene encoding troponin I have been found, but there may be other genes involved as well.

One of the problems with identifying a genetic cause is that although symptoms may appear in childhood, they also may not appear until the patient is between 50 and 60 years old. In addition, just as with the other forms of cardiomyopathy, there is reduced penetrance. In some families, patients also experience cardiac conduction problems and skeletal muscle weakness.

Arrhythmogenic Right Ventricular Dysplasia/Cardiomyopathy

Arrhythmogenic right ventricular dysplasia/cardiomyopathy (ARVD/C) appears to be underdiagnosed. The prevalence has been reported as between 1 in 1000 and 1 in 5000 (Lahtinen, 2011). In ARVD/C, there is a high risk of ventricular arrhythmias because of a fibro/fatty replacement of tissue in the ventricular myocardial wall. As the disease progresses, the left ventricle becomes more involved. This structural change makes it more likely that the patient will experience ventricular tachycardia and sudden cardiac death. It is difficult to know how many cases of sudden death are caused by ARVD/C, but it may be as high as 20% of sudden cardiac death in the young.

ARVD/C is transmitted as an autosomal dominant trait, and eight associated genes have been identified. These genes encode transmembrane proteins (TMEM43), calcium channels (RyR2), and the transforming growth factor beta-3 (TGFB-3). Five of the genes that are associated with ARVD/C code for proteins in the desmosomes or cell junctions. Other loci have been associated, so more genes will probably be identified in the future. Approximately 30% of cases are familial, and some occur in conjunction with systemic genetic diseases, such as Naxos disease, which is transmitted in an autosomal recessive manner. Autosomal recessive transmission of ARVD/C is much less common than autosomal dominant transmission. Just like the other forms of cardiomyopathy, penetrance is reduced, and getting a good family history is essential.

Summary

There are both single-gene and multifactorial causes of cardiovascular diseases. Single-gene disorders tend to be rare, and multifactorial disorders tend to be common. Even so, the number of people diagnosed with cardiomyopathy seems to be on the rise. Young athletes are at particular risk of sudden death due to undiagnosed HCM. Atherosclerosis is a major cause of coronary artery disease, stroke, and hypertension. Although the complete picture of the genes involved in these diseases has been elusive, association studies are providing important information about genes that are likely to be involved. Most multifactorial disorders, such as hypertension, are probably the result of the actions of several genes working together, each contributing a small effect, combined with environmental risk factors. We are starting to find polygenic risk factors for complex diseases such as atrial fibrillation, coronary artery disease, and stroke, but it is difficult to know when we will have a complete picture.

GENE GEMS

- About 50% of the risk for atherosclerosis can be attributed to genetics.
- Familial hypercholesterolemia is a single-gene problem that greatly increases the risk of coronary artery disease.
- There are genetic causes of both ischemic and hemorrhagic stroke.
- Less than 1% of strokes are caused by single-gene problems, and these occur primarily in people who have genetic disorders such as Marfan syndrome or Fabry disease.
- Most strokes are probably caused by several gene variants working together combined with environmental risk factors.
- Thrombophilias increase the risk of stroke, and these can be caused by single-gene genetic diseases such as factor V Leiden.
- Hypertension is caused by several gene variants working together with environmental risk factors.
- Mutations of genes involved in the RAAS pathways are often implicated in hypertension.
- Different mutations in ion channel genes can cause different arrhythmic phenotypes.
- Atrial fibrillation seems to have high genetic heterogeneity.
- The heart rhythm and conduction problems caused by genetic variations in genes that code for ion channel proteins are called channelopathies.
- There are at least eight different types of LQTS.
- The gene involved in LQTS affects the likelihood of certain triggers, causing torsade de pointes.
- Some drugs can lengthen the QT interval and cause an "acquired" LQTS.
- Private mutations are common in LQTS.
- Familial hypertrophic cardiomyopathy (FHCM) is transmitted as an autosomal dominant trait.
- Hypertrophic and dilated cardiomyopathy are caused by mutations in genes that code for proteins in the sarcomere.
- Young people and athletes with HCM are at an increased risk of sudden cardiac death during exercise.
- Familial dilated cardiomyopathy is usually transmitted as an autosomal dominant trait, but it can also be transmitted as either an autosomal recessive or an X-linked recessive trait.
- Arrhythmogenic right ventricular dysplasia/cardiomyopathy is often caused by mutations in genes that code for proteins in cell junctions.

Self-Assessment Questions

1. Your 40-year-old patient is hospitalized for a myocardial infarction, but her lipid levels are normal. She says that she would like to have a genetic test to see why she was affected at such a young age. What do you say?
   a. "Heart attacks seem to be caused by a combination of many affected genes working together as well as environmental factors. There is no single gene test that will be able to identify why this happened to you."
   b. "Let's talk with your nurse practitioner about scheduling a test for familial hypercholesterolemia."
   c. "You really shouldn't be concerned about your genetic risk. Because you are female, it is very low."
   d. "It was just bad luck combined with the fact that you were once a smoker."

2. The process in which gene variants interact with other gene variants to cause disease can be described by what word/phrase?
   a. Phenotype variation
   b. Reduced penetrance
   c. Epistasis
   d. Variable expressivity

3. What is true about the gene variants that cause hypertension?
   a. A few genes with major contributions have been identified.
   b. Genes that code for proteins in the RAAS pathways are often involved.
   c. Hypertension is always secondary to another genetic disease.
   d. Polymorphisms have little or no impact on the hypertensive phenotype.

4. Your patient has been diagnosed with long QT syndrome (LQTS). What do you know about this heart rhythm problem?
   a. LQTS is a congenital genetic disease that will be evident during the first 2 years of life.
   b. LQTS is treated in the same way, no matter the cause.
   c. Cardiac events are triggered by various environmental factors, depending on what gene is involved.
   d. Deafness always accompanies LQTS.

5. Why is it important that an adolescent with a history of hypertrophic cardiomyopathy (HCM) in the family have an echocardiogram before playing high-intensity sports?
   a. HCM is transmitted as an autosomal dominant trait and can cause sudden cardiac death during exercise.
   b. HCM is transmitted as an autosomal dominant trait, and it is most likely to cause a problem during swimming.
   c. Teens with HCM are counseled to play only pickup games of basketball.
   d. Having HCM in the family makes it more likely that one will have Ehlers-Danlos syndrome.

6. The mitochondrial disease MELAS results in strokelike episodes in addition to encephalopathy and lactic acidosis. It is transmitted from a mother to her children but is not transmitted by an affected father. Why is this so?
   a. The mitochondria are in the cytoplasm, and virtually all the cytoplasm comes from the egg.
   b. This is an X-linked recessive condition, so the father cannot transmit the disease to his sons, and his daughters will only be carriers.
   c. This is an X-linked dominant condition, so men are not affected.
   d. MELAS causes male infertility.

7. How does factor V Leiden increase the likelihood of stroke?
   a. Factor V Leiden activates protein C.
   b. Factor V Leiden increases thrombin formation.
   c. People affected with factor V Leiden have increased blood viscosity.
   d. Affected people have a type of factor V that is resistant to activated protein C.

CASE STUDY

John is a 16-year-old who loves to play soccer. His 18-year-old brother, Andre, passed out while playing basketball and has now been diagnosed with long QT syndrome (LQT1). The cardiologist suggests that all Andre's siblings should have a cardiac examination before they play sports, including an electrocardiogram. John's ECG shows a borderline QT prolongation during activity, so the cardiologist recommends genetic testing. John tests positive for the same mutation in the gene *KCNQ1* (LQT1) that Andre has and is told that he must stop playing soccer. He is counseled to take up a less intense sport, like golf. John is clearly upset and wants to know why this is happening to him. He feels just fine and does not understand why he cannot play his favorite sport.

1. What is the connection between sports restrictions and long QT syndrome?
2. How can understanding genetics help to predict who might be affected with long QT syndrome if someone in the family is already affected?
3. How and with what terms will you explain to John why these modifications in exercise are necessary?
4. Can you think of any way John could remain involved with his soccer team?

References

AHA. (2009). Hypertension. Retrieved April 9, 2010, from http://americanheart.org.

AHA. Heart disease and stroke statistics. Dallas, TX: American Heart Association, 2010.

Alberts, M. Stroke genomics. In Roden, D. Cardiovascular genetics and genomics. Dallas, TX: American Heart Association, 2009, 177–192.

Arizona Center for Education and Research on Therapeutics (AZCERT). Retrieved from www.qtdrugs.org.

Arnett, D. K. Hypertension. In Roden, D. Cardiovascular genetics and genomics. Hoboken, NJ: Wiley-Blackwell, 2009, 167–176.

Baird, A. E. (2010). Genetics and genomics of stroke: novel approaches. *Journal of the American College of Cardiology, 56*(4), 245–253.

Bierut, L. J. (2009). Nicotine dependence and genetic variation in the nicotinic receptors. *Drug and Alcohol Dependence, 104*(Suppl 1), S64–69.

Consortium, W. T. C. C. (2007). Genome-wide association study of 14,000 cases of seven common diseases and 3,000 shared controls. *Nature, 447*(7145), 661–678.

Darbar, D., and MacRae, C. A. Genomics and atrial arrhythmias. In Roden, D. Cardiovascular genetics and genomics. Dallas, TX: American Heart Association, 2009, 67–79.

Elliott, P., and McKenna, W. J. (2009). How should hypertrophic cardiomyopathy be classified? Molecular diagnosis for hypertrophic cardiomyopathy: Not ready for prime time. *Circulation: Cardiovascular Genetics, 2*(1), 87–89; discussion 89.

Helgadottir, A., Thorleifsson, G., et al. (2007). A common variant on chromosome 9p21 affects the risk of myocardial infarction. *Science, 316*(5830), 1491–1493.

Hershberger, R. E., Lindenfeld, J., et al. (2009). Genetic evaluation of cardiomyopathy—a Heart Failure Society of America practice guideline. *Journal of Cardiac Failure, 15*(2), 83–97.

Hobbs, H. H., Russell, D. W., et al. (1990). The LDL receptor locus in familial hypercholesterolemia: Mutational analysis of a membrane protein. *Annual Review of Genetics, 24*, 133–170.

Horne, B. D., Carlquist, J. F., et al. (2008). Association of variation in the chromosome 9p21 locus with myocardial infarction versus chronic coronary artery disease. *Circulation: Cardiovascular Genetics, 1*(2), 85–92.

Lahtinen, A. M., Lehtonen, E., et al. (2011). Population-prevalent desmosomal mutations predisposing to ARVCM. *Heart Rhythm. 8*, 1214-1221.

Ikram, M. A., Seshadri, S., et al. (2009). Genomewide association studies of stroke. *New England Journal of Medicine, 360*(17), 1718–1728.

Marks, D., Thorogood, M., et al. (2003). A review on the diagnosis, natural history, and treatment of familial hypercholesterolaemia. *Atherosclerosis, 168*(1), 1–14.

Maron, B. J. (2003). Sudden death in young athletes. *New England Journal of Medicine, 349*(11), 1064–1075.

Maron, B. J., Carney, K. P., et al. (2003). Relationship of race to sudden cardiac death in competitive athletes with hypertrophic cardiomyopathy. *Journal of the American College of Cardiology, 41*(6), 974–980.

Maron, B. J., and Salberg, L. Hypertrophic cardiomyopathy for patients, their families, and interested physicians. Malden, MA: Blackwell Futura, 2006.

Maron, B. J., Seidman, C. E., et al. (2009). How should hypertrophic cardiomyopathy be classified? What's in a name? Dilemmas in nomenclature characterizing hypertrophic cardiomyopathy and left ventricular hypertrophy. *Cardiovascular Genetics, 2*(1), 81–85; discussion 86.

Roberts, R., McPherson, R., et al. (2009). Genetics of atherosclerosis. In Roden, D. Cardiovascular genetics and genomics. Hoboken, NJ: Wiley-Blackwell, 2009, 151–166.

Roy, H., Bhardwaj, S., et al. (2009). Molecular genetics of atherosclerosis. *Human Genetics, 125*(5–6), 467–491.

Self-Assessment Answers

1. a **2.** c **3.** b **4.** c **5.** a **6.** a **7.** d

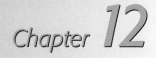
The Genetics of Cancer

Learning Outcomes

1. Use the genetic terminology associated with cancer development.
2. Compare the characteristics and growth regulation of benign tumor cells and cancer cells.
3. Examine genetic factors influencing cancer development, including mutational events in suppressor genes and oncogenes.
4. Compare the cancer development processes of initiation and promotion.
5. Compare the cancer development processes of progression and metastasis.
6. Analyze families for the presence of sporadic, familial, and hereditary cancer.
7. Indicate who within a kindred is at an increased genetic risk for hereditary cancer.

KEY TERMS

Benign tumor	Initiation	Primary tumor
Cancer	Latency period	Progression
Carcinogen	Malignant transformation	Promotion
Familial cancer	Metastasis	Sporadic cancer
Inherited cancer	Neoplasia	

Introduction

Cancer is a type of unregulated cell growth that has no useful purpose and is invasive and that without intervention would lead to death. Cancer is also called a *malignancy*. Cancer is a common, worldwide health problem that has always afflicted humans and, more rarely, other mammals. The types of cancers seen today vary somewhat from those that occurred thousands of years ago. Predominant cancer types also vary between industrialized nations and developing nations. A key concept in cancer development is that cancer cells arise from normal cells through changes in genes that control cell division. Understanding the genetic basis for cancer development and its progression involves applying concepts previously presented for basic DNA structure and function, control of cell division, protein synthesis, mutational events, and mendelian inheritance.

"All cancer is genetic." Is this a true statement? Yes, it is a true statement because cancer development involves changes in the genes that regulate cell division. "All cancer is inherited." Is this a true statement? The answer is more complex. Yes, cancer is inherited from one cell generation to the next. No, most cancers and the risk for cancer development are not inherited from one's parents; however, there are exceptions.

For many decades, scientists and clinicians involved in cancer research and care have considered the possibility that gene activity could be related to cancer development. Some of the early evidence supporting a possible interaction between genetics and cancer include the following observations:

- People who have known chromosome abnormalities (such as Down syndrome [trisomy 21] and Turner syndrome [monosomy X]) have an increased incidence of certain cancers.
- People with broken or fragile chromosomes (Fanconi anemia or Bloom syndrome) have an increased incidence of certain cancers.
- Some cancer types (such as breast cancer), in addition to occurring in people who do not have a family history of cancer, also occur within families and at times appear to follow an autosomal dominant pattern of inheritance.
- Some families have a much higher incidence of either one type of cancer or many types of cancer than can be accounted for by chance alone.
- Cancer cells often have abnormal numbers and/or structures of chromosomes.
- More malignant cancer cells usually have more abnormal chromosomes.

The influence of genetic changes that affect cell growth and cancer development are becoming clearer. Such changes result in conferring cancer cells with characteristics, responses, and growth advantages that optimize the survival of cancer cells over normal cells. The genes most affected by mutations that result in cancer development are those genes regulating normal cell growth—the oncogenes and suppressor genes. Recall from Chapter 3 that *oncogenes* are a large group of genes that produce proteins that promote cells to enter and complete the cell cycle. *Suppressor genes* are a set of master control genes that produce proteins that restrict cells from entering the cell cycle and that inhibit movement of a cell from one phase to the next within the cell cycle.

Benign Tumor Cells

Neoplasia is any new or continued cell growth that is not needed for normal development or for the replacement of dead and damaged tissues. It can be benign or malignant. **Benign tumors** are a type of neoplasia that does not share most of the characteristics of cancer cells. Although benign tumors are abnormal, they arise from normal cells and retain most normal cell characteristics. Their growth is not invasive; however, depending on location, they can cause death. Some examples of benign tumors include uterine fibroids (leiomyomas), fat tumors (lipomas), colon polyps (intestinal epithelial adenomas), and skin moles (nevi).

Characteristics of Benign Tumor Cells

APPEARANCE

Benign tumors arise from normal cells and retain a normal differentiated appearance. Their specific morphology is the same as that of the parent cells, even if their location is not. They also retain a small nuclear-to-cytoplasmic ratio.

FUNCTION

Benign tumors usually retain the differentiated function or functions of the parent cell. For example, not only do the cells of intestinal adenomas look like normal intestinal cells, but they also produce the same substances.

ADHERENCE

Benign tumors may grow in the wrong place within the body, such as the growth of endometrial tissue on an ovary and not in the uterus, but they do produce most cell adhesion molecules. As a result, these cells adhere tightly to one another and do not migrate.

PLOIDY

With few exceptions, tumor cells that are totally benign are diploid and do not display abnormal chromosome numbers or structures. Exceptions include benign meningiomas, which are often missing a number 22 chromosome, and lipomas, which often have structural rearrangements of chromosomes 6, 12, or 13.

CELL GROWTH

Benign tumors have continuous or inappropriate cell growth not needed for normal function. They serve no useful purpose. Benign tumor cells do grow by hyperplasia but do not have the ability to invade other tissues or organs. Their growth occurs by simple, nonessential expansion. Although growth may continue beyond an appropriate time, the rate of growth is normal.

Pathologic Potential

The mere existence of benign tumor cells indicates that the strict regulation of growth has been overcome to some degree. In many benign tumors, growth is slow and may even stop eventually. For other benign tumors, however, there is a risk that growth regulation will continue to deteriorate and a malignant tumor (cancer) will result. For example, intestinal adenomas have a high potential to become malignant, although considerable time passes before this happens. (This is why everyone over 50 years of age should have a colonoscopy so that polyps can be removed and colon cancer prevented.) When benign tumor cells become cancerous, it is the result of inhibited suppressor gene function and/or enhancement of oncogene function.

Cancer Cells

Cancer is a disease of cells, although it is often addressed as an organ problem (e.g., lung cancer, colon cancer, breast cancer). As explained earlier, cancer cells arise from normal cells. Humans are constantly exposed to personal and environmental conditions that can mutate the genes and alter the normal regulation over cell growth. Such changes can transform a normal cell into a cancer cell. This type of transformation that causes cancer development is termed *carcinogenesis, oncogenesis,* or **malignant transformation**. Substances capable of causing genetic mutations that lead to cancer development are **carcinogens.** Cancer cells are always abnormal, have no useful purpose, and invade normal body tissues and organs. Without treatment, most cancers lead to death.

Characteristics of Cancer Cells

APPEARANCE

Cancer represents a continuum of progression from just barely malignant, in which a normal cell has been transformed into a cancer cell, to as highly malignant as a cell can become. Thus, there are degrees of malignancy. Over time, cancer cells eventually lose all the specific differentiated appearance of the cells from which they arose and become *anaplastic* as small, round cells with a large nuclear-to-cytoplasmic ratio. Early in the cancer continuum, cancer cells may still show some normal cell appearance features, but these are later lost until no parental cell features are retained.

FUNCTION

In the progression of cancer from nearly normal to highly malignant, cancer cells gradually lose most or all differentiated functions that the parent cells performed. They become less differentiated in both appearance and function.

ADHERENCE

The ability to produce cell adhesion molecules (CAMs) is usually lost in cancer cells. They adhere poorly to each other and can easily break off from a formed tumor. This loss of adherence allows cancer cells to migrate into surrounding tissues and enter blood vessels in order to migrate to distant sites. The invasion of nearby and distant tissues is unique to cancer cells and is a common cause of death. For example, if breast cancer remained only within the breast, a nonvital organ, it would not kill the patient. However, breast cancer does invade vital organs (e.g., brain, bone marrow, lungs, liver) and disrupts their functions enough to cause death.

PLOIDY

Early in the cancer process, the cancer cell's chromosomes may be normally diploid. As they become more malignant, they usually become aneuploid, with gains or losses of whole chromosomes, chromosome breakage, and the structural rearrangements of chromosomes. Often, the more malignant a cancer cell becomes, the greater the degree of aneuploidy it has. Some chromosomal rearrangements are unique to a cancer type and can be used to identify it as a specific cancer type. These unique types of aneuploidy may indicate which oncogenes are overexpressed in a tumor and may be able to be controlled through targeted therapy. For example, a chromosome rearrangement in which the ends of the q arms of chromosome 22 are translocated to the q arms of chromosome 9 results in the activation of a special tyrosine kinase (TK) that converts bone marrow cells into chronic myelogenous leukemia. This special TK is inhibited by the targeted therapy drug imatinib mesylate (Gleevec). This drug works only on cancer cells that overexpress this special TK.

CELL GROWTH

Cancer cells no longer respond to external or internal signals, which indicates that cell division is not needed. They are not contact inhibited and continue to divide even when too many cells are already present and nutrition stores are low. Without treatment, they persist in cell division until the host dies. This loss of contact inhibition allows the persistence of cancer cell division regardless of how many cancer cells are occupying a given space.

Cancer cells also do not respond to signals for apoptosis. They do not experience a reduction of telomeric DNA with cell division, even though they may not have particularly long telomeres. Cancer cells have large amounts of telomerase, which maintains their telomeric DNA.

Suppressor gene regulation of cell division appears lost or defective in cancer cells, and oncogenes are then overexpressed, which leads to uncontrolled mitosis. They may not go through the cell cycle more rapidly than do normal cells; they just reenter the cell cycle quickly, spending very little time in the reproductive resting state of G_0. Cell cycle checkpoints are not effective, and promitotic forces are unopposed. Usually, one or more suppressor genes are disabled and cannot restrict oncogene expression. With excessive oncogene expression, cyclins and CDKs are overproduced and cell division occurs inappropriately and continually. (Using the car example described in Chapter 3, the driver and/or the car's brakes are nonfunctional, so acceleration goes wild.) Because highly malignant cancer cells divide almost continually, their *mitotic index* (the percentage of cells within a block of tissue that are actually in the cell cycle at any point in time) is relatively high, usually greater than 50%.

Immortality

Cancer cells are considered *immortal* because they do not respond to apoptotic signals and are resistant to natural cell death. There is no preprogrammed number of cell divisions for them, and they can tolerate very low levels of nutrients. One feature of cancer cells is that additional gene changes continue to occur that alter the plasma membrane to enhance uptake of all needed nutrients. When limited nutrients are present in the environment, cancer cells can take them in more efficiently than normal cells, leaving normal cells in a starved and weakened condition.

Cancer Development

Malignant Transformation

Other names for malignant transformation, the process of changing a normal cell into a cancer cell, are *carcinogenesis* and *oncogenesis*. This process takes time and involves many steps to overcome the body's natural resistance to cancer (Fig. 12–1). The steps of the process are initiation, promotion, progression, and metastasis, as shown in Figure 12–2.

Initiation

Normal cells may become cancer cells when their oncogenes are overexpressed, which results in poorly controlled cell division. The initial step in malignant transformation is mutating the DNA in such a way that either suppressor genes cannot perform their cell growth regulation functions or oncogenes become resistant to suppressor gene control. Any substance or event that can damage DNA has the potential to mutate suppressor genes or oncogenes and is a carcinogen. For cancer development, this type of mutation is termed **initiation.** It is an irreversible event that can lead to cancer development if the cell's mitotic ability remains intact. If a cancer cell cannot divide, it cannot progress to widespread malignant disease. However, when conditions favor the continuing growth of even one transformed cell, widespread malignant disease can occur. This is known as the *monoclonal* (from one cell) *origin* of cancer. Initiation is a required step in carcinogenesis. Without initiation, even if the remaining steps occur, cancer does not develop.

In general, most cancers arise in tissues that have retained mitotic ability. This does not mean that all the cells within one organ type have retained mitotic ability. Rather, it means that of the mixture of cells composing an organ, those that retain mitotic ability are much more likely to undergo carcinogenesis than those that have not. For example, the three main types of normal cells in the uterine

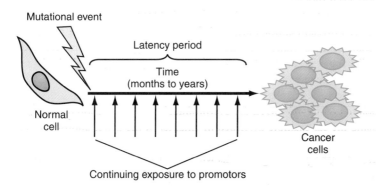

Figure 12–1. Malignant transformation from a normal cell to cancer cells after exposure to a mutational event.

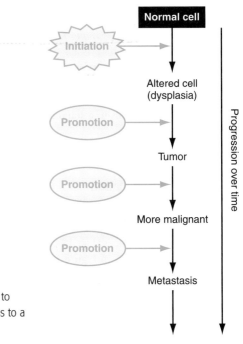

Figure 12–2. The steps of initiation and continued promotion to transform a normal cell to a cancer cell and allow it to progress to a highly malignant, metastatic state.

cervix are squamous epithelial cells, glandular cells that secrete mucus, and neuroendocrine cells. Only the squamous epithelial cells retain mitotic ability, and about 90% of cervical cancer arises from these cells. Although cancer can arise from cardiac muscle cells, which are nonmitotic, this is a very rare type of cancer. Table 12–1 lists the most common cancer types and their incidence in North America.

Carcinogenic substances capable of initiation include a wide variety of chemicals, physical agents, and viruses. Initiation can also occur through spontaneous DNA replication error, which is more likely when cells are dividing more frequently, such as during inflammation or after injury. When initiation has occurred in germ line cells (ova or sperm), the risk for cancer development can be passed on to one's children. Children who are born as a result of conception in which one of the two germ line cells has been initiated essentially have all their cells already past the initiation step of carcinogenesis. These people have a greatly increased risk for cancer development if the other steps of carcinogenesis occur at any time throughout their life spans.

It is important to remember that cell initiation occurs much more frequently than does cancer development. We are constantly exposed to environmental carcinogens and may have some cells initiated daily. However, we do not develop cancer daily, and most people will never develop cancer at all. Only about one out of every three people in North America will develop cancer at some point in their lives. Not only are the other steps of carcinogenesis needed for initiated cells to become malignant, personal factors also make some people more resistant to cancer development than others.

Promotion

Although a cell initiated by a carcinogen can develop into cancer, it will do so only if promotion occurs after initiation. **Promotion** is the process of enhancing the growth of initiated cells over time (see Figs. 12–1 and 12–2). It is a long, slow process for an initiated cell to form a malignant tumor. No one develops an identifiable cancer the day after exposure to a carcinogen, even if it is an especially strong

TABLE 12–1

The Incidence of Common Cancers in North America

Cancer Type	Incidence (Estimates for 2010)
All cancers	1,703,360
Lung and bronchus	246,620
Prostate	242,330
Breast	232,460
Colorectal	165,070
Lymphomas (all types)	81,130
Urinary bladder	78,530
Melanoma	75,400
Kidney (and renal pelvis)	64,040
Thyroid	49,000
Uterine (corpus)	48,510
Pancreas	48,050
Leukemia	47,900
Ovary	25,090
Uterine cervix	14,200

Data compiled from: American Cancer Society. (2010). Cancer facts and figures 2010. Report No. 01-300M-No. 5008.10. Atlanta: Author; Canadian Cancer Society. (2010). Canadian Cancer Statistics, 2010.

or potent carcinogen. Time and continuing exposure to agents that cause promotion (promoters) are needed (note that promoters are different from the promoter regions of DNA for protein synthesis discussed in Chapter 2). The time between initiation and the development of an identifiable tumor is the **latency period,** which ranges from months to years. (People never get lung cancer 1 week after they smoke their first cigarette.) The length of the latency period varies depending on the following: the strength of the carcinogen (more powerful carcinogens result in a shorter latency period), whether the tissue is also exposed to additional carcinogens (cocarcinogens), the amount of exposure to promoters (greater exposures result in a shorted latency period), and the individual's resistance to cancer development (discussed later in the "Personal Factors Related to Cancer Development" section).

Promoters are substances or conditions that enhance (promote) the growth of the initiated cancer cell. Promotion can also shorten the latency period. Promoters include naturally occurring hormones, such as estrogen, testosterone, and insulin; drugs; and a wide variety of chemicals. For example, when cervical epithelial cells have been initiated by viral infection or exposure to cigarette smoke or another chemical, growth is enhanced by the presence of the woman's own naturally secreted estrogen or progesterone. Thus, the hormone is serving as a promoter.

Some carcinogens have both initiating ability and promoting ability. These are known as *complete carcinogens* because additional exposure to another promoter is *not* needed for cancer to develop. A few examples of complete carcinogens include radiation, benzopyrene, naphthylamine, and nitroquinoline.

Progression

After sufficient cancer cells have been promoted enough that an identifiable tumor exists, other conditions are needed for this tumor to become as malignant as possible. **Progression** is the continuing genetic changes that occur in cancer cells that alter their physical, biochemical, and metabolic processes, and confer survival advantages to these cells. The most important changes allow cancer cells and tumors to develop a separate blood supply and enhance cellular nutrition. In small tumors, nutrition occurs by diffusion, which is not efficient after a tumor is larger than 1 cm. With increased growth, tumor cells become hypoxic and begin to secrete *tumor angiogenesis factor (TAF),* which is similar to the angiogenesis factors that normal tissues may secrete under hypoxic conditions. TAF stimulates nearby blood vessels and capillaries to branch into the tumor, establishing a tumor blood supply and improving tumor nutrition.

Other changes brought about by progression include membrane permeability changes. Many normal cells require insulin and insulin receptors to allow glucose to enter them. Cancer cell membranes become directly permeable to glucose so that insulin and insulin receptors are not needed. However, glucose uptake is increased further in the presence of insulin. Cancer cell membranes become even more efficient at amino acid uptake. As a result of these changes, cancer cells are able to meet their increased metabolic needs quickly and often at the expense of normal cells.

Because cancer cells have no need for differentiated functions, changes through progression result in the loss of differentiated functions. This loss reduces the energy expenditure wasted on differentiated functions, which now can be used for even more efficient cell division. Thus, through progression, cancer cells and tumors acquire selection advantages that allow them to live and divide no matter how the conditions around them change. Over time, cancer cells become more and more malignant, expressing fewer and fewer normal cell features.

A **primary tumor** is the original tumor, usually identified by the tissue from which and in which it first arose (e.g., ovarian cancer, colorectal cancer, prostate cancer). When primary tumors are located in vital organs, such as the brain or lungs, their excessive growth interferes with the performance of vital functions and leads to death. When primary tumors are located in soft tissue, tumor expansion can occur with little or no damage to surrounding tissue. However, malignant tumors do not remain in the tissues in which they arise.

Metastasis

Metastasis is the spread of cancer cells from the primary tumor to other body areas, where they grow and damage additional tissues and organs, often leading to death. One of the advantages acquired by cancer cells with progression that allows metastasis to occur is the loss of cell adhesion molecules (CAMs), making cancer cells poorly adherent to each other. An additional advantage is the expression of enzymes on the cancer cell's surface that makes these cells able to penetrate other tissues and blood vessel walls. Cancer cells then form *secondary tumors (metastatic tumors)* by breaking off from the primary tumor. Secondary tumors can form by extension into nearby tissues and can enter the bloodstream and establish colonies in remote tissues. Even though the tumor is now in another organ, it is still a cancer from the original parent tissue. For example, when prostate cancer spreads to the bone and lymph nodes, it is prostate cancer in the bone and lymph nodes, not bone cancer and not lymphoma.

Metastasis is a complex process that requires many steps over time. Most steps result from continued genetic changes through progression. Many cancers have a predictable pattern of metastasis. Table 12–2 lists the secondary tumor sites for metastasis of common tumors. Although other mechanisms for metastasis to distant sites exist, the most common way cancers spread is through the bloodstream. Metastatic sites are often in organs with extensive capillary networks.

TABLE 12–2

The Usual Sites of Metastasis for Selected Cancers

Cancer Type	Sites of Metastasis
Prostate cancer	Bone (especially spine and legs)*
	Pelvic nodes
	Liver
Lung cancer	Brain*
	Bone
	Liver
	Lymph nodes
	Pancreas
Breast cancer	Bone*
	Lung*
	Liver
	Brain
Colorectal	Liver*
	Lymph nodes
	Adjacent structures
Melanoma	Gastrointestinal tract
	Lymph nodes
	Lung
	Brain
Pancreatic cancer	Liver*
	Lungs
	Bone
	Spleen
	Adrenal glands
	Lymph nodes
	Blood vessels

*Most common site of metastasis for the specific cancer

Cancer Causes and Risk

As discussed earlier, cancer development takes years and depends on several tumor and patient factors. The three factors influencing carcinogenesis and metastasis are environmental exposure to carcinogens (initiators and promoters), immune function, and genetic predisposition. These three factors explain some of the variation in cancer development from one person to another, even when each person has the same environmental exposure.

The main defect in carcinogenesis is inappropriate and excessive oncogene expression, regardless of the specific cause. In theory, mutating an oncogene could increase its activity, although such damage usually makes a gene lose its function rather than enhance it. One way mutation of an oncogene can lead to its increased expression is when mutation causes an increase in the number of copies of the oncogene in the affected cells (*amplification*). Instead of having one copy of the two alleles for a specific oncogene within one cell, perhaps there are as many as 500 copies. (In the car analogy, this would be like having a jet engine in a small car but having just the normal brakes for the car. Just a little pressure on the gas pedal would make the car go very fast and not be able to stop with the existing brakes.) Another way is to move the oncogene (translocate it) to an area of the genome not under suppressor gene control. (Think about putting a car's engine on a grocery cart that has no brakes.)

The more common way initiation leads to excessive oncogene expression is by damaging any one of many suppressor genes. When a suppressor gene is damaged, it can no longer express its products in the proper amounts to control oncogene expression. Suppressor genes, like most single genes, have two alleles. When one allele is damaged and nonfunctional, the amount of suppressor gene product in the affected cells is reduced by about 50%, and there is less strict control over oncogene expression (Fig. 12–3; using the car analogy, if the front brakes are nonfunctional, the car can still be stopped before crashing, but it takes more planning by the driver and longer distances for the remaining brakes to perform this function). When both suppressor gene alleles are nonfunctional, oncogene expression is unopposed and mitosis occurs continually. (When both sets of brakes are nonfunctional, the engine runs without controls and the driver cannot stop the car before it crashes.)

External Factors Related to Cancer Development

External factors, including environmental exposure to carcinogens, are responsible for at least 80% of cancer in North America. Chemical carcinogens vary in how great their carcinogenic potential is. For example, tobacco and alcohol appear to be only mildly carcinogenic, requiring long-term exposure to large amounts of these substances before cancer develops. (These two substances can act as *cocarcinogens* so that when they are used together, they enhance each other's carcinogenic potential.) Chemicals with carcinogenic potential can be found almost anywhere in the environment, including in the food chain. Dietary influences on cancer development include chemicals in food and diets that are deficient in substances that are antioxidants, which tend to repair damaged cells and reduce the effects of mutational events on mitosis.

Physical carcinogenesis occurs through direct gene damage and mutation by physical agents. Two common physical agents that can result in cancer development are radiation and chronic irritation. Radiation can directly mutate DNA. Potential sources of radiation include exposure to rocks and soil that contain varying amounts of uranium and radium; x-rays for the diagnosis and treatment of disease; cosmic radiation; solar radiation from the sun; tanning beds; and germicidal lights. Chronic irritation greatly increases mitosis in affected tissues, increasing the likelihood of unrepaired spontaneous DNA replication error.

The infection of cells with certain types of viruses, known as *oncoviruses,* can lead to carcinogenesis. These infecting viruses break the DNA of the cells they infect and then insert their own genetic material into the human DNA. The result of breaking the DNA and inserting viral genes mutates the normal cell's DNA. These mutations can damage suppressor genes and can allow the overexpression of oncogenes.

Personal Factors Related to Cancer Development

The personal factors of age, immune function, and genetic risk, along with environmental exposures to carcinogens, influence cancer development. Aging is a major factor in cancer development. Just think about how many more women over the age of 60 develop breast cancer than women between the ages

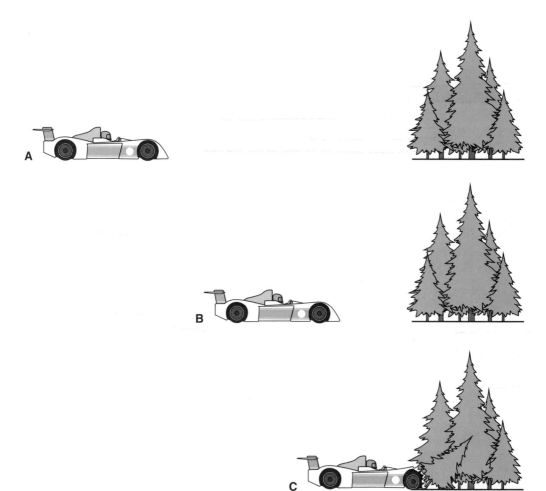

Figure 12–3. (A) The car has both sets of brakes (suppressor gene alleles) working properly so that the car stops well in front of the trees. (B) The front brakes (one suppressor gene allele) are not functioning, and the car takes a longer distance to stop, but still does not hit the trees. (C) The front and rear brakes (both suppressor gene alleles) are both nonfunctional. The car cannot stop and hits the trees.

of 20 to 40 years! Advancing age allows for the effects of exposure to environmental carcinogens to accumulate, and at the same time results in reduced immune function.

A well-functioning immune system protects the body from cells that are no longer completely normal, such as damaged cells and cancer cells. Immune system cells, especially macrophages and natural killer cells, recognize unhealthy cells and attack and destroy them. This is most likely the protection that prevents those daily mutational events (which result in a few cells becoming initiated) from remaining in the body long enough to continue, preventing the rest of the carcinogenesis steps and the development of an identifiable tumor. Anyone whose immune function is less than optimal has an increased risk for cancer. Mutation and initiation do not occur more often; they are less frequently recognized and cancer gets a foothold. The role of immune protection against cancer development is supported by the increased cancer incidence seen among people who are immunocompromised, including the following groups:

- Children under age 2 whose immune systems are not yet fully developed
- Adults older than age 60 whose immune function is gradually declining
- Patients with any form of long-term immune deficiency (especially HIV/AIDS)
- Patients who are organ transplant recipients taking immunosuppressive drugs to prevent organ rejection
- Patients who have serious autoimmune or inflammatory disease and must take cortisol or other strong immunosuppressants to control the disease

Genetic Factors Related to Cancer Development

Although all cancer is "genetic," not all cancers are inherited. Cancers can be classified on the basis of how frequently they occur in a kindred and whether an inherited genetic mutation may be responsible for increased risk. These classes are sporadic cancer, familial cancer, and inherited cancer. A confounding factor is that some cancer types, such as breast cancer, colorectal cancer, and prostate cancer, can fall into any of these classes, and some families may have all three classes of one cancer type within a kindred.

SPORADIC CANCER

Sporadic cancer is cancer that occurs usually as a result of environmental exposure or unknown factors and does not have any observable pattern of inheritance within a kindred. At the cell level, mutations through carcinogenesis have occurred, disrupting the normal regulation of cell division, usually among somatic cells. These cancers are not present in higher-than-expected levels within three or more family generations. Although the cause of the cancer is not always known (making primary prevention difficult), there is no predisposition for it. For example, breast cancer is a common cancer, occurring in one out of eight women in North America over the age of 60 years. In Figure 12–4, the family history of a 72-year-old woman recently diagnosed with breast cancer is examined. There are a grand total of 15 female relatives in three generations on the paternal and maternal side. Only three other women, none of whom is a first-degree relative, have been diagnosed with breast cancer, and all were older than age 60 at the time of diagnosis. An important feature of sporadic cancers among somatic cell tissues is that the person cannot pass on a predisposition for the cancer to his or her children because these mutations are acquired *only* in the tissues that develop the cancer. (Children do not inherit somatic cells from their parents. They inherit only germ line cell genes that are then used to develop somatic cells.)

Mutations of different suppressor gene and oncogene somatic cells are associated with different cancer types. Table 12–3 lists known cancers associated with specific gene mutations in somatic cells.

FAMILIAL CANCER

Familial cancer is cancer that occurs at a higher-than-expected frequency within a kindred but does not demonstrate any observable pattern of inheritance. The family may have a higher-than-expected incidence of other cancer types as well. However, most family members who develop cancer do so at older ages. Breast cancer can also be familial. Figure 12–5 shows a typical pedigree for familial breast cancer. Five of 15 women in the kindred have had breast cancer, and all were older than 60 years at the time of diagnosis (a little higher than expected by chance alone). In addition, four other family members have had cancer, some of whom were or are first-degree relatives to each other. At this time, no specific pattern of inheritance emerges, and no specific genetic testing is recommended. Eventually, there may be a genome-wide association study (GWAS) that can provide insight into risk for familial cancer. (For more information on genome-wide association studies, refer to Chapter 14.)

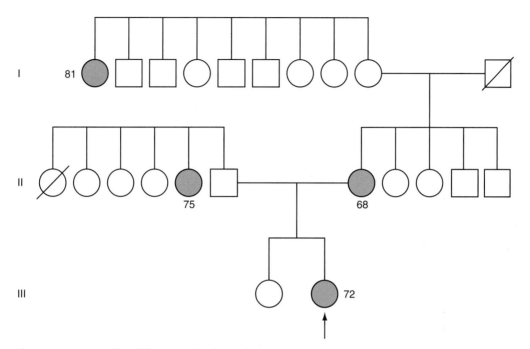

Figure 12–4. A typical family history and pedigree showing sporadic breast cancer.

INHERITED CANCER

Inherited cancer is cancer that occurs with an observable autosomal dominant pattern of inheritance among much younger-than-expected individuals in a kindred. Figure 12–6 shows a pedigree for a family with familial breast and ovarian cancer as a result of a *BRCA1* suppressor gene mutation. This is a germline mutation and is present in one *BRCA1* allele in *all* of a person's cells. These cells essentially have already gone halfway through initiation at conception and require only one additional allele mutation followed by promotion for a malignancy to occur. This is why the cancer tends to appear at earlier ages than expected. Although its presence does not absolutely mean that the person will go on to develop breast and/or ovarian cancer, the risk is very high. In addition, each person with one mutated *BRCA1* allele in every cell has a 50% chance of passing on the mutated allele and its predisposition to his or her children.

There are a number of inherited germ line mutations of suppressor genes or oncogenes that greatly increase the risk for cancer development. In addition, the mutations of genes that regulate DNA repair also increase the risk for cancer. Other family characteristics, in addition to an autosomal pattern of inheritance, that indicate the possibility of a *BRCA1* mutation include the following:

- Cancers occurring at ages several decades younger than the national average
- Breast cancer in male relatives
- Breast cancer in both breasts
- The presence of a second primary cancer in the same patient
- The presence of family members with rare types of genitourinary or gastrointestinal cancers

TABLE 12–3

Examples of Cancers Caused by Mutations in Suppressor Genes, Oncogenes, and DNA Repair Genes

Mutated Gene	Cancer Types
Suppressor Genes	
APC	Colorectal, stomach, and pancreatic carcinomas
ATM	Breast, stomach, bladder, pancreas, lung, and ovarian carcinomas
BRCA1	Breast, ovarian, genitourinary, and gastrointestinal carcinomas
BRCA2	Ovarian, breast, and prostate carcinomas
DCC	Colorectal carcinomas
Rb1	Retinoblastoma, sarcomas, bladder, breast, esophageal, and lung carcinomas
PTEN	Breast, prostate, and uterine carcinomas; melanomas; brain tumors (glioblastomas, astrocytomas)
Tp53	Bladder, breast, colorectal, esophageal, liver, lung, ovarian, and CNS sarcomas; lymphomas; and leukemias (Li-Fraumeni syndrome)
WT1	Wilms tumor
Oncogenes	
abl	Chronic myelogenous leukemia and other leukemias
c-myc	Burkitt lymphoma; other lymphomas; breast, stomach, and lung carcinomas
Hras	Many carcinomas and sarcomas
Kras	Colorectal and pancreatic carcinomas, a wide variety of other carcinomas and sarcomas
Nras	Neuroblastoma
met	Osteosarcoma
myb	Colorectal carcinomas, leukemias
PTCH	Bladder and breast carcinomas
ret	Thyroid tumors
trk	Colorectal carcinomas and thyroid tumors
DNA repair genes	
MLH1	Hereditary nonpolyposis colon cancer (Lynch syndrome); endometrium, ovary, stomach, small intestine, liver, gallbladder duct, and upper urinary tract cancers
MSH2	Hereditary nonpolyposis colon cancer (Lynch syndrome); endometrium, ovary, stomach, small intestine, liver, gallbladder duct, upper urinary tract, brain, and sebaceous skin cancers
MSH6	Hereditary nonpolyposis colon cancer (Lynch syndrome); endometrium, ovary, stomach, small intestine, liver, gallbladder duct, upper urinary tract, brain, and skin cancers; neurofibromatosis, leukemia, and lymphoma
PMS1	Hereditary nonpolyposis colon cancer (Lynch syndrome)
PMS2	Hereditary nonpolyposis colon cancer (Lynch syndrome); glioblastomas, leukemias, and lymphomas

Data compiled from the National Cancer Institute (http://ghr.nlm.nih.gov/gene/)

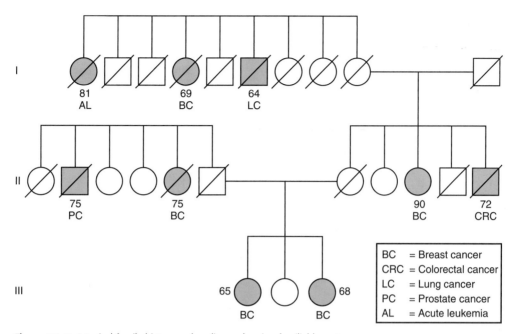

Figure 12–5. A typical family history and pedigree showing familial breast cancer.

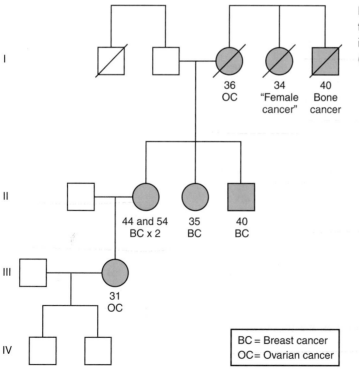

Figure 12–6. A pedigree showing the autosomal dominant pattern of inheritance for inherited cancer (*BRCA1* positive).

Overall, the percentage of cancers that occur as a result of the inheritance of a germ line gene mutation ranges between 5% and 15%. Although this is a low percentage, people who have these mutations are at great risk for cancer development. Genetic testing for cancer predisposition is available to confirm or rule out a person's genetic risk for a few specific inherited cancer types. These tests do not diagnose the presence of cancer nor are they 100% predictive; they merely demonstrate increased risk. Therefore, predisposition testing for inherited cancer should not be performed unless a family history clearly indicates the possibility of increased genetic risk and the patient wants to have the test results. More information on predisposition testing and its associated issues or potential problems is presented in Chapter 14.

Summary

All cancers arise from normal cells that have mutations in either suppressor genes or oncogenes. These mutations result in loss of the strict control of mitosis that normal cells have. Although all cancer is "genetic," only 5% to 15% of cancers are inherited. Whether a person develops cancer is related to his or her age, exposure to carcinogenic substances or events, the degree of efficient immune function, and genetic composition and predisposition.

GENE GEMS

- Cancer cells arise from normal cells.
- Suppressor gene products limit cell division by controlling the expression of oncogenes so that mitosis occurs only when and to the extent it is needed.
- Oncogenes are normal genes, and their products are promitotic.
- Benign tumors grow by simple, nonessential expansion.
- The transformation of a normal cell into a cancer cell is caused by genetic mutations.
- Whenever oncogenes are overexpressed after normal growth and development are complete, the person is at risk for cancer development.
- Tissues that retain mitotic ability are far more likely to undergo carcinogenesis than those that do not continue to replace dead or damaged cells through mitosis.
- Malignant tumors have physical, biochemical, and metabolic advantages that allow them to survive and invade other tissues (metastasis).
- If conditions are right, widespread cancer can develop as a result of initially having only one cell undergo malignant transformation.
- Secondary tumors are still designated as tumors of the parent tissue.
- The major factors that interact to influence cancer development are advancing age, exposure to environmental carcinogens, the effectiveness of immune function, and genetic predisposition.
- Somatic cell mutations that lead to cancer development cannot be passed on to one's children as a predisposition for cancer.
- Germ line cell mutations that lead to cancer development have a 50% risk for being transmitted to one's children and predisposing them to cancer.
- Only about 5% to 15% of all cancers result from inherited mutations.

Self-Assessment Questions

1. Which pathologic description of a tumor would you interpret as being the "most malignant" cancer?
   a. Undifferentiated; 60% mitotic index; aneuploid
   b. Highly differentiated; 10% mitotic index; aneuploid
   c. Poorly differentiated; 25% mitotic index; euploid
   d. Moderately differentiated; 50% mitotic index; euploid

2. Why is malignant cell growth (cancer cell growth) considered "uncontrolled"?
   a. Cancer cells always divide more rapidly than do normal cells.
   b. The mitosis of malignant cells usually produces more than two daughter cells.
   c. Malignant cells reenter the cell cycle more often, so cell division is a continuous process.
   d. Malignant cells are able to bypass one or more phases of the cell cycle during mitotic cell divisions.

3. Which theory of carcinogenesis has the most support?
   a. DNA damage, which permits overexpression of oncogenes
   b. RNA damage, which results in incomplete protein formation
   c. Autoantibodies, which attack specific "self" tissues and organs
   d. The failure of embryonic tissues to undergo normal differentiation

4. By which process does "promotion" assist in cancer development?
   a. Inflicting mutations at specific sites on the exposed cell's DNA
   b. Stimulating or enhancing cell division of cells damaged by a carcinogen
   c. Increasing the transformed cell's capacity for error-free DNA repair
   d. Making cancer cells appear more normal and escaping immunosurveillance

5. How is progression different from metastasis?
   a. Progression cannot occur unless the process of metastasis occurs first.
   b. Metastasis occurs in both benign and malignant cells, whereas progression is a feature that is unique to malignant cells.
   c. Metastasis is dependent on gene mutations in suppressor genes, and progression is dependent on gene mutations in oncogenes.
   d. Progression involves continual gene changes in a cancer cell that enhance its degree of malignancy, whereas metastasis is the ability of the cell to invade other tissues.

6. An 85-year-old patient tells you she does not perform breast self-exams because there is no history of breast cancer in her family. What is your best response?
   a. "You are correct. Breast cancer is an inherited type of malignancy and your family history indicates a low risk for you."
   b. "Breast cancer can be found more frequently in families; however, the risk for general, sporadic breast cancer increases with age."
   c. "Because your breasts are no longer as dense as they were when you were younger, your risk for breast cancer is now decreased."
   d. "Examining your breasts once per year when you have your mammogram is sufficient screening for someone with your history."

Continued

7. A 36-year-old patient who has a suspicious mammogram tells you that her mother died of bone cancer when she was 40 years old. What should be your next question for this patient?
   a. "Have any other members of your family had bone cancer?"
   b. "Did your mother ever have any other type of cancer?"
   c. "How old were you when you started your periods?"
   d. "Did your mother have regular mammograms?"

CASE STUDY

A 28-year-old client, Leslie, has been diagnosed with benign breast disease. She is worried about the possibility of developing breast cancer because of her family history. At age 64, her mother, Margaret, was diagnosed with unilateral breast cancer (in situ) 2 years ago by mammography. Margaret had a lumpectomy followed by radiation. Margaret has two sisters and two brothers who do not have any cancer diagnosis. Margaret's mother and aunt (two of nine siblings) were both diagnosed with unilateral breast cancer at age 70. Both had mastectomies. The aunt is now 81 and has recently had a recurrence. Margaret's mother is 97 and remains disease-free. Leslie's father died of melanoma at age 54. He had five sisters. One sister died at age 60 in an automobile accident. The youngest sister, age 64, was treated for cervical cancer 2 years ago. She is currently considered to be disease-free. The oldest sister was diagnosed with unilateral breast cancer 5 years ago at age 75. Treatment included lumpectomy and an antiestrogen receptor agent. She remains disease-free. There are no other identified cases of cancer in this kindred.

1. Draw the pedigree for the family.
2. What specific pattern of inheritance (if any) is indicated by the pedigree for the cancer in this family?
3. What pedigree criteria support your identified pattern of inheritance for this health problem?
4. Who in this family could benefit from genetic counseling and possible genetic testing? Explain your choices.

References

American Cancer Society. (2011). Cancer facts and figures 2011. Report No. 01-300M-No. 5008.11. Atlanta: Author.

Calzone, K., Masny, A., and Jenkins, J. (eds). Genetics and genomics in oncology nursing practice. Pittsburgh: Oncology Nursing Society, 2010.

Canadian Cancer Society. (2010). Canadian Cancer Statistics, 2010.

Feero, G., Guttmacher, E., and Collins, F. (2010). Genomic medicine—An updated primer. *New England Journal of Medicine, 362*, 2001–2011.

Markowitz, S., and Bertagnolli, M. (2009). Molecular origins of cancer: Molecular basis of colorectal cancer. *New England Journal of Medicine, 361*(25), 2449–2460.

Self-Assessment Answers

1. a 2. c 3. a 4. b 5. d 6. b 7. b

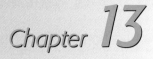

Chapter 13

Genetic Contributions to Psychiatric and Behavioral Disorders

KEY TERMS

Autism

Autism spectrum disorders (ASD)

Behavioral genetics

Behavioral phenotype

Biologically plausible

Copy number variants (CNVs)

Externalizing psychopathology

Introduction

Many psychiatric problems seem to run in families. However, most of the gene variants that contribute to major psychiatric problems provide us with only a glimpse of the heritability of these disorders. With new techniques such as genome-wide association studies (GWAS) and assessing **copy number variants** (usually either deletions or duplications of stretches of DNA) comes the promise that some of the mysteries of mental illness will be solved. For the health-care professional, advances in genetic knowledge will contribute to more effective diagnoses and treatment of patients with psychiatric problems.

Applications of Genetics for the Psychiatric Patient

Pharmacogenetics and Pharmacogenomics

Finding the right drug to treat a psychiatric illness can be extremely difficult, and often patients are prescribed multiple drugs before the right one is found—if it ever is! Prescribed psychotropic medications may be effective in only a small group of patients or may be only partially effective (Zandi and Judy, 2010). Even when a drug is working to alleviate symptoms of mental illness, it produces side effects that range from unpleasant to debilitating. In one study, schizophrenic patients were followed for up to 18 months. More than 74% of these patients stopped taking their medication because it was either not helpful or the side effects were not tolerable (Lieberman et al., 2005). Weight gain and *tardive dyskinesia* (repetitive involuntary ticlike movements, often of the lower face) can be a problem for genetically vulnerable people taking first-generation antipsychotics (Lencz and Malhotra, 2009).

Leukopenia (below-normal numbers of white blood cells responsible for fighting infection) is a life-threatening problem for people taking clozapine, a second-generation antipsychotic. Although newer second-generation antipsychotics cause fewer adverse reactions and tend to work better for more people, they do cause weight gain, metabolic syndrome, sedation, and diabetes in some (Zandi and Judy, 2010). Adverse reactions can result in nonadherence in some patients. Not taking antipsychotic medication as prescribed increases the risk of relapse to more than five times that of people who take their medication regularly (Lencz and Malhotra, 2009). Because of this ongoing problem, health-care professionals specializing in psychiatry have been at the forefront of investigations into using genetics to find the right drug for the right patient (Potash, 2010).

Even though using genetic information to personalize the medication selection for psychiatric patients is exciting, there is much work to be done before pharmacogenetic testing is used widely for this population. It is still unclear exactly how genetic variations affect the ways in which people respond to their medications. Studies have produced conflicting results. There are probably many different biological pathways (and many different genes) involved in processing and excreting these drugs. In addition, environmental variants such as smoking, drinking alcohol, or being obese could also interfere with accurate predictions of drug response based on genetics (Zandi and Judy, 2010). You can read more about pharmacogenetics and pharmacogenomics in Chapter 15. This includes a specialized form of genetic testing called *drug response testing*.

Genetic Testing

Genetic testing may also help clinicians find the best diagnosis for a patient and identify the genetic risk among family members. DNA-based testing has been used successfully to diagnose single-gene neuropsychiatric and developmental disorders such as Huntington disease or fragile X. Through the use of GWAS, locating susceptibility genes can lead scientists to biological pathways they never suspected would be involved in the cause of a disease. This can help clinicians develop a clearer understanding of the disease process itself and, perhaps, find new ways to treat a challenging disorder (Potash, 2010).

Recently, companies have marketed direct-to-consumer (DTC) diagnostic and predictive genetic tests for some psychiatric disorders. One DTC test reported on the presence or absence of a single nucleotide polymorphism that had been associated with a two to three times increased risk of having bipolar disorder. The problem is that this association was supported by only one study. The Web site advertising this test stated that if you have this version of the gene, you are "three times more likely to have bipolar disorder" (Psynomics, 2010). Such a statement is misleading and could have a devastating effect on a person who tested positive but did not have appropriate access to a counselor for interpretation of this result.

Most experts in psychiatry would welcome genetic tests to help confirm clinical diagnoses. However, there is strong disagreement about whether these tests are at all meaningful, and there is great concern about "diagnostic tests" for mental illness being sold directly to the consumer. The consensus is that genetic testing for mental illness is in the very early stages of development, and at this point, these tests have very little clinical utility or validity. That means that the information provided by currently available psychiatric genetic tests is unlikely to help clinicians care for patients any better than not testing them (Mitchell et al., 2010). A more complete discussion of genetic testing can be found in Chapter 14.

Behavioral Genetics

It is important to remember that genes do not directly control behavior. We cannot say that someone is a thief because he inherited the "stealing" gene from his father. We do know that genes are important in determining how people develop and how effectively proteins are made. The field that focuses on the way gene variants affect how people act is called **behavioral genetics**. Many genes can have a significant influence on behaviors, particularly if we take into consideration the environment in which a person interacts with others. The interaction of genes, environments, and behaviors are very complex, and a genetic predisposition for a certain behavior may be altered over time with changes in diet and parenting. Experts disagree about the implications of current knowledge in behavioral genetics (Baker, 2004).

Many health-care professionals consider mental illness a behavioral disorder. It may not seem obvious at first; however, the symptoms of illness such as schizophrenia, personality, and mood disorders do appear as behaviors. Scientists who specialize in the field of behavioral genetics study the impact that variations in our genomes have on our behaviors. In this chapter we will review genetic contributions to autism spectrum disorders (ASDs), attention-deficit hyperactivity disorder (ADHD), affective disorders, schizophrenia, addictive disorders, and personality disorders. For a clear understanding of the phenotypes and pathophysiology of each of these disorders, it is important that you consult a reference that is specifically focused on discussing psychiatric disorders. A thorough explanation of these important problems is beyond the scope of this text.

Autism

Autism means that a person has difficulty with social interactions and the development of language, often accompanied by a narrow range of repetitive behaviors and interests (El-Fishawy and State, 2010). Autism is one of several syndromes that are grouped together as pervasive developmental disorders (PDDs). These include Asperger disorder and a few other less well-known problems such as Rett disorder. The category of **autism spectrum disorders (ASDs)** describes collections of symptoms that are like autism but do not quite meet the definition of PDD. Autism is common worldwide. The prevalence is estimated at about 0.1% overall. The actual prevalence of the entire autism spectrum is very difficult to estimate because the phenotype is far from exact. However, many sources serving the lay community say the prevalence of ASD is 1 in 166 (El-Fishawy and State, 2010).

Autism itself is widely variable and is seen as a collection of symptoms in hundreds of syndromes with a neurological basis (Table 13–1). For example, between 1% and 3% of people with autism have fragile X syndrome. However, about 50% of people with fragile X syndrome demonstrate the behaviors associated with autism. A specific genetic cause, such as fragile X, can be identified in only about 25% of children with autism. Exposure to some *teratogen* (a substance, disease, or condition occurring during pregnancy that can cause an identifiable birth defect) can be identified in a few cases; however, the specific cause is unknown for up to 80% of affected people (Miles et al., 2010). The genetic causes for autism include chromosomal abnormalities, which account for about 5% of cases, and copy number variants (CNVs), such as very small deletions and duplications, which account for about 10% to 20% of cases. Single-gene neurological disorders that have features of ASD account for another 5%. It is clear that most cases of ASD are the result of variations in several genes working together, probably with an environmental trigger (El-Fishawy and State, 2010).

Males are about four times more likely to be affected with ASD than females. The male-to-female ratio of those affected with Asperger syndrome is even higher at about 14 males to 1 female. These statistics would certainly support that there is some biological, perhaps genetic, reason for the differences in the risk for men versus women for ASD. It has long been believed that the genetic contribution to risk for autism was larger than for any other neurodevelopmental disorder.

Studies have found that monozygotic (identical) twin concordance is between 70% and 90%. That means that about 90% of the time, if one twin is affected with autism, the other identical twin will also be affected. They will both have the **behavioral phenotype** of autism. That means that they will both show the behavioral signs and symptoms that are associated with autism. Dizygotic (fraternal) twin concordance is about 10%. This may not seem very high at first glance, but it is about 100 times higher than the risk of autism in someone from the general population. That is a huge difference and indicates that, for some people, autism is highly heritable. Unfortunately, very little about the specific gene variants that increase susceptibility to autism is known (El-Fishawy and State, 2010).

TABLE 13–1

Examples of Known Genetic Causes of Autism Spectrum Disorders

Chromosome abnormalities	Maternally derived duplications (Angelman syndrome and Prader-Willi syndrome)
	Trisomy 21 (Down syndrome)
	Sex chromosome aneuploidies (XYY, XXY, XO)
Copy number variants	16p11.2 deletion
	15q13.3 deletion
Single-gene disorders	Fragile X syndrome
	PTEN macrocephaly syndrome
	Sotos syndrome
	Rett syndrome
	Tuberous sclerosis complex
	Neurofibromatosis type 1
	Timothy syndrome
	Smith-Lemli-Opitz syndrome
Metabolic conditions	Mitochondrial disorders
	Phenylketonuria
	Adenylosuccinate lyase deficiency
	Creatinine deficiency syndrome

Source: Miles, J. H., McCathren, R. B., Stichter, J., and Shirawi, M. (2010). Autism spectrum disorders. Retrieved November 25, 2010, from www.ncbi.nlm.nih.gov/books/NBK1442/.

Environmental Contributions

Although autism appears to be a complex (multifactorial) disorder involving the actions of many genes and possibly the environment, exposure to chemicals such as valproic acid, terbutaline, or thalidomide during pregnancy has been identified as a cause of autism. There are likely to be a number of other environmental triggers for autism as well. Symptoms of autism develop slowly in most children. However, for about 30% of people who are affected, symptoms begin between 18 and 24 months of age. This is called *regressive-onset autism*. Unfortunately, this is also the age at which many children are receiving immunizations, and this shared time frame has led to a major controversy about whether childhood immunizations cause autism. Numerous studies have refuted this connection, and the original research studies that supported it have been retracted. Even so, many parents are fearful that immunizations can cause autism and have chosen not to immunize their children. This has led to outbreaks of measles and increases in deaths of unprotected children (Miles et al., 2010).

Finding Genetic Associations

GWAS have linked a number of different genes to ASD. These include genes coding for proteins that are important in synapse formation and function and in neuronal cell adhesion and regulation. A number of neurodevelopmental genes have also been associated with ASD. Genes coding for sodium and calcium channels and neurotransmitters have also been associated. These proteins are important in the transmission of electrical and chemical signals between neurons in the brain.

It is essential that at least a three-generation family history be recorded when a person is diagnosed with ASD. Ask the family if there are any relatives with behavioral or language problems that might suggest ASD. Because the origins of ASD for most people are still unclear, a family history of any disorders that might possibly be related should also be included. For example, ask about and record a family history of alcoholism or other addictive disorders and any other social or psychiatric problems (Miles et al., 2010). Gathering this information can be helpful as scientists and clinicians work to understand this very complex and increasingly common problem.

Attention-Deficit Hyperactivity Disorder

About 5% of children worldwide may have attention-deficit hyperactivity disorder (ADHD) or one of its forms. Three subtypes have been described. These include an inattentive subtype, a hyperactive/impulsive subtype, and a combined subtype. Each of these results in some degree of difficulty with social interaction and academic performance. Whereas children without ADHD may become restless and not pay attention, these problems are severe to debilitating for children with this diagnosis. For a diagnosis of ADHD to be made, the observed behaviors must be inappropriate for the child's age and developmental level and must be present in a variety of situations. For example, a child who shows signs of inattention at school but can easily focus on a television program of interest to him or her is probably not showing signs of ADHD. It can be difficult to determine whether a child is being hyperactive or is just full of energy. The diagnosis must be made by a professional with knowledge and experience caring for children with hyperactivity.

For most people who are affected, hyperactivity lessens as they age. However, for about 2% to 4% of people, the problem persists into adulthood. Some of these affected adults will report problems with addictions or personality disorders. Some have been involved with the criminal justice system. As we saw with autism, boys are almost twice as likely as girls to be affected. In fact, there is sometimes an overlap in diagnosis between autism and ADHD.

Finding Genetic Associations

ADHD runs in families, and people have long suspected that there is a genetic connection. However, the lack of an obvious pattern of transmission in a given family argues against ADHD being due to the action of a single gene. Only 25% of people who report a history of hyperactivity during their own childhoods have an affected child (Sharp, McQuillin, and Gurling, 2009).

GWAS support the idea that ADHD is a complex (multifactorial) disorder caused by the actions of many gene variants along with environmental contributions. GWAS have found regions on more than 10 chromosomes that are associated with ADHD in some people. The strongest evidence comes from a meta-analysis that combined and analyzed the results of seven different studies. There is strong support that gene variants located in a specific region on chromosome 16 contribute to ADHD susceptibility (Sharp, McQuillin, and Gurling, 2009).

Some large studies have found copy number variants, gene duplications or deletions that are associated with ADHD in some children. Many of the genes that have been associated play a role in learning and behavior, so they are considered **biologically plausible**. This means that it makes sense to consider that a given gene might be involved based on knowledge of the protein it encodes. (These are also known as *candidate genes*.) Some genes that have been associated with ADHD are involved in the development of neurons and transmission across the synapse. Some are the same genes that have been associated with autism. One study found an association in four different sections of a gene that has been associated with restless leg syndrome, a problem that is common among people with ADHD (Sharp, McQuillin, and Gurling, 2009).

Finding the specific genetic contributions to ADHD would be helpful for a number of reasons. There is treatment that is effective for many people diagnosed with ADHD; it is not effective for all. Furthermore, the treatment is not a cure, and the drugs used can have some unpleasant side effects. Finding the genes responsible for ADHD would help scientists understand the pathophysiological origins of the problem and may lead to improved and targeted treatment. Even when a clinical diagnosis is possible, genetic/genomic knowledge has much to contribute to our ability to provide effective care.

Schizophrenia

Schizophrenia is a potentially incapacitating chronic psychiatric disorder with a prevalence of about 4 in 1000 people. The symptoms include episodes of psychosis with hallucinations and delusions. Often, people with schizophrenia have dulled emotions and disorganized thoughts with language difficulty and sometimes manic and depressive symptoms (Gejman, Sanders, and Duan, 2010). Symptoms usually begin in adolescence or early adulthood, often interrupting lives that have begun with so much promise.

There is no laboratory test that can determine if someone has schizophrenia, and sometimes the variability in the phenotype makes diagnosis based on clinical observation and self-report tricky. Not being able to clearly and specifically define the phenotype makes studying the genetics of a problem much more difficult. To make things even harder, we do not completely understand the pathophysiology of schizophrenia or even all that much about higher brain function!

Once again, there is a disease that is complex (multifactorial) and is due to the interactions of many genes, each exerting a small effect, combined with environment. Epigenetic mechanisms have also been suggested as possibly important in the onset of schizophrenia. *Epigenetics* refers to variations outside of the DNA sequence itself, such as those that alter gene expression by altering methylation patterns or histone proteins. Epigenetic changes can also be inherited. Epigenetic differences may account for the fact that monozygotic twin concordance for schizophrenia is only 40% to 50%, even though the genetic contribution to schizophrenia risk is probably much higher. Table 13–2 shows the estimated risk of someone developing schizophrenia when a relative is affected. The *heritability estimate* for schizophrenia is about 80%. Heritability estimates are the cause of the variation of the phenotype within a population and not causes within a given family. For example, even though the heritability estimate is 80%, that does not mean that if a mother is schizophrenic that each of her children has an 80% risk of being schizophrenic. It does mean that if we look at the variations in phenotype in specific populations, about 80% can be attributed to genetics and about 20% can be attributed to environment.

Environmental Contributions

It is clear from epidemiological studies that environment does play a role in the risk of schizophrenia. For example, the risk of schizophrenia is higher under the following conditions:

- Obstetrical complications
- Birth in urban environments
- Birth during famines

Prenatal infections have also been implicated, as has advanced paternal age. Advanced paternal age is an important risk factor for the development of some autosomal dominant disorders. Of course, there may be more environmental factors that have not yet been identified. However, even though environmental factors clearly increase schizophrenia risk, their contribution is very small compared with the contribution of genetic susceptibility.

TABLE 13–2

The Estimated Risk of Getting Schizophrenia When a Relative Is Affected

Relationship to the Person With Schizophrenia	Degree of Relationship (Genes Shared)	Risk of Developing Schizophrenia
General population	None	1%
First cousins	Third-degree relatives (12.5%)	2%
Uncles or aunts	Second-degree relatives (25%)	2%
Nieces or nephews	Second-degree relatives (25%)	4%
Grandchildren	Second-degree relatives (25%)	5%
Parents	First-degree relatives (50%)	6%
Siblings	First-degree relatives (50%)	9%
Children	First-degree relatives (50%)	13%
Dizygotic twins	First-degree relatives (50%)	17%
Monozygotic twins	Identical twin (100%)	48%

Source: Gottesman, I. I. Schizophrenia genesis: The origin of madness. New York: Freeman, 1991.

Finding Genetic Associations

GWAS indicate that copy number variants (CNVs) probably play an important role in the risk of schizophrenia. Although CNVs are common throughout the genome, sometimes they are associated with disease. One large study found that the largest deletions, some longer than 2 million base pairs, are found only in people with schizophrenia and not in normal controls (people without schizophrenia). The authors of this study suggest that it is these rare variations in the genome, which are more likely to be CNVs, that contribute to schizophrenia, rather than single nucleotide polymorphisms. Genetic causes of schizophrenia may also be different from person to person. This could be a reason why it has been so difficult to find the genetic cause of this disease, even though it has such a high heritability (Need et al., 2009).

The major histocompatibility complex (6p22.1) has been associated with schizophrenia in some studies. The gene *NOTCH4,* which is important in neurodevelopment, is found in this region. It is biologically plausible that defects in *NOTCH4* could be related to risk of schizophrenia. Other associated genes are important in the formation of synapses; the signaling of dopamine, glutamate, and serotonin; the synthesis of glutamate; and catecholamine metabolism (COMT) (Tiwari et al., 2010). Just as there is some overlap of symptoms, there is also some overlap among the genes that have been associated with schizophrenia and those associated with bipolar disorder.

Affective Disorders

Major depression and bipolar disorder are affective, or mood, disorders. Typically, people who have only depression (unipolar depression) do not also have mania. However, most people who have mania have episodes of depression. This is called *bipolar disorder* (formerly called *manic-depression).* Both types of affective disorders seem to be related. Many families report a history of both depression and bipolar disorder among their relatives. We would expect to see some commonalities and some differences as we look into the genetics of both. One meta-analysis of several GWAS found a region on chromosome 3 that was associated with both depression and bipolar disorder in the people they studied (McMahon et al., 2010).

Major Depression

Major depression is very common, affecting one is six persons in the United States at some point in their lives. Depression affects women twice as often as men. Major depressive disorder (MDD) is defined as having a minimum of one 2-week episode of depression. First-degree relatives of people with MDD have almost three times the risk of having depression than the general population. There are a number of different subtypes, including anxious depression, melancholic depression, MDD with psychotic features, and postpartum-onset depression. Overall heritability is estimated at about 50%. Again, do not be confused by this statistic. It does not mean that in every family, half of the risk is genetic and half is environmental. In fact, if we looked at a population with depression, heritability of 50% could mean that in half the families, it was 100% genetic and in the other half it was 0% genetic! If your patient has a first-degree relative with major depression, she or he probably has about two to three times the risk of having depression of someone from the general population who does not have a first-degree relative with depression. If her or his first-degree relative has had multiple episodes of depression (recurrent depression), the risk is even higher.

Bipolar Disorder

Bipolar disorder (BPD) is a serious mental health problem with episodes of mania and depression that usually follow each other in cycles. It can be completely disabling and is associated with a high suicide rate. The risk of someone having BPD over his or her lifetime is about 1%, although some sources estimate it a bit higher than that. The manic episodes consist of at least 1 week of elated or irritable mood that is accompanied by racing thoughts and highly pressured speech. The affected person is easily distractible and agitated and may engage in high-risk behaviors, including hypersexuality and out-of-control spending. They may experience psychosis but will certainly have difficulty working or socializing as they normally do. Hypomania is a milder version, lasting at least 4 days (Barnett and Smoller, 2009).

The genetic contribution to BPD is quite high. It has been estimated at being between 60% and 85% heritability. First-degree relatives of a person with BPD have about ten times the risk of BPD than the general population. They also have a three to four times greater risk of having unipolar depression. Monozygotic twin concordance is about 40%. Clearly, BPD and major depression are complex (multifactorial) diseases.

Environmental Risk Factors

There is some controversy about what environmental exposures increase the risk for affective disorders. Use of recreational drugs, such as cannabis or alcohol, is common among people with psychiatric disorders, and it is difficult to determine whether the drug use triggered the illness or if the illness triggered the drug use. Patients may self-medicate to help them cope with distressing psychiatric symptoms. In addition, there are clearly genetic influences on addictive behaviors, as we will see in the next section. At this point, there is little clinically useful information about the link between use of drugs and the onset of affective disorders (Barnett and Smoller, 2009).

Some people suggest that DNA methylation (an epigenetic phenomenon) may be important in the onset of several different psychiatric disorders. For example, we know that BPD is more common among children born to older fathers (advanced paternal age). This increase in risk could be caused by epigenetic changes from the father's exposure to environmental stressors over time (Barnett and Smoller, 2009).

Finding Genetic Associations

GWAS have the potential to identify new pathways for the targeted treatment of BPD. Those doing research in this area report that BPD is highly polygenic, which means that BPD is caused by many genes, each contributing a small effect. This means that genome-wide studies must include very large populations of patients and controls in order to tease out all the genes that are involved in this disease process. The goal is not only to better understand why and how BPD happens, but, most importantly, to also find better ways to treat it.

One example of progress in our understanding of genetic contributions to BPD involves the association between variants in the dopamine D2 receptor (DRD2) and BPD. Dopamine is a neurotransmitter that is very important in regulation of emotion, motivation, and the ability to feel a sense of reward. It is also the most common catecholaminergic neurotransmitter in the brain. It is *biologically plausible* that a gene involved with dopamine production or use might play a role in the onset of mood disorders. For example, we know that depression is common among people who have Parkinson disease, which is caused by low levels of dopamine. Dopaminergic drugs have been used to treat people who have depression that is resistant to conventional antidepressants. Several investigators have looked for a connection between dopamine and BPD. A meta-analysis of 14 separate studies supported the association of DRD2 variants and BPD (Zou et al., 2010). Although this is not the whole picture, research like this is moving the science forward.

Improvements in technology have allowed analysis of CNVs and GWAS. There is a lot of information being produced by these studies, but some investigators have questioned the usefulness of finding these very rare variations and saying that they are associated with disease, because they are present in very few individuals (Alaerts and Del-Favero, 2009). The challenge of finding genetic links for affective disorders is similar to the challenges of finding genetic links for schizophrenia. Both certainly run in families; however, the phenotype is somewhat variable and there is overlap with other disorders. In addition, these are diseases that are complex and most likely involve the actions of many genes and environment. We look forward to learning more about the genetic contributions to these difficult diseases.

Addictive Disorders

A *substance use disorder* is described as out-of-control drug use that is not consistent with adaptation and continues in spite of serious adverse consequences. People are considered dependent when there are signs of developing tolerance, they require higher doses, and there are symptoms of withdrawal when the drug is stopped. Unfortunately, these disorders are very common. Both alcohol and nicotine dependence and abuse affect about 13% of Americans. Another 6% of people are dependent on some other drug (Hartz and Bierut, 2010).

People with addictive disorders often carry a dual diagnosis (comorbidity). In one study, people who were addicted to substances (other than nicotine) were almost three times more likely to have a psychiatric illness than people who were not addicted. About 13% of the U.S. population is addicted to nicotine. The percentage is much higher, between 30% and 70%, in people who have been diagnosed with psychiatric illnesses. The most common causes of death among people with mental illness are premature cancer and heart disease, both of which can be directly linked to cigarette smoking. These two problems are so clearly interwoven that completing genetic studies that tease out the differences in genetic causes can be challenging (Hartz and Bierut, 2010).

Alcohol Dependence

Alcohol dependence is a complex (multifactorial) problem. It combines the effects of genes and the environment. The environmental contribution is fairly obvious, because a person must consume alcohol in some form in order to become dependent. However, the genetic contributions are fairly clear as well. The heritability estimate for addiction to alcohol is between 50% and 60% in both males and females (Hartz and Bierut, 2010). If a person has a first-degree relative who is alcohol-dependent, his or her risk of being alcohol-dependent is between three and eight times the risk of the general population. Of course, separating out *nature* (genetic input) and *nurture* (environmental input) can make things a bit more complicated! Are family members of alcoholics using or abusing alcohol because of a genetic predisposition or because they learned that alcohol use or abuse is a readily available coping strategy?

The first genetic information related to alcohol use and abuse came from studies of people of Asian descent. A significant number of Asians experience an unpleasant facial flushing and sometimes vomiting when they drink alcohol. This reaction is caused by a deficiency of the enzyme aldehyde dehydrogenase (ALDH2), which is important in the body's ability to metabolize ethanol. This deficiency may actually protect people from the risk of alcohol addiction. A mutation causing a deficiency in this enzyme was found in 41% of Japanese people in the general population but in only 2% of Japanese alcoholics (Hartz and Bierut, 2010).

This finding led researchers to look closely at the genes that code for proteins involved in alcohol metabolism, which occurs in the liver in a two-step process. The first step involves the conversion of ethanol to acetaldehyde. The enzyme involved in this process is alcohol dehydrogenase (ADH). The second step is the breakdown of acetaldehyde into water and acetate. The enzyme used in this process is aldehyde dehydrogenase (ALDH). People carry different versions of the genes (alleles) that code for these enzymes. That means that some people produce enzymes that are more effective at breaking alcohol down than those carried by other people. Studies have found that people who carry alleles for the more powerful versions of these proteins are more likely to be alcoholic. There also seems to be an increase in addiction to other substances in people with more efficient versions of these enzymes. This is simply an observation that has been described. Unfortunately, investigators do not really understand why there is this connection (Dick and Agrawal, 2008).

Genes that encode neurotransmitter proteins, such as GABA (gamma-aminobutyric acid) or acetylcholine, have also been associated with alcohol dependence. GABA is the most important inhibitory neurotransmitter. If you have more GABA (or more GABA receptors), fewer impulses will be transmitted across the synapse. Evidence suggests that alteration in GABA levels are involved in some of the behavior changes that are associated with alcohol intoxication, such as a decrease in anxiety, decreased coordination, and increased sedation. The GABA$_A$ receptor is made up of five subunits, which means that there are a lot of genes involved in making an efficiently functioning GABA$_A$ receptor and many opportunities to make a receptor that does not work very well (Dick and Agrawal, 2008). Acetylcholine is a neurotransmitter involved with memory, reward, and learning. It is typically an excitatory function. One of the acetylcholine receptors is encoded by a gene with a variant linked with alcohol dependence.

Another group of genes that has been associated with drug dependence are those involved in the endogenous opioid system. This system is composed of molecules made by the body that produce responses similar to those produced by morphine and heroin. The drug naltrexone is useful in the treatment of alcohol dependence because it works by blocking the action of the endogenous opioid system. The gene *OPRM1* codes for the μ-opioid receptor, and variations in this gene have been associated with alcohol dependence. Some of the genes involved in the endogenous cannabinoid system have also been implicated.

Summary of Addictive Disorders

There is clearly a connection between some types of mental illness and addictive disorders. Some authors have suggested that there is an overarching category of what is called **externalizing psychopathology**. This includes problems such as alcohol and other drug dependence. It also includes conduct disorders and antisocial personality disorder. Experts propose there is a group of gene variants that can increase susceptibility to all of these categories; however, there are also other gene variants that are specific for alcohol and other drug dependence. We can expect lots more information about these connections as the number of large studies of people with addictive behaviors increases.

Personality Disorders

A personality disorder is a collection of socially distressing feelings and behaviors that are different from what is expected in a person's culture and result in difficulty managing activities of daily living. Personality disorders tend to have their onset during adolescence or young adulthood and have historically been considered entirely learned behaviors. These are lifelong problems that typically do not respond well to medications and therapy. The specific traits vary from person to person, but they tend to remain fairly consistent and inflexible over a person's lifetime. Between 10% and 15% of adult Americans meet the criteria for at least one personality disorder. There are ten classifications divided into three clusters in the *Diagnostic and Statistical Manual IV–TR* of the American Psychiatric Association (APA, 2000). These are listed in Table 13–3 along with the prevalence of each in the U.S. population (Shedler and Westen, 2004). Providing a thorough description of each personality disorder is well beyond the scope of this text.

TABLE 13–3

Personality Disorders and Their Prevalence in the United States

Cluster A (odd, eccentric)	• Paranoid personality disorder: 0.5–2.5%
	• Distrustful and suspicious
	• May have aggressive outbursts or appear cold
	• Schizoid personality disorder: 3%
	• Detachment
	• Limited range of emotions
	• Schizotypal personality disorder: 3%
	• Eccentric thoughts and behaviors
	• Odd beliefs and magical thinking
Cluster B (dramatic, emotional)	• Antisocial personality disorder: 3% of men, 1% of women
	• Lack of empathy
	• Manipulative
	• Problems with impulse control
	• Borderline personality disorder: 2%
	• Unstable moods
	• Impulsive behavior
	• Difficulty in relationships
	• Histrionic personality disorder: 2–3%
	• Highly emotional
	• Attention-seeking
	• Narcissistic personality disorder: less than 1%
	• Sense of entitlement
	• Grandiose ideas
	• Arrogance
Cluster C (anxious, fearful)	• Avoidant personality disorder: 0.5–1%
	• Uncomfortable in social situations
	• Fearful of rejection
	• Dependent personality disorder: 0.5%
	• Clinging behavior
	• Need to be cared for
	• Obsessive-compulsive personality disorder: 1%
	• Preoccupied with order, cleanliness, and control
	• Lack of flexibility

Source: APA. *Diagnostic and statistical manual of mental disorders,* 4th ed., text revision ed. Washington, DC: APA, 2000; Shedler, J., and Westen, D. (2004). Refining personality disorder diagnosis: Integrating science and practice. *American Journal of Psychiatry, 161*(8), 1350–1365.

As we have seen with the other psychiatric disorders, personality disorders are complex (multifactorial) and involve the contributions of many genes (each exerting a small effect) and the environment. Until recently, little was known about the genetics of personality disorders. With the increased application of GWAS, we are starting to learn a bit more. However, there is still a long way to go before the genetic contributions to personality disorders are truly understood.

One of the major problems is the difficulty with identifying a clear phenotype. This is always a challenge, but having the ability to accurately describe a phenotype is essential if genetic studies are going to make any sense at all. Specialists debate whether personality disorders should be seen as separate categories or considered as one category having differing dimensions. Seeing them as separate categories would make genetic studies much easier, because there would be clearer phenotypes. However, consensus supports viewing personality disorders dimensionally, with some core factors that are shared in common (Reichborn-Kjennerud, 2010).

Normal personality traits tend to be very heritable, with between 30% and 60% of the difference attributable to genetics. If your parents are shy and reserved, you are more likely to be shy and reserved than if your parents are loud and extroverted. Of course, things are never simple; there are many families with wide variations in the normal personality traits of their children. Children in the same family also share environmental factors. Many experts believe that environmental factors may not have a major impact on the personality of the children (Reichborn-Kjennerud, 2010). Others strongly disagree, noting the social environment can produce stressors that require coping support that may be unavailable. This could result in a psychological vulnerability and learned behaviors that are dysfunctional (Eccles et al., 1993).

Some personality disorders have been studied far more than others. For example, there are significant genetic contributions to the Cluster A personality disorders. These are paranoid, schizoid, and schizotypal personality disorders. Heritability has been reported to be between 30% and 60%, which is about the same as the heritability of normal personality traits. The heritability of antisocial personality disorder has been reported as being between 75% and 80% (Gunter, Vaughn, and Philibert, 2010). As with autism spectrum disorders, antisocial personality is sometimes considered to be a spectrum of disorders with a common set of traits, which makes comparing studies less useful.

Some personality disorders have big differences in prevalence between the sexes. For example, *antisocial personality disorder* is three times more common among men than women, and *borderline personality disorder* is three times more common among women than men. It is difficult to know if these differences have cultural or biological roots, and it may be a bit of each.

Be cautious when looking at statistics about the prevalence of personality disorders, particularly borderline and antisocial personality disorders, which can be challenging to diagnose. Diagnosis is based on behaviors and does not necessarily follow criteria strictly. When a person is labeled with a particular diagnosis, it tends to follow them around, whether it is accurate or not. Clinicians note that, to clearly diagnose a personality disorder, the affected person must be seen for a considerable period of time, and an accurate history must be collected (Dr. Connie Wilson, personal communication, December 20, 2010).

Overall, there seems to be a significant genetic contribution to the risk of developing a personality disorder. There are also nongenetic and probably environmental risk factors that play a lesser but still important role. The number of people who have multiple problems, such as substance abuse, conduct disorders, and antisocial personality disorder, makes finding specific genetic links challenging. Nevertheless, we anticipate results from GWAS will make significant contributions to our understanding of the pathophysiology and susceptibility to personality disorders.

Summary

Psychiatric disorders are challenging for a variety of reasons. They are difficult to treat because people respond differently to drugs, and sometimes they are difficult to diagnose because of variations in the phenotype. Genetic/genomic studies have great promise in helping clinicians with both diagnosis and treatment. Pharmacogenetics and pharmacogenomics promise to provide drug response information that can be combined with clinical knowledge to improve patient care. However, there is a long way to go before we see significant clinical application of genetic testing for the diagnosis and treatment of psychiatric disorders. Studies are in process, and as genetic/genomic technologies improve, we can expect to see much useful genetic information reach the bedside.

GENE GEMS

- In the future, pharmacogenetics may help clinicians find a safe and effective psychotropic drug with minimal side effects to better treat patients.
- Complex biological pathways and the contributions of environmental factors make predicting responses to psychotropic drugs difficult.
- A few neuropsychiatric disorders, such as Huntington disease and fragile X, are caused by problems with single genes.
- Most psychiatric problems are complex (multifactorial), combining the effects of several genes working together with the environment.
- Genome-wide association studies (GWAS) can be helpful in identifying genes with variations that increase susceptibility to psychiatric disorders.
- Direct-to-consumer genetic tests exist; however, as with genetic testing to diagnose mental illness in general, their clinical usefulness is questionable.
- Behavioral genetics is the field that focuses on the ways in which gene variants affect how people act.
- Autism is a disorder of social interaction and language use that is often viewed as a pervasive developmental disorder called *autism spectrum disorder* (ASD). These disorders may have some genetic risk factors in common.
- Monozygotic twin concordance for autism is between 70% and 90%, meaning that the genetic contribution is very high.
- Symptoms of regressive-onset autism begin between 18 and 24 months of age, which is the age when many children receive childhood immunizations; however, there is no evidence linking immunizations and autism.
- Genes coding for proteins important in the generation and transmission of neural impulses have been associated with susceptibility to autism.
- Attention-deficit hyperactivity disorder (ADHD) seems to run in families; however, it does not follow an obvious pattern of transmission.
- When there is a lot of variety in the phenotype (e.g., schizophrenia), genetic studies are more difficult.
- Epigenetic factors may be important in psychiatric disorders such as schizophrenia.
- Both genetics and environment are important in determining susceptibility to schizophrenia.
- The heritability of major depression and bipolar disorder is very high, and both can be found in the same family.
- Addictive disorders are closely linked to other psychiatric problems, and they have both genetic and environmental contributions to susceptibility.
- Variations in genes that encode neurotransmitters such as GABA have been associated with alcohol dependence.
- The difficulty in placing personality disorders in discrete categories makes genetic studies more difficult.
- Personality disorders are highly heritable, much like normal personality traits.

Self-Assessment Questions

1. Schizophrenia is reported to have a heritability estimate as high as 80%. What does this mean?
   a. If a parent has schizophrenia, each child has an 80% risk of getting schizophrenia.
   b. If we look at a population, 80% of the risk for schizophrenia comes from genetics.
   c. If your patient's sibling has schizophrenia, her risk of getting schizophrenia is 80%.
   d. Genetics contributes 20% to the risk of schizophrenia.

2. Which statement best describes a major barrier to finding the genetic causes of psychiatric problems?
   a. Most psychiatric problems are single-gene disorders that follow standard modes of transmission.
   b. Psychiatric disorders are rare, making study recruitment difficult.
   c. For diseases such as schizophrenia and personality disorders, the phenotype varies widely.
   d. Most of these diseases are primarily due to environmental factors, with genetics contributing only a small percentage of risk.

3. Why is it so common for people with mental illness to also have addictive problems?
   a. They are caused by the same small group of genes.
   b. These disorders may share some genetic and/or environmental factors in common.
   c. The neurotransmitter GABA has been linked to nicotine dependence and schizophrenia.
   d. Opioid receptors are involved in both affective disorders and alcohol dependence.

4. How is it that personality disorders seem to run in families?
   a. Personality traits in general tend to be highly heritable.
   b. This is clearly due to shared environment.
   c. There is no environmental contribution to personality disorders.
   d. Twin concordance for Cluster A personality disorders is close to 100%.

5. How is the concept of "externalizing psychopathology" useful in explaining the genetics of psychiatric and addictive disorders?
   a. Conduct disorders include addictive behaviors.
   b. Antisocial personality disorder is highly heritable.
   c. All genes for these disorders are shared in common. It is environment that decides which disorder will occur.
   d. There are gene variants that increase susceptibility to all these disorders, and there are others that are specific to each individual disorder.

CASE STUDY

Margaret is a psychiatric nurse who has suffered from depression on and off throughout her life. Her father was an alcoholic and verbally abusive during her childhood. Margaret is doing well in adulthood. She is happily married to a very understanding man, and antidepressants are successfully treating her depression. She has not had a major episode in more than 5 years. Margaret has two young adult daughters. The younger daughter also has episodes of depression, which are treated with short-term antidepressants. Margaret is most concerned about her older daughter, who shows signs of cycling between being abnormally lively and spending irresponsibly and being down and not communicating for weeks at a time. The daughter is not interested in seeing a therapist and does not acknowledge that anything might be wrong. Margaret is afraid that her daughter has bipolar disorder and feels guilty about "causing" her older daughter's problem.

1. Do you think that there could be a genetic link between the problems of Margaret's dad, Margaret, and her daughters?

2. Would referral for genetic counseling benefit this family? Why or why not?

3. Do you think that an antidepressant that is successful in treating Margaret's depression might be useful for her daughter with depression? Why or why not?

4. How might genetic information help Margaret's older daughter agree to seek diagnosis and treatment for her problems?

References

Alaerts, M., and Del-Favero, J. (2009). Searching genetic risk factors for schizophrenia and bipolar disorder: Learn from the past and back to the future. *Human Mutation, 30*(8), 1139–1152.

APA. Diagnostic and statistical manual of mental disorders, IV-TR, 4th ed., text revision ed. Washington, DC: APA, 2000.

Baker, C. *Behavioral genetics.* Washington, DC: American Association for the Advancement of Science, 2004.

Barnett, J. H., and Smoller, J. W. (2009). The genetics of bipolar disorder. *Neuroscience, 164*(1), 331–343.

Dick, D. M., and Agrawal, A. (2008). The genetics of alcohol and other drug dependence. *Alcohol Research & Health, 31*(2), 111–118.

Eccles, J. S., Midgley, C., Wigfield, A., et al. (1993). Development during adolescence. The impact of stage-environment fit on young adolescents' experiences in schools and in families. *American Psychologist, 48*(2), 90–101.

El-Fishawy, P., and State, M. W. (2010). The genetics of autism: Key issues, recent findings, and clinical implications. *Psychiatric Clinics of North America, 33*(1), 83–105.

Gejman, P. V., Sanders, A. R., and Duan, J. (2010). The role of genetics in the etiology of schizophrenia. *Psychiatric Clinics of North America, 33*(1), 35–66.

Gunter, T. D., Vaughn, M. G., and Philibert, R. A. (2010). Behavioral genetics in antisocial spectrum disorders and psychopathy: A review of the recent literature. *Behavioral Sciences & the Law, 28*(2), 148–173.

Hartz, S. M., and Bierut, L. J. (2010). Genetics of addictions. *Psychiatric Clinics of North America, 33*(1), 107–124.

Lencz, T., and Malhotra, A. K. (2009). Pharmacogenetics of antipsychotic-induced side effects. *Dialogues in Clinical Neuroscience, 11*(4), 405–415.

Lieberman, J. A., Stroup, T. S., McEvoy, J. P., et al. (2005). Effectiveness of antipsychotic drugs in patients with chronic schizophrenia. *New England Journal of Medicine, 353*(12), 1209–1223.

McMahon, F. J., Akula, N., Schulze, T. G., et al. (2010). Meta-analysis of genome-wide association data identifies a risk locus for major mood disorders on 3p21.1. *Nature Genetics, 42*(2), 128–131.

Miles, J. H., McCathren, R. B., Stichter, J., et al. (2010). Autism spectrum disorders. Retrieved November 25, 2010, from www.ncbi.nlm.nih.gov/books/NBK1442/.

Mitchell, P. B., Meiser, B., Wilde, A., et al. (2010). Predictive and diagnostic genetic testing in psychiatry. *Psychiatric Clinics of North America, 33*(1), 225–243.

Need, A. C., Ge, D., Weale, M. E., et al. (2009). A genome-wide investigation of SNPs and CNVs in schizophrenia. *PLoS Genetics, 5*(2), e1000373.

Potash, J. B. (2010). Preface: Promises kept: robust discovery in psychiatric genetics. *Psychiatric Clinics of North America, 33*(1), xiii–xvi.

Psynomics. (2010). Psynomics, genetics for the new psychiatry. Retrieved December 10, 2010, from www.psynomics.com/.

Reichborn-Kjennerud, T. (2010). Genetics of personality disorders. *Clinics in Laboratory Medicine, 30*(4), 893–910.

Sharp, S. I., McQuillin, A., and Gurling, H. M. (2009). Genetics of attention-deficit hyperactivity disorder (ADHD). *Neuropharmacology, 57*(7-8), 590–600.

Shedler, J., and Westen, D. (2004). Refining personality disorder diagnosis: Integrating science and practice. *American Journal of Psychiatry, 161*(8), 1350–1365.

Tiwari, A. K., Zai, C. C., Muller, D. J., et al. (2010). Genetics in schizophrenia: Where are we and what next? *Dialogues in Clinical Neuroscience, 12*(3), 289–303.

Zandi, P. P., and Judy, J. T. (2010). The promise and reality of pharmacogenetics in psychiatry. *Psychiatric Clinics of North America, 33*(1), 181–224.

Zou, Y. F., Wang, F., Feng, X. L., et al. (2010). Association of DRD2 gene polymorphisms with mood disorders: A meta-analysis. *Journal of Affective Disorders.*

Self-Assessment Answers

1. b **2.** c **3.** b **4.** a **5.** d

Genomics and Disease Management

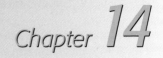

Chapter *14*

Genetic and Genomic Testing

Learning Outcomes

1. Use the genetic terminology associated with genetic testing.
2. Compare the different types of genetic tests.
3. Explain how differing frequencies of carriers in populations might affect the validity of genetic test results.
4. Discuss the implications of direct-to-consumer genetic testing.
5. Discuss the risks and benefits of genetic testing.
6. Identify dependable Internet-based resources for current information about genetic testing.

KEY TERMS

Carrier test

Cytogenetic test

Diagnostic test

Direct-to-consumer (DTC) genetic testing

DNA sequencing

Fluorescent in situ hybridization (FISH)

Genetic test

Genome-wide association study (GWAS)

Newborn screening

Polymerase chain reaction (PCR)

Predictive test

Predispositional test

Preimplantation genetic diagnosis (PGD)

Prenatal test

Presymptomatic test

Introduction

Genetic testing is the analysis of DNA, RNA, chromosomes, proteins, and protein metabolites to identify heritable variations in genes and/or chromosomes. Traditionally, genetic testing has been done for clinical and research purposes only, but with the advent of direct-to-consumer (DTC) offerings, genetic testing is also being done recreationally! We will spend some time at the end of this chapter discussing DTC testing and the risks and benefits, but first we will cover the types of genetic tests.

Currently, clinical genetic testing can be done for well over 2000 disorders (GeneTests, www.genetests.org), but getting a positive result for a genetic test can mean many different things, depending on the purpose of the test and the relationship of the gene variant or mutation to the disorder. Some gene variants have been shown to cause particular diseases. The ΔF508 mutation in the *CFTR* gene causes cystic fibrosis (CF). Other variants are merely *associated* with a disorder, which means that they are often found in people with the disorder, but we do not know if they *cause* the disease. For example, several polymorphisms located on chromosomes 1, 10, and 15 have been associated with coronary artery disease. That does not mean that everyone who has one, or even all, of these polymorphisms will get CAD (Samani et al., 2007).

The most up-to-date information about the availability of genetic testing can be found at www.genetests.org. This Web site is funded by the National Institutes of Health and is administered by the University of Washington, Seattle. In addition to information about genetic testing, gene.tests.org provides expert-authored, peer-reviewed articles about diseases with a genetic component and has a wealth of other educational materials on genetics in general.

Accurate patient information about genetic testing is available from a number of medical centers. Table 14–1 provides an example of patient information about genetic testing for hemophilia provided by Cincinnati Children's Hospital Medical Center. It includes information about how the disease is inherited and how carrier testing is done.

The Sample for Genetic Testing

If you watch television procedural crime dramas, you know that genetic material can be obtained from the most unlikely sources and that not a lot of genetic material is required to identify the killer. DNA from blood, saliva, skin, hair follicles, tissue blocks obtained in surgery, or biopsy samples from living or deceased persons can be extracted. The most commonly used samples are genetic samples of epithelial cells from cheek (buccal) swabs or saliva and leukocytes from blood. There are several categories of clinical genetic testing.

Types of Genetic Tests

Diagnostic Testing

Diagnostic testing is done to confirm or rule out a particular diagnosis in a symptomatic person. For example, Marfan syndrome (MFS), which is transmitted in an autosomal dominant fashion, is usually diagnosed based on clinical features, but some healthy patients have a body type similar to patients with Marfan syndrome (*marfanoid physique*). In some cases, even specialists are not certain that MFS is the correct diagnosis. Doing a genetic test for the gene variants known to cause MFS can make the diagnosis clear. For some diseases, standard clinical or biochemical tests may be a better choice than genetic testing. For example, in the case of cystic fibrosis, a sweat chloride test is still considered the best way to provide an accurate diagnosis, even though we know the gene that causes CF when it is defective.

Diagnostic genetic testing provides information about other family members as well as the person being tested. For example, your patient's parents may request genetic testing to confirm her diagnosis of CF. If she tests positive, then both of her biological parents are almost certain to be cystic fibrosis carriers, and each of her current or future siblings has a 50% risk of being a carrier and a 25% risk of being affected. Testing only one person in the family told us something about the genetic risk of several family members.

Predictive Testing

Predictive testing is for asymptomatic people who want information about their risk of getting a genetic disease in the future. There are two types of predictive testing. When a **presymptomatic test** is positive, the individual will get the disease he was tested for at some point in his future, as long as he

TABLE 14–1

Genetic Testing for Hemophilia

How It's Inherited

Hemophilia results from a defect in the genetic material of the body. This genetic material is called *deoxyribonucleic acid* or *DNA*. Any part of the DNA that controls an inherited trait is called a *gene*. Examples of inherited traits are eye color, hair color, and blood type. The most common forms of hemophilia result from defects in the genes that control the production of clotting factors VIII or IX.

Genes are present within the cell in packages called *chromosomes*. Most of the body's cells contain a complete copy of chromosomes and their genes. Among the chromosomes people inherit from their parents are two sex chromosomes, labeled X and Y. All males receive the X chromosome from their mother and the Y chromosome from their father. Females have two X chromosomes, one inherited from each parent.

The genes that control the production of the clotting factors VIII and IX are located in the X chromosome. Males (XY) have hemophilia when the gene for clotting factor VIII (hemophilia A, classical hemophilia) or clotting factor IX (hemophilia B, Christmas disease) on the single X chromosome is affected. Women (XX), who are carriers, generally don't have symptoms of hemophilia because only one X chromosome has a copy of the hemophilia gene. The other gene of the other X chromosome allows for normal production levels of clotting factors VIII or IX. Those women who have only one affected gene are called *hemophilia carriers*. Not all males with hemophilia have mothers who are carriers. Sometimes a mutation (a genetic change) occurs resulting in hemophilia. Currently, it is not known why this mutation happens.

Sons of women who carry the hemophilia gene have a 50% chance of inheriting the gene and having hemophilia. Daughters of women who are carriers have a 50% chance of also being carriers of hemophilia. In families where only one male is known to have hemophilia, it is usually possible to determine whether the hemophilia gene was passed from a mother who carries the gene or whether a new mutation occurred in the person with hemophilia.

Carrier Testing Procedure

The Hemophilia and Thrombosis Center at Cincinnati Children's Hospital Medical Center can perform genetic testing and counseling for hemophilia.

As part of genetic counseling, a physician or genetic counselor will take a family history and draw a family tree, called a pedigree. The pedigree generally includes three generations: children, parents, aunts, uncles, cousins, and grandparents. The pedigree helps identify people within the family who could be carriers of the gene. Women who are possible carriers of hemophilia could then choose to be tested.

Direct Mutation Testing

For hemophilia A and B, it is possible to look for mutations within the gene. This approach is called direct DNA testing and is the most accurate method for identifying carriers. A blood sample from the male family member with hemophilia is checked first. In about 98% of cases, a mutation can be identified. Next, a blood sample from the woman desiring carrier testing is obtained, and her DNA is checked for the specific mutation. Such testing is performed at specialized laboratories. Results are generally available in several weeks.

Linkage (Indirect) Testing

In some cases of hemophilia A and hemophilia B, a mutation cannot be identified. However, it may be possible to use indirect or linkage tests to determine the gene carrier status of females by tracking the gene in the family. Blood samples are obtained from the male with hemophilia and other family members. Patterns of linked DNA in the person with hemophilia are compared to the DNA in family members to check for the same pattern. Linkage testing is not as accurate as direct testing and does not provide information for all families. The genetic counselor will discuss these issues individually with families.

Continued

Who Should Have Carrier Testing for Hemophilia?

Because women rarely show symptoms of hemophilia, they can be carriers of the disorder without knowing it. Women related to a male with hemophilia, such as a mother, sister, aunt, or cousin on the mother's side, can be carriers and may want to have carrier testing. The daughters of a male with hemophilia are always carriers of hemophilia.

A women's decision about carrier testing or how she chooses to use that information can be influenced by many factors. These factors include the severity of the hemophilia that occurs in her family and her own desires and beliefs, as well as those of her partner. Women who are considering having children may find it most beneficial to have carrier testing before becoming pregnant. Females typically are tested for carrier status when they are old enough to make an informed decision, normally in the late teens or older.

Prenatal Testing

A woman with a family history of hemophilia A or B may wish to have the fetus tested during pregnancy. Making the decision to pursue prenatal screening is a personal choice and involves many factors. The risks and benefits of prenatal screening should be discussed with an obstetrician or genetic counselor.

During the 10th or 12th week of pregnancy, an outpatient test called *chorionic villus sampling* can be performed. A small amount of the developing placenta is obtained for testing. Another outpatient procedure called an *amniocentesis* can be performed after week 13 of pregnancy. During the amniocentesis, a small amount of fluid containing fetal cells is removed and tested for hemophilia if the fetus is male (XY).

Contact Us

For additional information about genetic testing or genetic counseling, contact the Division of Human Genetics, 513-636-4760.

Last Updated: October 2010

does not die from something else first! Testing for Huntington disease (HD) is a presymptomatic test. When a person tests positive for the disease-causing number of triplet repeats in the Huntington gene, that person will get HD if he lives long enough. Of course, HD has age-related penetrance, and usually symptoms appear between the ages of 35 and 55. HD has virtually 100% penetrance by age 80. This has made having genetic testing for HD a very difficult choice for those at risk. We will revisit some of the legal and ethical issues of HD testing in a later chapter.

Predispositional testing is done when having a gene variant increases the *likelihood* that a person will get a genetic disease, but that does not mean that the person is certain to get it. Testing for the breast cancer risk alleles (mutations in *BRCA 1* and *2*) is predispositional. Testing positive for a documented mutation confers an 85% risk of getting breast cancer over a person's lifetime. While this risk is high, it is not 100%, so something else must be happening (environment or additional gene variants) in those men and women who actually get sick.

Inconclusive Results

Unfortunately, there is another possible result besides positive or negative. If the person tested is found to have a gene variant, but it has not yet been linked to the disease in question, the results are considered "inconclusive." For example, if your patient is at risk for breast cancer and has a variation in *BRCA1* or *BRCA2* that has not been documented as increasing the risk of breast cancer but has also not been identified as a benign common variation, the results would be reported as "inconclusive." When a patient receives this result after a genetic test, he or she is often confused. We expect that persons with inconclusive results would continue high-risk monitoring according to recommendations, but it is essential that they receive appropriate counseling to help them understand what their results actually mean.

Carrier Testing

Carrier testing is done when persons have family members affected by a heritable disease, but they themselves are not affected. Carrier testing can also be done for persons who are at high risk of a genetic disease based on their ethnicity. Table 14–2 shows carrier frequencies of some genetic diseases in particular ethnicities. Most carrier testing is done for couples considering having children. For example, when two people of Ashkenazi Jewish (Eastern European) background plan to have children, they are often counseled to have carrier testing for diseases with risk alleles common in this population. Because these diseases are autosomal recessive or X-linked recessive, finding out if one or both persons in the couple carries the risk allele can be helpful in deciding whether to have children, to use technologically assisted reproduction (see the "Preimplantation Genetic Diagnosis" section), or to prepare for the possibility of having a sick child. Table 14–3 lists diseases that are common in people with Ashkenazi background. Carrier testing for this group of diseases can be done at the same time and is called an "Ashkenazi Panel" by some clinical laboratories.

Some genetic testing panels are targeted to people of specific ethnicities. For example, there are more than 1000 different mutations that can cause cystic fibrosis. Genetic testing for CF looks for the most common mutations. Many of these mutations are more common among people of some ethnicities than others. Mutation testing for CF varies based on a person's race and ethnicity. If an Asian patient is tested for the mutations that are most common among people of European descent, the Asian patient who is a CF carrier may receive a negative test result, because the mutation he or

---

TABLE 14–2

Carrier Frequencies in Selected Genetic Conditions

Disease	Population	Carrier Frequency
Cystic fibrosis	European American	1 in 29
	Ashkenazi Jewish	1 in 29
	Hispanic	1 in 46
	African American	1 in 65
Sickle cell disease	African American	1 in 10
	Mediterranean	1 in 40
Tay-Sachs disease	Ashkenazi Jewish	1 in 30
	French Canadian/Cajun	1 in 30
B-Thalassemia	Mediterranean	1 in 25
	African American	1 in 75

Data from: Basic Ashkenazi Genetic Disease Screen (Tay-Sachs, Canavan disease, familial dysautonomia, cystic fibrosis). Emory University, 2005; http://genetics.emory.edu/pdf/Emory_Human_Genetics_Basic_AJ_Panel.PDF; Jorde, L. B., Carey, J.C., and Bamshad, M. J. Medical genetics, 4th ed. Philadelphia: Elsevier, 2010.

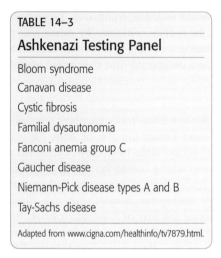

she carries is uncommon among Europeans. Thus, it is important to include information about ethnicity when requesting some tests.

Prenatal Testing

Once a woman is pregnant, **prenatal testing** can be done to determine if the fetus carries a specific gene variant or a chromosomal disorder. There are a number of different kinds of prenatal genetic tests. These tests vary by when they can be done, the disorders tested for, and the invasiveness of the procedure. The simplest are blood tests, commonly referred to as the first-trimester (done between 9 and 13 weeks of pregnancy) or quadruple-marker screens (done between 14 and 20 weeks of pregnancy). Screening maternal serum alpha-fetoprotein (MSAFP) can indicate the risk of neural tube defects. MSAFP is also used in Down syndrome screening, along with unconjugated estriol and human chorionic gonadotropin levels (NHGRI, 2006).

It must be remembered that many prenatal tests are not diagnostic—they are screening tests. Therefore, they will not provide a conclusive answer as to whether the baby is affected. Instead, they provide information that indicates if further testing is needed to confirm or rule out the presence of a disorder.

During the second trimester, an ultrasound can be done to visualize the fetus. Although an ultrasound does not provide specific genetic information, it does allow the baby to be evaluated for features consistent with a known genetic disorder. Fetal echocardiography, magnetic resonance imaging, and fetoscopy can also be done when attempting to diagnose a possible genetic problem in the fetus.

Tissue sampling and actual genetic testing can be done by chorionic villi sampling (CVS) between 10 and 12 weeks of pregnancy or by amniocentesis, which is generally done after week 14. Both procedures carry a small risk of causing a spontaneous abortion or intrauterine infection, but they allow direct evaluation of the baby's chromosomal complement.

Preimplantation Genetic Diagnosis

Preimplantation genetic diagnosis (PGD) is a process done in conjunction with in vitro fertilization. A group of embryos are tested prior to implantation when one or two cells are removed from the eight-cell blastocyst. Cells from each embryo can be tested to find gene variants causing single-gene disorders, chromosomal problems, or to determine sex. One or two "healthy" embryos are then selected for implantation. If the parents are concerned about an X-linked recessive disorder, which affects primarily boys, they may choose to implant only female embryos. Persons using PGD may also be older and concerned about the impact of advanced maternal or paternal age on the health of their baby. PGD is expensive and available in only a few cities. In addition, PGD may not be ethically acceptable to all families, because unwanted embryos are often discarded, but it offers an alternative to prenatal testing and pregnancy termination for couples willing and able to have the procedure.

Newborn Screening

Newborn screening is done to identify those infants at high risk of a variety of disorders for which immediate treatment or intervention is available. The tests are usually biochemical rather than gene-based, but results can indicate the likelihood of a genetic disorder being present. Newborn screening has been done since the 1960s, when Dr. Robert Guthrie developed the test to screen for phenylketonuria (PKU). Screening programs vary somewhat from state to state in the United States. Newborn screening programs are designed to protect the public health, and each state screens for up to 30 disorders, including hearing problems, heart problems, and infectious diseases. With the advent of tandem mass spectrometry, screening for more disorders has become easy and is a frequent addition to state screening programs. The four disorders screened for most commonly are PKU, congenital hypothyroidism, galactosemia, and sickle cell disease. All of these disorders are autosomal recessive. States are also responsible for follow-up on any positive result, so when a state adds a newborn screen to its list, the decision also has a financial impact (NNSGRC, 2009).

Other Types of Genetic Testing

There are several other types of genetic testing used by consumers to answer questions that are unrelated to disease risk. Zygosity testing is used to determine if twins are *monozygotic* (identical) or *dizygotic* (fraternal). Sometimes dizygotic twins look so similar that it is difficult to tell without testing their genotypes! Parentage testing has become very popular on daytime talk shows. It is used to determine whether family relationships are biological in nature. Knowing one's biological parents allows a person to report an accurate medical family history. Table 14–4 lists the types of genetic testing, interpretation, and follow-up.

Oversight of Genetic Testing

The stakes are high when considering genetic testing. False negatives from a prenatal test could result in the unexpected birth of a critically ill child, while false positives could result in the termination of a normal pregnancy. All laboratories performing such tests must be certified under the Clinical Laboratory Improvement Act (CLIA). Sometimes families choose to participate in research studies that incorporate genetic testing. It is important for them to find out if they will receive their genetic test results and if the laboratory doing the testing is CLIA certified. Many research laboratories are not CLIA certified, and the results they provide should not be used to make health-care decisions (NHGRI, 2006).

Genetic testing in the United States is overseen by four different federal agencies: the Centers for Disease Control, the Centers for Medicare and Medicaid Services, the Food and Drug Administration, and the Office for Human Research Protections. The United States Department of Health and Human Services is working to improve the oversight of clinical laboratories that offer genetic tests. Not just the accuracy but also the clinical usefulness of all genetic tests must be established, and the ways in which these tests are done must be monitored. The Secretary's Advisory Committee on Genetics, Health, and Society (SACGHS) released a report in 2008 that recommended improvements in the oversight of genetic tests (2008).

TABLE 14–4

Types of Genetic Testing, Interpretation, and Follow-up

For Positive Test Results

If the test purpose was . . .	The interpretation is . . .	And follow-up includes genetic counseling* and . . .
Diagnostic testing	Clinical diagnosis is confirmed.	Medical management and treatment
Predictive testing	The likelihood of showing disease symptoms is increased.	Counseling for life planning; medical management if available
Carrier testing	The patient is a carrier.	Testing offered to partner; prenatal testing offered if indicated
Prenatal testing	A fetus is diagnosed with a specific condition	Pregnancy treatment/management or termination
Newborn screening	Disease in a newborn is suggested; carrier status in a newborn may be identified.	Confirmatory testing—if positive, medical management and treatment; carrier testing offered to parents

*Genetic counseling includes discussion of expected course of the disorder, possible interventions, underlying cause, risks to family members, reproductive options, support.

For Negative Test Results

If the test purpose was . . .	The interpretation is . . .	And follow-up may include . . .
Diagnostic testing	Clinical symptoms are unexplained.	Further testing and/or follow-up genetic consultation
Predictive testing	The likelihood of showing symptoms is decreased.	Counseling for survivor guilt and long-range life planning; no high-risk surveillance needed
Carrier testing	High likelihood that the individual is not a carrier; low risk of having a child affected with the condition in question	Testing offered to other family members if indicated
Prenatal testing	If fetus was symptomatic (e.g., by ultrasound findings), clinical symptoms remain unexplained and may need further investigation. If fetus was not symptomatic, the chance of the condition tested for is very small.	If fetus was symptomatic, further testing and/or pregnancy management; if fetus was not symptomatic, no follow-up
Newborn screening	The newborn is not expected to have the condition tested for.	No follow-up

(Revised March 4, 2009)
www./genetests.org; University of Washington, Seattle

Laboratory Methods Used for Genetic Testing

DNA Sequencing

DNA sequencing refers to the analysis of the bases in a stretch of DNA. Laboratories most commonly look at the sequence of nucleotides in the regions that code for protein (exons) and the intron/exon boundaries, or splice sites. Now, the introns themselves and the regions between genes (intergenic regions) are sometimes being considered because they may contain sequence variations in regulatory sequences like promoters or silencers. DNA sequencing is the most accurate and most specific test used in identifying gene variants.

To evaluate a sequence, a DNA sample is extracted from some body fluid or tissue. Laboratories usually use leukocytes from blood or epithelial cells from saliva or buccal samples. Any cell with a true nucleus can be used (as any fan of television procedural crime dramas knows). The process of **polymerase chain reaction (PCR)** is used to amplify (greatly increase the quantity of) tiny amounts of DNA for examination. While the process is not complex, it does take some time.

An electropherogram is a graphic illustration of the nucleotide sequence in a stretch of DNA amplified by PCR. Different colored spikes correspond to one of the four DNA bases (A is green, T is red, C is blue, and G is black). The lab technician can read the electropherogram and report any variations between the sequence found in the patient sample and the order that is reported to be the common sequence (or *wildtype*).

Cytogenetic Testing

Cytogenetic testing involves the evaluation of whole chromosomes for variations in structure or number. Cytogenetic testing is done in a variety of situations. For example, a chromosome study is often done when evaluating a possible genetic cause for infertility or developmental disability. Cancer tumor cells can also be evaluated by cytogenetic testing. For example, if a person has chronic myelogenous leukemia, finding a 9:22 translocation (Philadelphia chromosome) can help clinicians choose a targeted therapy. Cytogenetic testing is also used if a prenatal screen shows that a fetus may have Down syndrome. In such a case, the fluid from amniocentesis can be tested to determine if cells have an extra chromosome 21.

In order to observe and identify individual chromosomes, cells must first be cultured and stopped during the stage of metaphase in cell division. During metaphase, chromosomes are condensed and it is easier to identify them individually. The chromosomes are spread out on a slide and are stained for better visibility under a microscope. Persons trained in cytogenetics can look at the banding pattern and the size of the chromosomes and determine which one is which. The result is a karyotype, such as those you saw in Chapter 5, Figures 5–1 and 5–3.

Fluorescent In Situ Hybridization (FISH)

Fluorescence in situ hybridization (FISH) is a laboratory test that uses a string of fluorescently labeled nucleic acids (DNA bases) that are complementary to the bases in an area of interest on a section of a chromosome or on a strand of DNA or mRNA. The string of bases is called a *probe*, and they are designed to glow (or fluoresce) in the presence of a specific dye. The probe is attached or hybridized to the sequence of interest, which is most commonly a string of single-stranded DNA. When a cell containing the probe hybridized to the complementary strand of DNA is examined under a fluorescence microscope, the region of interest will glow.

For example, a laboratory technician can use FISH to determine whether a cell taken from the amniotic fluid contains two or three copies of chromosome 21. To do this, a fluorescent probe that is complementary to a region on chromosome 21 would be designed and allowed to hybridize (bind) with the patient's chromosomes. The number of chromosomes glowing would be counted. If there were three chromosomes glowing in each cell, the test would be positive from trisomy 21.

FISH can be used to determine whether a person carries a translocation. Probes for each chromosome are dyed with different colors of fluorescent dye. If chromosome 9 shows a region the color of chromosome 22, and chromosome 22 shows a region the color of chromosome 9, a 9:22 translocation has occurred. FISH is also used to detect deletions, microdeletions, or duplications of chromosomal material.

Genome-Wide Association Studies

Genome-wide association studies (GWAS) are used by researchers to find areas of the genome that are associated with disease. The process involves the use of genetic markers or, more commonly, single nucleotide polymorphisms (SNPs). The genomes of large numbers of people (often about 1000) with a given disease are compared with the genomes of people (also about 1000) without the disease, to look for gene variations that are more common in the people who have the disease. Once regions of interest are identified, they are said to be "associated" with the disease, and the genes located in those regions can be examined further. This technique is possible because of contributions from the Human Genome Project, which was completed in 2003, and the Human HapMap Project, in 2005.

GWAS are most useful in studying genetic variations that contribute to complex or multifactorial diseases such as diabetes mellitus type 2, Parkinson disease, heart disease, obesity, or asthma. It is very difficult to establish the genetic risk factors for complex diseases, because they usually involve many genes that each contribute a small amount of risk combined with environmental risk factors. Studies are ongoing and some have produced exciting results.

In 2005, scientists used GWAS to find a genetic risk factor that contributed to age-related macular degeneration (AMD), the most common vision disorder in older people. AMD blurs "straight-ahead vision," often making reading difficult and driving unsafe. Three separate studies found a variation in the gene for complement factor H, which produces a protein that regulates inflammation. The idea that inflammation played an important part in the onset of macular degeneration was new to people investigating this disease (NHGRI, 2010).

Direct-to-Consumer Genetic Testing

During the last few years, many companies have begun to offer **direct-to-consumer (DTC) genetic testing**, most commonly over the Internet. A wide range of tests are available, including tests for single-gene disorders, such as heritable breast cancer, and some for multifactorial diseases. Some companies offer limited contact with a genetic counselor, while others do not. Making genetic testing available without extensive counseling by genetic professionals raises some interesting concerns. While some people believe they have the right to learn about their genetic risk on their own, whether or not they have enough information to properly understand their results is another matter entirely.

The American College of Medical Genetics (ACMG, 2008) and the American Society of Human Genetics (ASHG, 2007) have issued statements on DTC genetic testing. Both organizations are adamant that a knowledgeable professional be involved in ordering and interpreting genetic tests. The ACMG lists concerns such as "lack of informed consent, inappropriate testing, misinterpretation of results, testing that is inaccurate or not clinically valid, lack of follow-up care, (and) misinformation . . ." (ACMG, 2008). Other concerns include the strength of the scientific evidence on which the tests are based and whether the companies are sufficiently protecting their customers' privacy. Clinicians fear that inaccurate or misunderstood results could lead people to take health and lifestyle risks by doing things such as continuing to smoke because they think their risk of cardiovascular disease is low or choosing not to have screening mammograms because they think that having no sequence variations in *BRCA1/2* means they have no risk of getting breast cancer. Furthermore, DTC genetic testing is not cheap, costing between $300 and $3000 (or much more), depending on the extensiveness of the test (Brody, 2009).

It is important for you to guide your patients to genetics professionals rather than the Internet when they are considering genetic testing. There is currently no federal oversight of genetic testing, and only 11 states require that the consumer sign a consent form (Brody, 2009). The companies that offer these tests often imply that they are being offered for recreational use and that they should not be used for clinical decision-making, but it is unclear about how consumers view these test results and what actions they might take based on them.

The Risks and Benefits of Genetic Testing

There are potential risks and benefits when having genetic testing. For example, knowing that you do not carry the family's gene variant for colon cancer means that you can adhere to the general recommendations for colonoscopy screening rather than the more frequent screenings recommended for those who have a genetic risk. Being tested can reduce uncertainty. A positive predictive test can allow the patient time to prepare for the likelihood of becoming ill, and a negative test can relieve his or her worry. Table 14–5 shows two sample laboratory reports for genetic tests provided courtesy of Cincinnati Children's Hospital Medical Center. One reports the results of mutation analysis for cystic fibrosis. The second reports test results for mutations that can result in an autosomal recessive form of nonsyndromic hearing loss. These reports would be provided to the health-care practitioner ordering the tests.

Counseling is essential before undergoing a genetic test. The meaning of positive, negative, and inconclusive results should be discussed with a genetics professional prior to testing. Genetics professionals include genetic counselors, genetic nurses, or medical geneticists. There are currently only 1200 genetic counselors in the United States, so having access to quality genetic counseling may be difficult, but its importance cannot be overemphasized. Patients and their families should be led through a discussion of options for managing the range of possible results. Genetic counselors have training that allows them to explain the many different types of genetic tests and what tests are appropriate given the family history. Most importantly, they can guide a family through the difficult decisions both before and after genetic testing is done.

Genetics services are usually provided through major medical centers or private clinics that specialize in genetics. They are often organized by specialty, so you may find genetic counselors or genetics nurses that specialize in prenatal, pediatrics, adult, or cancer genetics. You can help your patients locate genetics professionals in your area by consulting the Clinic Directory at genetests.org (NCBI, 2009). More information about the types of services offered by genetics professionals can be found in Chapter 16.

Important issues such as the right to privacy, informed consent, and confidentiality are crucial when considering genetic testing. These topics will be discussed in Chapter 17.

Summary

Genetic testing is becoming much more common. It is being used clinically to help predict or diagnose genetic disease. Advanced reproductive technologies are being used to screen embryos for sex or genetic traits in the process of preimplantation genetic diagnosis. Genetic tests are even being sold directly to

TABLE 14–5

Sample Laboratory Reports Courtesy of Cincinnati Children's Hospital Medical Center: Mutation Analysis for Cystic Fibrosis and GJB2 (Connexin 26) Gene Mutation Analysis

Cystic Fibrosis

RESULT: Positive Findings—Carrier

Cystic fibrosis (CF) is a common autosomal recessive disease affecting primarily Caucasians of Northern European descent, with an incidence of approximately 1 in 2500 to 3300 live births and a carrier rate of 1 in 25 to 29. Cystic fibrosis is caused by mutations in the cystic fibrosis transmembrane conductance regulator (CFTR) gene located on the long arm of chromosome 7 (7q31.2).

METHODOLOGY–MUTATIONS ANALYZED:

DNA was isolated from the sample and screened for the 23 ACMG/ACOG CF mutations listed below. The analysis was performed using polymerase chain reaction (PCR)–amplified segments of the CFTR gene and allele-specific oligonucleotide hybridization.

2184delA	G551D	3659delC	R117H	1898+1G>A
A455E	R553X	N1303K	621+1G>T	711+1G>T
ΔI507	R560T	W1282X	2789+5G>A	3120+1G>A
ΔF508	1717-1G>A	R334W	3849+10kbC>T	
G542X	R1162X	R347P	G85E	

RESULT SIGNIFICANCE:

This individual has a self-reported positive family history of cystic fibrosis (CF). Using the methodology described above for the 23 mutation screening panel recommended by the American College of Obstetrics and Gynecology (ACOG), we have found that this patient has one copy of the following mutation, indicating that this individual is a carrier for CF: INSERT MUTATION

CLINICAL RECOMMENDATIONS:

The above interpretation and findings assume that the individual is NOT clinically affected with CF. Genetic counseling is strongly recommended for this patient and for carrier screening analysis to be offered to relatives and reproductive partners of known CF mutation carriers. You can arrange for further testing and genetic counseling by calling (513) 636-4760.

Detailed methodologies available on request. Should you have any additional questions regarding these findings or their implications, please do not hesitate to contact us.

REFERENCES

1. Bobadilla J. L., et al. (2002) *Human Mutation, 19*, 575–606.
2. Grody, W. W., et al. (2001). *Genetics in Medicine 3*(2), 149–154.

This test was developed and its performance characteristics determined by the Molecular Genetics Laboratory. It has not been cleared or approved by the United States Food and Drug Administration. The FDA has determined that such clearance or approval is not necessary. This laboratory is certified under the Clinical Laboratory Improvement Amendments of 1988 (CLIA) as qualified to perform high-complexity clinical laboratory testing.

TABLE 14–5

Sample Laboratory Reports—cont'd

GJB2 (Connexin 26) Gene Mutation Analysis

RESULT: AFFECTED

As part of the comprehensive hearing loss detection program at the Molecular Genetics Laboratory and the Center for Hearing and Deafness Research (CHDR), GJB2 sequence analysis has been completed in (name of patient). This patient has two mutations in GJB2.

The GJB2 finding is: Allele 1: _ Allele 2: _

Mutation nomenclature is based on the recommendation by American College of Medical Genetics that nucleotide +1 is designated the A of the ATG-translation initiation codon.

CLINICAL SIGNIFICANCE:

The most likely cause of hearing loss in this patient is DFNB1 (autosomal recessive nonsyndromic hearing loss locus #1). At this point, further diagnostic evaluation is most likely not warranted (Preciado et al., 2004).

According to our research from the CHDR, hearing loss associated with DFNB1 is generally more severe than for patients without DFNB1.

Particularly, if both alleles have nonsense mutations, 70% to 90% of patients will have severe to profound hearing loss. If at least one of the mutations is a missense mutation, almost 80% of patients will have mild to moderate hearing loss (Lim et al., 2003).

The audiogram shows _____. If not already done, a consultation with an experienced pediatric audiologist for amplification should be considered.

GENETIC SIGNIFICANCE:

Genetic counseling is strongly recommended for family-specific assessment of genetic risks. Hearing loss secondary to GJB2 mutations is inherited as an autosomal recessive condition. The parents of this child are obligate carriers of DFNB1 related hearing loss. Confirmation of their heterozygous carrier status by mutation analysis is recommended. The recurrence risk of hearing loss in each full sibling of this patient is 25% (one in four). Carrier testing of at-risk family members is available by mutation analysis.

CLINICAL RECOMMENDATIONS:

There are no further clinical recommendations at this time. If you have any further questions or concerns about this testing or any other issues relating to hearing loss, including treatment such as hearing aids and cochlear implantation, please feel free to contact me, Dr. John Greinwald, at the Center for Hearing and Deafness Research (513-636-4870). Likewise, I would be glad to see this patient in consultation.

Genomic DNA was isolated from the above stated specimen. The coding region and exon 1/intron 1 boundary of the GJB2 gene (13q12) was analyzed by PCR and sequencing using the reference M86849. Sensitivity of DNA sequencing is over 99% for the detection of nucleotide base changes, small deletions and insertions in the regions analyzed. Multiple exon deletions and insertions may not be identified by this methodology. Detailed methodologies are available on request.

References:

1. Preciado, D. A., et al. (2004).
2. *Otolarnygol Head Neck Surg, 131*(6), 804–809.
3. Lim, L. H., et al. (2003). *Arch Otolarnygol Head Neck Surg, 129*(8), 836–840.
4. Scott, D. A., Kraft, M. L., et al. (1998). *Human Mutation, 11*, 387–394.

This test was developed and its performance characteristics determined by the Molecular Genetics Laboratory. This test utilizes the Applied Biosystems 3730xl Genetic Analyzer operated by the Cincinnati Children's Hospital Medical Center Genetic Variation and Gene Discovery Core Laboratory. It has not been cleared or approved by the United States Food and Drug Administration. The FDA has determined that such clearance or approval is not necessary. This laboratory is certified under the Clinical Laboratory Improvement Amendments of 1988 (CLIA) as qualified to perform high-complexity clinical laboratory testing.

Source: Reports courtesy of Cincinnati Children's Hospital Medical Center

consumers over the Internet. Many genetics professionals are concerned that people will choose to have genetic tests without receiving counseling from health-care professionals who have genetic expertise. This could result in people taking tests they do not need or in misinterpreting the results. It could have negative implications for family dynamics because genetic tests often tell us something about the family, as well as the person being tested. Advances in genetic testing have brought with them many new and challenging ethical dilemmas.

GENE GEMS

- Genetic testing includes the testing of DNA, RNA, chromosomes, protein products, and protein metabolites.
- Clinical genetic testing is available for more than 2000 different diseases.
- Some gene variants may be found in many people with a disease, while not necessarily being the cause of the disease.
- Updated information about genetic testing can be found at www.genetests.org.
- A sample for genetic testing can be taken from many body fluids or tissues, but the most common sources are buccal swabs, saliva, and blood.
- Predictive genetic testing is used to find out how likely it is that an asymptomatic person will get a genetic disease.
- Carrier testing is used to find out if a person who has a genetic disease in his or her family can pass the disease on to his or her children.
- Carrier frequencies for genetic diseases vary in populations.
- Preimplantation genetic diagnosis can be used to screen and select unaffected embryos for implantation.
- Direct-to-consumer genetic testing is controversial.
- There are potential risks and benefits of genetic testing.
- Genetic counseling is essential before having a genetic test.

Self-Assessment Questions

1. Genetic testing that examines an *asymptomatic* person's DNA sequence, looking for mutations that increase a person's susceptibility to a disease, is an example of which type of testing?
   a. Diagnostic testing
   b. Predispositional testing
   c. Presymptomatic testing
   d. Cytogenetic testing

2. Which of the following types of testing is most likely to be done when a healthy couple would like to know if they might pass on a recessive condition to their baby?
   a. Prenatal screening via chorionic villa sampling
   b. Prenatal screening via amniocentesis
   c. Carrier genetic screening
   d. Multiple marker screening

3. Which of the following types of genetic testing will confirm that the individual will *eventually* develop the disease if she or he lives long enough?
   a. Diagnostic
   b. Carrier testing
   c. Presymptomatic
   d. Predisposition

4. A woman with a family history of a breast cancer gene mutation is tested for variations in *BRCA1* or *BRCA2*. How would you explain her results?
   a. If she has a negative result, she will not develop breast cancer in her lifetime.
   b. If she has a negative result, she has a lower risk of developing breast cancer than the general population.
   c. If she has a positive result, she will definitely develop breast cancer in her lifetime.
   d. If she has a positive result, she has a much greater risk of developing breast cancer than the general population.

5. Which of the following is *true* about access to genetic testing?
   a. A person cannot get a genetic test without a doctor's order.
   b. Genetic counseling is a requirement before a person can get a genetic test.
   c. Genetic testing is inexpensive and fun!
   d. In many states, genetic testing can be obtained from companies that advertise directly to consumers.

6. Where can you find up-to-date information about the availability of genetic testing for clinical and/or research purposes?
   a. http://genetictestsforyou.com
   b. www.genetests.org
   c. Your textbook
   d. From an Internet search for "genetic testing"

CASE STUDY

Your patient Marge and her husband met at a support group for the siblings of persons with sickle cell disease (SCD). They want to have children but are afraid of having a child who has SCD. They ask you what you think about preimplantation genetic diagnosis (PGD) for their situation.

1. Is PGD an appropriate test for them?

2. Should they wait until Marge is pregnant to have prenatal testing?

3. Is there any danger in having a PGD?

4. Is there another kind of testing they could use to determine their carrier status?

References

ACMG. ACMG Statement on direct-to-consumer genetic testing. Bethesda, MD: American College of Medical Genetics, 2008.

ASHG. (2007). ASHG statement on direct-to-consumer genetic testing in the United States. *American Journal of Human Genetics, 81*, 635–637.

Brody, J. E. (2009). Buyer beware of home DNA tests. *New York Times.*

GeneTests/University of Washington, Seattle, 1993–2010; www.genetests.org.

NCBI. (2009). GeneTests.org. Retrieved August 10, 2009, from www.ncbi.nlm.nih.gov/sites/GeneTests/?db=GeneTests.

NHGRI. (2006). Reproductive genetic testing. Retrieved August 6, 2009, from www.genome.gov/10004766.

NHGRI. (2010). Genome-wide association studies. Retrieved March 17, 2011, from www.genome.gov/20019523.

NNSGRC. (2009). National newborn screening professional resources. Retrieved August 5, 2009, from http://genes-r-us.uthscsa.edu/index.htm.

SACGHS. (2008). Report of the Secretary's Advisory Committee on Genetics, Health, and Society. Retrieved July 15, 2010, from http://oba.od.nih.gov/oba/SACGHS/reports/SACGHS_oversight_report.pdf.

Samani, N. J., Erdmann, J., et al. (2007). Genome-wide association analysis of coronary artery disease. *New England Journal of Medicine, 357*(5), 443–453.

Self-Assessment Answers

1. b **2.** c **3.** c **4.** d **5.** d **6.** b

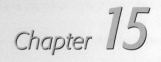

Chapter *15*

Assessing Genomic Variation in Drug Response

Learning Outcomes

1. Use the genetic terminology associated with pharmacogenetics.
2. Identify the goals of pharmacogenetics.
3. Explain the variation in drug responses when an agonist drug binds to the receptor and when an antagonistic drug binds to the receptor.
4. Compare the expected outcomes for drug responses among poor metabolizers, extensive metabolizers, and ultrametabolizers.
5. Describe the known effects of specific ethnicities as a factor in drug effectiveness.
6. Explain why some individuals experience no pain relief from high doses of codeine but do obtain relief with lower doses of morphine.
7. Explain why genotyping is not always accurate in predicting drug responses.
8. Describe variation in response to specific drugs related to differing levels in metabolizing enzymes.

KEY TERMS

Absorption

Agonist

Antagonist

Bioavailability

Elimination

Enterohepatic circulation

First-pass loss

Intended action

Metabolism

Minimum effective concentration (MEC)

Pharmacodynamics

Pharmacogenetics

Pharmacogenomics

Pharmacokinetics

Prodrug

Receptors

Side effects

Targets

Therapeutic effect

Introduction

Pharmacogenetics or pharmacogenomics is the study of how inherited variations in DNA affect the ways people respond to medications. Technically, **pharmacogenetics** refers to the effects of single-gene variations, and **pharmacogenomics** refers to the genome-wide effects. Although many people use the terms interchangeably, single genes do not work in isolation. Also, we are learning more and more about the complex pathways that lead to protein production and use, so *pharmacogenomics* (PGx) is usually the preferred term.

Pharmacogenetics is not a new idea. In fact, the term was first used in the 1950s after a physician discovered that people responded differently to medications because they had varying levels of metabolic enzymes. These variations in drug response were first written about by Pythagoras more than 2000 years ago, so although PGx seems like a new and exciting field, the ideas that form its basis have been around for a very long time.

The variations in individual drug response are based on polymorphisms in genes coding for metabolizing enzymes, transporters, and receptors (Fig. 15–1). The clinical responses to these differences can range from life-threatening adverse reactions (ADRs) to a complete lack of therapeutic effect. About 20% of drugs produce adverse reactions that were unknown when the drugs first came to market, and adverse drug reactions are considered one of the leading causes of death.

Many things alter the way our bodies use the drugs we take. Some examples are age, body mass index (BMI), tobacco or alcohol use, comorbid conditions, and alterations in organ function. Polymorphisms in genes involved in the drug response account for the largest portion of variation from person to person (Table 15–1). Genetic polymorphisms may lead to nonfunctional, super-functional, or absent proteins. The phenotype is often recognized before the genetic basis responsible for the drug response variation is known. If a patient develops a toxic reaction to a drug when the standard dose is

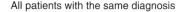

All patients with the same diagnosis

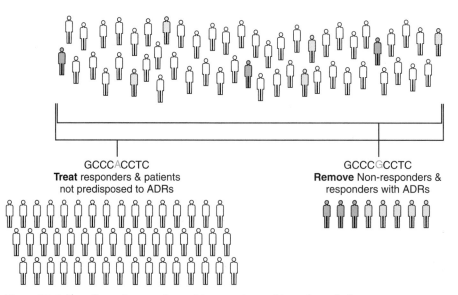

GCCCACCTC
Treat responders & patients
not predisposed to ADRs

GCCCGCCTC
Remove Non-responders &
responders with ADRs

Figure 15–1. The effects of gene polymorphisms on drug activity and metabolism.

> **TABLE 15–1**
>
> ## Personal Factors Affecting Drug Metabolism
>
> | Category | Factor |
> | --- | --- |
> | Physiological | Genetic polymorphisms in enzymes responsible for drug metabolism and elimination* |
> | | Age |
> | | Albumin and prealbumin blood levels |
> | | Cardiovascular function |
> | | Circadian rhythm variation |
> | | Disease |
> | | Fever |
> | | Gender |
> | | Gastrointestinal activity |
> | | Immunological activity |
> | | Infection |
> | | Kidney function |
> | | Lactation |
> | | Liver function |
> | | Pregnancy |
> | | Psychological status |
> | Environmental | Alcohol intake |
> | | Barometric pressure variation |
> | | Behavior |
> | | Dietary intake |
> | | Drugs (therapeutic, recreational, illicit) |
> | | Exercise level |
> | | Occupational exposures |
> | | Season variation |
> | | Sunlight exposure |
> | | Stress |
> | | Tobacco use |
> | | Weight and fat-to-lean ratio |
>
> *Degree of influence on personal variation of drug responses

given, it is likely that he or she has some variation in the way his or her body is using that drug or has a true allergy to it. It is important to review the physiological processes that lead to drug responses.

A drug is prescribed to produce a patient response, a desired and expected change in the function of one or more tissues or organs, known as its **intended action** or **therapeutic effect.** Although the intended action of a drug is expected to occur in any patient who receives it, not all patients respond to the drug as intended or to the same degree. This variation in patient response results from personal genetic differences that influence both the target of the drug and drug metabolism (how long the active drug remains in the body in contact with its target).

Pharmacodynamics

Pharmacodynamics is the body responses induced by a drug. These responses include both the intended action and side effects of the drug. A person's genetic differences can influence a drug's pharmacodynamics.

All cells have specific individual functions or actions that contribute to proper whole-body function. Drugs induce their responses by changing the activity level of different cellular functions. The function of any tissue or organ can be decreased, halted, or increased by exposure to a specific drug. The mechanism of action for any drug is how, at the cellular level, it acts to change cell and tissue function. For many drugs, the mechanism of action involves interaction of the drug with cellular receptors that normally control cell function. Although not all drugs exert their intended actions through a receptor, many do.

Receptors and Intended Actions

Receptors are sites on a cell surface or within a cell where naturally occurring substances can bind and control cell function. For example, binding of epinephrine or norepinephrine to beta$_1$-adrenergic receptors on smooth muscle cells in blood vessels causes internal cell responses that result in smooth muscle contraction (an increase in this cellular functional activity) and blood vessel constriction. When more norepinephrine is bound, the vessel constricts to a greater degree; when less norepinephrine is bound, the vessel is more relaxed. In this case, when the receptor is properly activated, cellular function (smooth muscle constriction) is increased. This response continues as long as norepinephrine remains bound to the receptor. Any drug that binds to a cell's receptor sites and causes the same response as the naturally occurring hormone or substance is known as an **agonist** (Fig. 15–2).

It is important to remember that different cell types may respond differently to the same substance. This difference is related to the receptor type. For example, when epinephrine or norepinephrine bind to beta$_2$-adrenergic receptors in bronchiolar smooth muscle, the internal cell responses cause smooth muscle relaxation and dilation of the airways. The drug is still acting as an agonist in this case because the cellular function of bronchiolar smooth muscle is to help maintain a patent airway through muscle relaxation. The substance is the same, but the cellular response is different because the receptors are different.

For a drug to stimulate a cell's function, it must bind correctly and tightly to the cell's receptors. This is known as a *functional fit* or *functional binding*. Some drugs bind incorrectly to a cell's receptors,

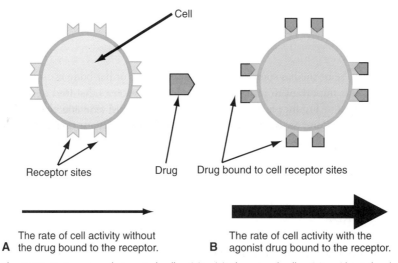

Cell

Receptor sites   Drug   Drug bound to cell receptor sites

The rate of cell activity without
A the drug bound to the receptor.

The rate of cell activity with the
B agonist drug bound to the receptor.

Figure 15–2. Receptors that control cell activity. (A) The rate of cell activity without the drug bound to the receptor. (B) The rate of cell activity with the agonist drug bound to the receptor.

blocking the cell's function (a *nonfunctional fit*). These drugs are known as **antagonists,** because they cause the opposite responses of an agonist and inhibit the expected cell function by preventing receptor interaction with agonist substances. Thus, when a beta-adrenergic antagonist drug (beta blocker), such as propranolol (Inderal), binds to $beta_1$ receptors in the heart, cardiac muscle contraction is less vigorous. When this drug binds to $beta_2$ receptors in the bronchiolar smooth muscle, the muscle constricts and the airways narrow. Most cells have more than one type of receptor, allowing different drugs to affect the same cell in different ways.

Cells with receptors that can bind with a drug (functionally or nonfunctionally) are the **targets** of the drug. For example, the targets of insulin are those cells that have insulin receptors. When insulin binds to insulin receptors, the membranes of those cells become more permeable (open) to glucose, allowing glucose in the blood to enter the cells. This action leads to reduced blood glucose levels. The targets of morphine, an opioid, are the receptors of neurons in the brain responsible for pain perception. These cells have opioid receptors, and when morphine binds to these receptors, the person's perception of pain is reduced. This response is enhanced when more opioid receptors are present and when the drug remains tightly bound to them. For example, hydromorphone (Dilaudid), an opioid for pain control, is an opioid agonist that binds more tightly to the opioid receptors and remains bound longer than morphine. As a result, hydromorphone can provide greater pain relief at lower doses than morphine.

The number of receptors cells have can vary from person to person, which affects the intended drug action. For example, a person may have 5000 beta-adrenergic receptors per cardiac muscle cell, whereas another person may have as many as 100,000 beta-adrenergic receptors per cardiac muscle cell. The person with higher receptor numbers will have a greater response to an agonist for those receptors and a lesser response to an antagonist for those receptors. Variation in the gene or genes coding for the receptors is one factor responsible for the differences in receptor numbers from one person to another.

Receptors and Side Effects

A perfect drug would affect only its target and result in the intended drug action. No drug is perfect, and all drugs have side effects in addition to their intended actions. **Side effects** are drug effects that are not the main purpose of the intended action. They are expected patient responses to the drug's mechanism of action and are usually mild, although not every person taking a drug experiences all expected side effects. For example, a person who uses an inhaled beta-adrenergic agonist for asthma, such as albuterol (Proventil), should have the intended action of bronchiolar smooth muscle dilation, resulting in reduced asthma symptoms. This person may experience side effects of the drug because beta-adrenergic receptors also are present on other tissues. Expected side effects include an increased heart rate and increased blood pressure, and these occur in nearly everyone taking this drug. Such side effects may be uncomfortable and may result in the patient choosing to avoid a specific drug. Additional side effects of albuterol can include feeling faint; developing a skin rash; swelling of the face, lips or tongue; developing an irregular heart beat; and experiencing chest pain. These side effects are less common, and when they occur with usual drug dosages, they may be related to a genetic variation that increases personal sensitivity to the drug.

When a known side effect is present to an exaggerated degree in a patient or an unusual response occurs, the reaction is called an *idiosyncratic response*. Genetic differences can result in increased personal sensitivity to the drug and in idiosyncratic responses. For example, nearly everyone who takes an opioid pain reliever for 2 days or longer becomes constipated to some degree. People who develop more severe constipation tend to be those who become constipated easily; however, very few people develop a paralytic ileus as a result of taking or receiving opioid pain medications. Some idiosyncratic reactions are unexpected effects that are unique to the patient and may not be related to the drug's mechanism of action. For example, people who have genetic variation that results in a glucose-6-phosphate dehydrogenase (G6PD) enzyme deficiency develop hemolytic anemia when they take primaquine to prevent malaria.

Pharmacokinetics

Most drugs must enter the body to produce their intended actions. Once inside the human body, the drug is distributed to different body fluid compartments. As a result of a drug coming into contact with a variety of cells, it is changed or processed by some of these cells. Thus, at the same time a drug is exerting one or more effects on the body, body cells are affecting the drug's chemistry. The actions of the body that change the physical and chemical properties of a drug are known as the process of **pharmacokinetics.** Because drugs are "foreign" substances in the body, most of the processes involved in pharmacokinetics focus on preparing the drug for eventual elimination. These processes include drug absorption, drug metabolism, and drug elimination.

Because most drugs exert their effects on body tissues and organs, drugs first have to enter the body and then enter the bloodstream so they can reach their targets. For the intended action to occur, the drug must reach and maintain a high enough constant level in the blood or target tissue to produce the action. The lowest blood or tissue level required to cause the intended action is known as the **minimum effective concentration** (**MEC**; Fig. 15–3). If the drug is eliminated faster than it is absorbed, the blood or tissue drug level will not be sufficient to produce the intended action. If the drug is eliminated more slowly than it is absorbed, the drug blood or tissue level may reach toxic concentrations and result in serious adverse reactions. For drugs to produce intended actions without becoming toxic, blood drug levels must be maintained at the MEC by balancing drug absorption with drug elimination, a condition known as a *steady-state* drug level (Fig. 15–4).

Although an average MEC has been calculated for every approved drug, genetic variation in drug absorption, drug metabolism, and drug elimination may make the MEC for a specific drug in one person very different from the "average MEC." (In addition to genetic difference, other factors that change drug MEC include age; general health; organ health; and the ingestion of additional drugs, food, alcohol, and herbal substances.)

Figure 15–3. The minimum effective concentration (MEC) of drug in the blood or tissue needed for the intended action.

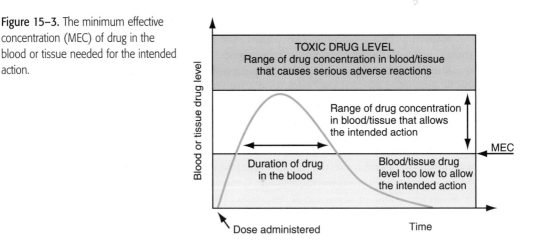

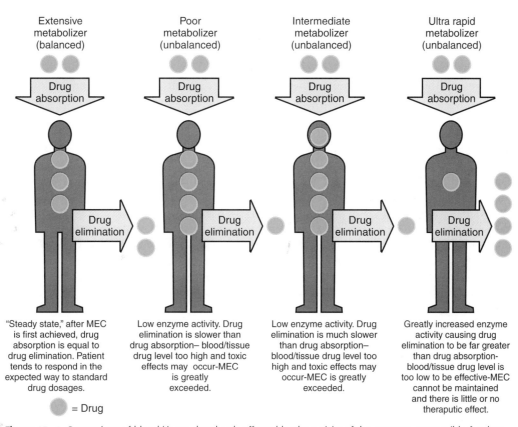

| Extensive metabolizer (balanced) | Poor metabolizer (unbalanced) | Intermediate metabolizer (unbalanced) | Ultra rapid metabolizer (unbalanced) |

"Steady state," after MEC is first achieved, drug absorption is equal to drug elimination. Patient tends to respond in the expected way to standard drug dosages.

Low enzyme activity. Drug elimination is slower than drug absorption– blood/tissue drug level too high and toxic effects may occur-MEC is greatly exceeded.

Low enzyme activity. Drug elimination is much slower than drug absorption– blood/tissue drug level too high and toxic effects may occur-MEC is greatly exceeded.

Greatly increased enzyme activity causing drug elimination to be far greater than drug absorption-blood/tissue drug level is too low to be effective-MEC cannot be maintained and there is little or no theraputic effect.

● = Drug

Figure 15–4. Comparison of blood/tissue drug levels affected by the activity of the enzymes responsible for drug metabolism and elimination.

Drug Absorption

Drug **absorption** is the entering of a drug from its route of administration into the bloodstream. The amount of an administered drug dose that actually reaches the bloodstream, regardless of the method of administration, is its **bioavailability.** When the entire drug dose administered reaches the bloodstream, the bioavailability is 100%. When only part of the drug dose administered reaches the bloodstream, drug bioavailability is less than 100%. Drugs can be administered by the percutaneous route (through skin or mucous membranes), the enteral route (through the gastrointestinal route), and the parenteral route (through injection into the bloodstream, subcutaneous tissue, or muscle). Only when a drug is administered intravenously or intra-arterially is its immediate bioavailability always 100%. For most other methods of drug delivery, less than the administered dose is absorbed into the bloodstream, resulting in lower percentages of bioavailability. The drug administration method with the least predictable bioavailability and the one that is most highly influenced by genetic variation is the enteral route, which is also the most common route for drug entry.

Enteral drugs are swallowed as liquids, tablets, or capsules (the enteral route does not include drugs that are absorbed through oral mucous membranes directly into the bloodstream) and are absorbed elsewhere in the gastrointestinal tract into the bloodstream. After a drug is swallowed, it is acted on by stomach acids, enzymes, and other secretions. Only a few drugs are absorbed into the bloodstream directly from the stomach. Each person's stomach secretions are unique in amount, which means that each person's stomach processing of a drug is unique. After leaving the stomach, most enteral drugs enter the small intestine, where they undergo further processing, especially dissolving, before the drugs can be absorbed into the bloodstream. This processing is the result of mechanical mixing and the action of various enzymes on the drug. Again, each person's intestinal enzyme concentration is unique. The innermost lining of the small intestinal is the major site of drug absorption. When drugs in the intestines are poorly absorbed, the drugs remain in the stool and are eliminated without exerting their intended actions.

Drugs absorbed through the small intestine into venous blood are quickly exposed to the liver before entering the rest of venous blood flow in the inferior vena cava back to the heart, where the drug is then distributed throughout the circulatory system. This circulatory detour, known as **enterohepatic circulation,** is a result of all the venous blood from the last half of the mouth, the esophagus, the stomach, the intestines, and the higher part of the rectum draining first into the portal vein and circulating to the liver before entering systemic circulation. As a result, the liver has a chance to metabolize drugs absorbed from the gastrointestinal tract *before* they reach target tissues or organs. Although this detour is generally a helpful process, allowing the liver to remove any microorganisms that remain in nutrients that enter the GI tract as food (after all, we do not sterilize our food before we eat it), the extensive enzyme systems in the liver can and do alter drug function. In addition to genetic differences in digestive enzyme function and anatomical variation in circulation to the intestinal tract, nongenetic factors that alter intestinal absorption of drugs include intestinal pathology and the presence of additional drugs, food, and herbal substances in the tract at the same time the drug is present.

Drug Metabolism

Drugs are considered foreign chemicals in the body, which triggers the normal response of processing the drug for elimination through metabolism. **Metabolism** is a chemical reaction in the body that changes the chemical shape, size, content, and activity of the drug. The liver enzyme systems, especially the cytochrome P450 (CYP, pronounced "sip") systems of enzymes, are most responsible for metabolism. These enzymes also are present in white blood cells, both those that circulate and those that are embedded within various body tissues. A few other organs, such as the adrenal glands, lungs, kidneys, intestinal mucosa, and skin also have enzymes that can participate in metabolizing drugs.

The cytochrome P450 system of enzymes is coded for by a gene family currently known to be composed of 51 main genes and hundreds of subfamilies. Each cytochrome P450 gene name begins with CYP, indicating that it is part of the cytochrome P450 gene family. The gene name also has a number indicating its assignment into a specific group within the main gene family and a letter that represents the gene's specific subfamily. The last number in the name indicates the gene's assignment to the specific gene within the subfamily. For example, the cytochrome P450 gene that is in group 2, subfamily D, gene 6 is written as CYP2D6 (National Institutes of Health, 2011). These genes are large, and there are many variations in the exact sequence of them. These variations make some genes and gene products more active and others less active than "average." This group of enzymes is extremely important in drug metabolism. Although these enzymes are present in several body sites, the liver has the greatest concentration of them and thus is the tissue in which drug metabolism is most active.

Metabolizing a drug is usually considered how it is inactivated and prepared for elimination. Although this is often true, it is important to remember that metabolism is a multistage action and that some stages can actually *activate* drugs as well as inactivate them.

The first stage or phase of drug metabolism is one in which the enzymes add specific groups to the original drug (parent compound, the actual chemical composition of the drug as it was when it entered the body), which usually results in making the drug express a negative charge. These groups may include hydroxyl groups (OH), amine or amide groups (NH), and sulfhydryl groups (SH). The reaction also can change the amount of oxygen or hydrogen present in the drug. These changes form drug metabolites that can bind more easily to body proteins and DNA. The metabolites may be active or inactive, or they may undergo more metabolism to make them easier to eliminate from the body.

When a drug enters the body as an active parent compound, it is capable of exerting the intended action in this form, and first-stage metabolism forms inactive metabolites. For example, when the lipid-lowering drug fluvastatin (Lescol) is swallowed, the drug is already active. It is rapidly absorbed from the stomach and enters the bloodstream at that point. When it is metabolized by one of the CYP enzymes, it becomes inactive and ready for elimination. On the other hand, the lipid-lowering drug atorvastatin (Lipitor) is a **prodrug,** meaning that it is ingested as an inactive parent compound and cannot exert its intended action in this form. When atorvastatin is metabolized by one of the CYP enzymes, five separate active drug metabolites are formed, each of which can help lower blood lipid levels. So, in this case, first-phase metabolism activates this drug rather than prepares it for elimination. For these active metabolites to be eliminated, they must then undergo second-stage metabolism, which then alters the chemical structure further to add substances to the now-active drug metabolites that enhance their excretion through the intestinal tract or in the urine by the kidney. (These substances include glucuronic acid, sulfuric acid, acetic acids, amide groups, and methyl groups.)

Because there are a variety of CYP enzymes and their activities are affected by their gene sequences, people often have differences in how well a drug works for them. For example, the opioid drug codeine is often given for pain relief. Codeine is a prodrug, and for it to alter a person's perception of pain, it must undergo first-stage metabolism by the specific enzyme CYP2D6. This action converts codeine to morphine, which then can bind to opioid receptors and reduce the perception of pain. For a person who has a deficiency of CYP2D6 or a gene mutation that makes it less active, codeine is not converted to morphine and the person does not have any pain relief from the drug (however, if he or she received morphine, the pain is relieved). A different enzyme (not CYP2D6) is responsible for second-stage morphine metabolism for elimination (Fig. 15–5).

Think about how variation in the activity of different metabolizing enzymes would affect a drug's intended action and a patient's response to that drug. If a person had higher-than-normal levels of the enzyme that prepared morphine for elimination (or a more active version of this enzyme), the patient would need higher or more frequent doses of morphine to maintain a good level of pain relief. On the other hand, if a person had lower-than-normal levels of the enzyme that prepared morphine for elimination,

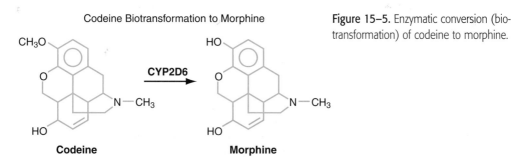

Codeine Biotransformation to Morphine

Figure 15–5. Enzymatic conversion (biotransformation) of codeine to morphine.

Codeine   **Morphine**

any morphine administered would remain active in the system longer. Although this would enhance the pain relief effect of morphine, it could also increase the side effects of the drug.

Elimination

Elimination is the inactivation and final removal of drugs from the body. Although many tissues and organs eliminate drugs to some degree after they have been prepared for elimination by metabolism, the most active elimination routes are the gastrointestinal tract, the kidneys, and the lungs. Drugs can be eliminated in the feces, urine, exhaled air, sweat, tears, saliva, breast milk, and semen.

Drugs that were metabolized by the liver for elimination are either sent to the gastrointestinal tract or to the blood and then to the kidney for elimination. As a result, even parenteral drugs can be eliminated through the gastrointestinal tract. When a drug is given orally, some of the drug is metabolized very quickly by the liver and rapidly eliminated from the body. This rapid inactivation and elimination of enteral drugs is called **first-pass loss.** For some drugs, first-pass loss can be so great that the enteral form of the drug has practically no intended action. For example, the drug nitroglycerin has a first-pass loss of 95%. This means that if the drug were administered orally, only 5% of it is bioavailable and able to exert its intended action (dilation of the coronary arteries). To avoid first-pass loss with this drug, it is administered as a sublingual (under the tongue) spray or tablet. This works because blood vessels under the front of the tongue are not part of enterohepatic circulation, and the venous blood drains from here without going through the liver before entering systemic circulation.

Drugs that are small and dissolved in the blood may leave the body in the urine. The drugs may change the color or smell of the urine. (This is why urine tests are accurate in determining the presence of some illegal drugs.)

Drugs that are small and easily vaporized (become gaseous) are metabolized and eliminated by the lungs with exhaled air. (This is why a breathalyzer test is accurate in determining a blood-alcohol level).

Genetic/Genomic Variations

People can be grouped according to variations in metabolic enzyme activity. Some people are considered "poor metabolizers." They have little if any of a specific enzyme activity and would have difficulty clearing an active drug that requires processing by this specific enzyme. They would be likely to have high blood levels of a drug given at a standard dose and might have adverse reactions or toxicity. Some people are considered intermediate metabolizers. They have low enzyme activity and have an even more difficult time clearing a drug. Most people are "extensive metabolizers," and they tend to respond in the expected way to drugs given at standard doses.

People who are "ultrarapid metabolizers" often have duplications of the gene coding for the enzyme responsible for metabolism. They have greatly increased enzyme activity and will clear an active drug very quickly. This can result in little or no therapeutic effect when standard doses are given (see Fig. 15–4). For example, tricyclic antidepressants (active drugs) are metabolized by the CYP2D6 enzyme. A person who has a variation in the gene coding for the enzyme CYP2D6 that makes him or her a poor metabolizer could have toxic plasma concentrations and side effects such as dry mouth, hypotension, sedation, tremor, or even cardiotoxicity. A person who has a variation, making the person an ultrarapid metabolizer, would not experience either the expected therapeutic effect or side effects.

When you are giving a prodrug that requires biotransformation before it can be used (e.g., codeine, which must be converted to morphine to have a therapeutic effect), things are quite different. A CYP2D6 enzyme poor metabolizer who takes codeine would not be able to efficiently convert the drug to morphine and so would have little or no plasma concentration of morphine, no analgesia, and of course, no constipation. An ultrarapid metabolizer would be rapidly and efficiently converting codeine to morphine and so might experience severe abdominal pain, constipation, and possibly respiratory depression.

It is important to remember that many enzymes may be involved in the metabolism of a given drug and that drugs are rarely given in isolation. There is a long list of drugs that are metabolized by the CYP2D6 enzyme (e.g. quinidine, fluoxetine, propanolol, etc.). With a set amount of enzyme present, giving two drugs that are both metabolized by it, means that the activity is spread over two drugs, which then reduces the rate of metabolism for both drugs. The normal amount of the enzyme would be insufficient to fully metabolize either drug. Thus, giving these drugs together increases the effects of both drugs because neither drug is fully metabolized and remains active in the system longer or to a higher concentration.

Not all drugs that are metabolized by CYP2D6 work as inhibitors when they are given together. Taking an inhibitor along with another drug metabolized by CYP2D6 could result in adverse reactions in someone who was genetically an extensive metabolizer (Table 15–2). While many drugs inhibit the activity of CYP2D6, there are no drugs that induce or increase its activity. Up-to-date information about CYP450 enzyme substrates, inhibitors, and inducers is available from the Indiana University Division of Clinical Pharmacology (http://medicine.iupui.edu/clinpharm/ddis/ClinicalTable.asp; see also Tables 15–3 and 15–4).

TABLE 15–2

Selected Clinically Relevant CYP450 Substrates

CYP2C9	CYP2C19	CYP2D6	CYP3A4,5,7
NSAIDs: Diclofenac, Ibuprofen, Piroxicam	**PPIs:** Lansoprazole, Omeprazole2, Pantoprazole, Rabeprazole	**Beta Blockers:** S-metoprolol, Propafenone, Timolol	**Macrolide Antibiotics:** Clarithromycin, Erythromycin2 (not 3A5), NOT azithromycin, Telithromycin
Oral Hypoglycemics: Glipizide, Tolbutamide	**Antiepileptics:** Diazepam, Phenobarbitone, Phenytoin	**Antidepressants:** Amitriptyline, Clomipramine, Desipramine, Imipramine, Paroxetine	**Antiarrhythmics:** Quinidine→3-OH (not 3A5)
Angiotensin II Blockers: Losartan, Irbesartan	**Others:** Amitriptyline, Clomipramine, Clopidogrel, Cyclophosphamide, Progesterone	**Antipsychotics:** Haloperidol, Risperidone, Thioridazine	**Benzodiazepines:** Alprazolam, Diazepam→3OH, Midazolam1, Triazolam2
Others: Celecoxib, Fluvastatin, Naproxen, Phenytoin, Rosiglitazone, Sulfamethoxazole, Tamoxifen, Tolbutamide, Torsemide, Warfarin		**Others:** Aripiprazole, Codeine, Dextromethorphan1, Duloxetine, Flecainide, Mexiletine, Ondansetron, Tamoxifen, Tramadol	**Immune Modulators:** Cyclosporine, Tacrolimus (FK506)
			HIV Antivirals: Indinavir, Ritonavir, Saquinavir
			Prokinetics: Cisapride

Continued

TABLE 15–2

Selected Clinically Relevant CYP450 Substrates—cont'd

CYP2C9	CYP2C19	CYP2D6	CYP3A4,5,7
			Antihistamines: Astemizole Chlorpheniramine
			Calcium Channel Blockers: Amlodipine Diltiazem Felodipine Nifedipine2 Nisoldipine Nitrendipine Verapamil
			HMG CoA Reductase Inhibitors: Atorvastatin Lovastatin NOT pravastatin NOT rosuvastatin Simvastatin
			Others: Aripiprazole Buspirone Gleevec Haloperidol Methadone Pimozide Quinine Sildenafil Tamoxifen Trazodone Vincristine

From http://medicine.iupui.edu/clinpharm/ddis/ClinicalTable.asp.

The CYP450 enzymes are responsible for metabolism of many drugs. The *CYP2* family contains 16 genes that code for the enzymes needed to metabolize approximately 50% of currently available prescription drugs. The *CYP3* family contains only 4 genes, but CYP3 enzymes metabolize 120 frequently prescribed drugs (see Table 15–2).

The CYP2D6 enzyme alone is responsible for metabolism of 25% to 30% of prescribed drugs, including many beta blockers, antiarrhythmics, antidepressants, antipsychotics, and opioids. The percentages of poor, extensive, and ultrarapid metabolizers vary with the geographical origin of one's ancestors, as well as by personal gene changes. For example, poor CYP2D6 enzyme metabolism is seen in 5% to 10% of European Americans but in only 2% to 4% of African Americans. Differences are even greater when we look at other ethnicities. About 0.7% of Chinese are poor metabolizers, compared

TABLE 15–3

Some Inhibitors of CYP450 Enzymes

CYP2C9	CYP2C19	CYP2D6	CYP3A4,5,7
Fluconazole	Ketoconazole	Bupropion	Indinavir
Amiodarone	Omeprazole Fluoxetine	Fluoxetine	Nelfinavir
		Paroxetine	Ritonavir
		Quinidine	Clarithromycin
		Duloxetine Amiodarone	Itraconazole
		Cimetidine	Ketoconazole
			Nefazodone
			Erythromycin
			Grapefruit juice Verapamil
			Diltiazem

Adapted from http://medicine.iupui.edu/clinpharm/ddis/ClinicalTable.asp.

TABLE 15–4

Some Inducers of CYP450 Enzymes

CYP2C9	CYP2C19	CYP2D6	CYP3A4,5,7
Rifampin	—	—	Carbamazepine
Secobarbital			Phenobarbital2
			Phenytoin2
			Pioglitazone
			Rifabutin
			Rifampin1
			St. John's wort
			Troglitazone1

Adapted from http://medicine.iupui.edu/clinpharm/ddis/ClinicalTable.asp.

to 19% of South Africans. There are also wide variations in the percentages of ultrarapid metabolizers. About 2% of both African Americans and European Americans are ultrarapid metabolizers, but 20% of Saudi Arabians and 30% of people from geographically nearby Ethiopia are as well (Table 15–5). Remember that the United States is an ethnically diverse country with considerable reproductive mixing of races and ethnicities. Although the numbers given may apply to people whose ancestors came from one geographic area, they cannot be relied upon to select an appropriate dose for a particular patient (see the "Genetic Testing for Drug Response" section).

TABLE 15–5

Estimated Ethnic Distribution of CYP2D6 Phenotype

Phenotype	CYP2D6	Estimated Ethnic Distribution
Poor metabolizers	None	Caucasians, 6%–10% Mexican Americans, 3%–6% African Americans, 2%–5% Asians, 1%
Intermediate metabolizers	Low	Not established
Extensive metabolizers	Normal	Most people
Ultrarapid metabolizers	High	Finns and Danes, 1% European Americans, 4% Greeks, 10% Portuguese, 10% Saudis, 20% Ethiopians, 30%

Adapted from: www.pharmacytimes.com/issue/pharmacy/2008/2008-7/2008-0.

Clinical Applications of Pharmacogenomics

Pharmacogenomics (PGx) is being used clinically in a variety of ways, including helping to predict the most appropriate dose for a given patient. Dose alterations in the chemotherapeutic agent 6-mercaptopurine (6MP) can be made based on genetic test results; however, it is not just the patient's genome that can be tested. For example, some clinical applications of PGx testing are based on genomic variation in tumors or viruses. Genetic testing of tumor cells has resulted in the development of targeted therapy designed to treat a subset of a disease. Examples include imatinib (Gleevec) for chronic myeloid leukemia, erlotinib (Tarceva) for lung cancer, and trastuzumab (Herceptin) for *Her2-neu* positive breast cancers. Testing of viral genomes has been used to help select the best treatments for HIV infection based on the drug resistance of the virus.

PG may have its greatest impact when drug doses are highly individualized and life-threatening adverse reactions are a common concern. The anticoagulant drug warfarin (Coumadin) is such a drug. People who have a polymorphism in the gene coding for the enzyme CYP2C9 take longer to stabilize the dose, have an increased risk of above-range INR, bleed earlier, and have more serious or life-threatening bleeding, but there are other proteins that play a part in the way people use warfarin.

Vitamin K epoxide reductase complex 1 (*VKORC1*) is a warfarin target gene, and variations in the genetic sequence coding for this gene product have resulted in resistance to warfarin. The VKORC1 enzyme recycles endogenous vitamin K, which aids with synthesis of coagulation factors that depend on vitamin K. Common polymorphisms in *VKORC1*, the gene coding for the VKORC1 enzymes, have been found to affect the dose response to vitamin K antagonists, like warfarin. Warfarin dosage genetic tests (testing both *CYP2C9* and *VKORC1*) can be purchased for between $50 and $500 from major medical centers or from Internet-based companies that offer genetic testing.

In 2007, the FDA placed precautions of the warfarin label, reminding physicians that people with genetic variations require a lower starting dose, but Medicare has refused to pay for warfarin response genetic testing, saying that there is little evidence that having a genetic test results in better outcomes for patients compared to the way in which warfarin is currently prescribed. Standard procedures of starting with a dose based on the patient's age, weight, organ function, and so on, and then adjusting that dose based on INR test results is thought to be more cost-effective.

The *CYP3A* family is responsible for metabolism of about 50% of drugs, including most calcium channel blockers, most benzodiazepines, most statins, and acetaminophen. Inhibitors of the *CYP3A* enzyme include grapefruit juice, ketoconazole, cimetidine, and erythromycin. Drugs that speed up metabolism by the *CYP3A* enzyme include St. John's wort, rifampin, and ritonavir. One of the challenges in the application of PGx is that for some enzyme families (e.g., *CYP3A*), studies have not shown consistent genotype/phenotype concordance; in other words, we have not been able to predict clinical response based on genetic tests.

The phase II liver enzyme N-acetyltransferase (NAT) is needed for metabolism of some drugs. NAT adds an acetyl group onto drugs in the process of acetylation. Sulfamethoxazole, hydralazine, procainamide, isoniazid, and caffeine all require acetylation to facilitate elimination. People can be grouped into two categories according to their ability to perform acetylation. Fast acetylators are similar to ultrarapid metabolizers in the CYP450 enzyme system. They tend to need larger and more frequent doses of drugs that require acetylation, but they can efficiently detoxify carcinogenic compounds in tobacco smoke. Slow acetylators may need a 10% to 15% reduction in dose and are at increased risk of side effects, including hepatotoxicity.

Drugs such as azathioprine (Imuran), mercaptopurine, and thioguanine, used to treat childhood leukemias, rheumatoid arthritis, or inflammatory bowel disease require metabolism by the enzyme thiopurine methyltransferase (TPMT). Activity of TPMT is trimodal, meaning there are three different levels of enzyme activity among groups of people. About 90% of people have high TPMT activity. They have faster drug metabolism, which results in lower exposure of leukemic cells to active thiopurines. About 10% of people have intermediate activity, and a very small fraction of people (maybe about 0.3%) have low activity. Those who have low TPMT activity are homozygous for variations in the gene coding for TPMT, so they produce nonfunctional protein. People with low TPMT activity risk myelosuppression, secondary cancers, and possibly fatal toxicity when they are given chemotherapeutic agents requiring metabolism by TPMT. They may need to have the dose of their chemotherapeutic agents reduced eight- to tenfold. Fortunately, testing for TPMT levels is available.

Glucose-6-phosphate dehydrogenase (G6PD) deficiency was one of the first pharmacogenomic variations discovered. This X-linked recessive disorder is common in the Middle East, Africa, and Southeast Asia and found in about 10% of black males (in the United States). Affected persons risk hemolytic anemia when they are given antimalarials, aspirin, probenecid, or vitamin K, or if they eat fava beans (favism). G6PD is necessary for erythrocytes to maintain cytoskeletal integrity in the presence of oxidative stress. Unfortunately, there is not a perfect correlation between genotype and phenotype, so genetic testing does not always predict clinical response.

Less is known about genetic variations in drug transporters. One example is the gene *ABCB1* coding for P-glycoprotein-MDR1, which is a membrane efflux transporter that is responsible for moving drugs, including such drugs as paclitaxel (Taxol) and digoxin (Lanoxin), from the intestine into the blood. When duodenal expression of *ABCB1* results in low levels of P-glycoprotein-MDR1, less drug can be transported across the membrane.

Genetic Testing for Drug Response

Laboratories at major medical centers offer genetic testing for drug response, and many provide excellent patient education materials on what PGx testing is, what it means, and how the results could improve patient care. But genetic testing for drug response can also be purchased from direct-to-consumer companies that market over the Internet. (Chapter 14 provides more information about direct-to-consumer genetic testing.) Small devices for bedside sample collection and rapid turnaround (about 8 hours) are now being marketed and can be used to identify polymorphisms quickly. As technology advances, more will be seen.

Health-care professionals treating people with mental health disorders have been particularly interested in PGx, largely because it is difficult to find the right drug and dose for each patient. Only 35% to 45% of patients respond sufficiently to their psychotropic drugs to return to a desired functional level. While there is an expanding base of studies involving psychotropic medications, the Evaluation of Genomic Applications in Practice and Prevention (EGAPP) panel decided that there was insufficient evidence to support the link between testing for CYP450 polymorphisms and improved clinical outcomes.

Summary

Drug response is a complex trait influenced by many genes and the environment. You have seen examples of increased or decreased drug metabolism in the CYP450s, acetylation, and TPMT enzyme systems. We have also seen genetic variants cause unexpected responses such as the hemolytic anemia seen when a person with G6PD deficiency takes an antimalarial drug. Despite some very promising studies, there has been little reported improvement in clinical outcomes using PGx testing for drug administration. That means that our understanding of the impact genetic variations have on the way we use drugs is incomplete. There are probably polymorphisms in modifier genes, or major genes that have not been identified that have an undiscovered impact on the ways that our patients process drugs such as warfarin or serotonin reuptake inhibitors. Much must be learned before pharmacogenomics will be in use at every bedside, but that day will come.

GENE GEMS

- Pharmacogenetics and pharmacogenomics are similar concepts, but pharmacogenomics has a more in-depth scope.
- We know most about genetic/genomic differences in the way people metabolize drugs.
- Drugs often work in the same way the body hormones, enzymes, and other proteins do.
- Most drugs exert their effects by binding to a cell receptor.
- At the same time that a drug is changing the body's activity, the body is processing the drug for elimination.
- Drugs have to reach a high enough level in the blood to exert their effects.
- Taking more than one drug at the same time can change the effectiveness of each drug.
- Drug metabolism reduces its bioavailability.
- The most important organs for drug metabolism and elimination are the liver, kidneys, and white blood cells.
- The CYP450 enzyme system is responsible for metabolism of many of the most frequently prescribed drugs.
- People can be classified as slow, intermediate, extensive, or ultrarapid metabolizers, depending on CYP350 enzyme activity.
- N-acetyltransferase (NAT) is required for phase II metabolism of many drugs.
- People can be classified as slow or fast acetylators.
- Genetic testing is available for some variations in the way people respond to drugs.
- There is a debate about the clinical efficacy of drug response genetic testing, but PGx testing is currently being used clinically.

Self-Assessment Questions

1. Which statement about agonist and antagonist drugs is true?
   a. The target tissues for these types of drugs are invading bacteria and viruses.
   b. Both agonist drugs and antagonist drugs must interact with receptors to produce their intended responses.
   c. Antagonist drugs produce only intended responses, and agonist drugs produce both intended responses and side effects.
   d. These types of drugs are less likely to cause allergic responses than drugs that are neither agonists nor antagonists.

2. Which of the following is a goal of pharmacogenetics?
   a. Making "blockbuster drugs" that will work equally well for everyone
   b. Bringing down the cost of pharmaceutical manufacturing
   c. Developing drugs that will treat very rare diseases
   d. Reducing adverse reactions

3. What is the expected response on heart rate when a patient is taking a drug that is an adrenaline antagonist?
   a. Heart rate is unchanged.
   b. Heart rate decreases.
   c. Heart rate increases.
   d. Heart rate is louder.

4. Your patient has been identified as a *poor metabolizer* of a drug that has just been ordered, and the drug is formulated as an active compound. What will be the most likely result if you give this active drug at the standard dose?
   a. No therapeutic response
   b. Adverse reactions and possible toxicity
   c. Therapeutic response as expected in the general population
   d. Drug inactivation occurs more rapidly, and the therapeutic response is limited.

5. Your patient waits tables at his family's Ethiopian restaurant. He has been taking the recommended dose of a tricyclic antidepressant but reports that he still feels very down and is not socializing with friends. What might be the problem?
   a. He is probably not taking his medication.
   b. He may be metabolizing the medication too fast and getting no effect.
   c. He may be skipping doses because of the level of undesirable side effects.
   d. He may be experiencing a problem due to interactions between Ethiopian spices and the tricyclic drug.

6. You are caring for a patient who is of German descent. She reports that she has no pain relief with the codeine that was ordered, and she asks for something stronger. Any ideas?
   a. Check the local emergency departments, because this is clearly drug-seeking behavior.
   b. Suggest that she use guided imagery after she takes her pain medication.
   c. Ask her nurse practitioner to consider switching her to another analgesic since she may have a CYP2D6 polymorphism that prevents her from converting codeine to morphine.
   d. Switch her to another drug since she may be an ultrarapid metabolizer of codeine.

Continued

7. Genotyping consistently and accurately predicts whether a patient will have a therapeutic response to a drug.
   a. True
   b. False

8. You are caring for a child with acute lymphoblastic leukemia. She has been genotyped and is homozygous for a TPMT polymorphism, producing very little of the enzyme needed for this drug's metabolism. How would you expect this to affect dosing of the drug 6-mercaptopurine?
   a. This child should receive only a small fraction of the standard dose.
   b. This child should receive the drug intravenously rather than orally.
   c. This child should receive more than the standard dose.
   d. This child should receive the standard dose.

Discussion Questions

1. What might happen if an active drug metabolized by CYP2D6 was developed in China and found to have very few adverse reactions and then marketed in South Africa?

2. What impact do you think PGx will have on your day-to-day patient care?

3. If your patient shows you a PGx test result (ordered over the Internet) and requests that her drug dose be altered, what will you do?

References

Eckman, M. H., Rosand, J., Greenberg, S. M., and Gage, B. F. (2009). Cost-effectiveness of using pharmacogenetic information in warfarin dosing for patients with nonvalvular atrial fibrillation. *Annals of Internal Medicine, 150*(2), 73–83.

FDA. (2008). Pharmacogenomics and its role in drug safety. Retrieved October 6, 2009, from www.fda.gov/Drugs/DrugSafety/DrugSafetyNewsletter/ucm119991.htm.

Indiana University Division of Clinical Pharmacology. (2010). CYP450 enzyme substrates, inhibitors, and inducers. Retrieved May, 2010 from http://medicine.iupui.edu/clinpharm/ddis/ClinicalTable.asp.

Kudzma, E., and Carey, E. (2009). Pharmacogenomics: Personalizing drug therapy. *Asian Journal of Nursing, 109*(10), 50–57.

Monsen, R. *Genetics and ethics in health care.* Silver Springs, MD: American Nurses Association, 2009.

National Institutes of Health. (2011). Home genetic reference: CYP gene family. Retrieved March 2011 from: http://ghr.nlm.nih.gov/geneFamily/cyp.

Prows, C. A., and Prows, D. R. (2004). Medication selection by genotype: How genetics is changing drug prescribing and efficacy. *American Journal of Nursing, 104*(5), 60–70.

Schwarz, U. I., Ritchie, M. D., Bradford, Y., et al. (2008). Genetic determinants of response to warfarin during initial anticoagulation. *New England Journal of Medicine, 358*(10), 999–1008.

Weinshilboum, R., and Wang, L. (2004). Pharmacogenomics: Bench to bedside. *Nature Reviews. Drug Discovery, 3*(9), 739–748.

Self-Assessment Answers

1. b **2.** d **3.** b **4.** b **5.** b **6.** c **7.** b **8.** a

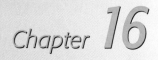

Chapter 16

Health Professionals
and Genomic Care

Learning Outcomes

1. Use the terminology associated with genetic counseling.
2. Describe the educational preparation and general roles of various genetic professionals.
3. Explain the role of general registered nurses in providing genomic care.

KEY TERMS

Certified genetic counselor (CGC)

Clinical geneticist

Clinical laboratory geneticist

Genetic counseling

Genomic care

Medical geneticist

Nondirective

Research geneticist

Introduction

Genomic care is ensuring that the influence of a person's genetic history on health and disease is considered as part of general assessment information for all patients and families. This information must be put into perspective for health status as much as personal environmental considerations of disease development and for responses to therapy. This does not mean that all patients should have some sort of genetic testing. Rather, it means that all health-care professionals are obligated to avoid overlooking genetic issues that may affect an individual's health or risk for health problems.

So, now you are taking a genetics course or discussing genetic issues in one of your clinical courses. Perhaps you also had a genetics focus in your college biology course. Does this make you a genetic professional? Is your family physician or nurse practitioner a genetic professional? Who has the responsibility for working with families and individuals at increased genetic risk for a health problem or problems? What is your role as a direct care provider in the era of "genomic medicine"? This chapter addresses these issues.

Genetic Professionals

The title of *genetic professional* implies that the individual has extensive education and, often, special credentialing in some aspect of the broad genetics field. Such a professional is an expert in one or more areas of genetics. By this criterion, a person with an entry-level degree in a health-care profession, such as a registered nurse, registered dietitian, physical therapist, pharmacist, or physician, is *not* a genetics professional, because genetics was not the focus of her or his professional education. However, according to the National Coalition for Health Professional Education in Genetics (NCHPEG), all health-care professionals are expected to have at least a basic understanding of the general patterns of inheritance and genetic terminology, as well as to be able to construct an accurate three-generation pedigree from assessment information (see Appendix C). This is not to say that a professional, such as a registered dietitian or registered nurse who works within a specialty area that deals with one type of genetic problem such as cystic fibrosis or phenylketonuria, is not very informed about the genetic issues associated with the disorder, but this on-the-job acquired knowledge is limited in scope. That person is still not a genetics professional.

Genetic counseling is defined as "the process of helping people understand and adapt to the medical, psychological and familial implications of genetic contribution to disease occurrence or recurrence" (National Society of Genetic Counselors, 2006). A variety of genetic professionals are credentialed to perform genetic counseling to varying levels.

Regardless of education level and credentialing, any level of genetic counseling must be performed in a nondirective manner. **Nondirective** means that the person providing genetic information and counseling presents all facts and available options in a way that neither promotes nor excludes any decision or action (within legal boundaries). Remaining nondirective can sometimes be very difficult, because patients and families may feel overwhelmed and want someone else to make decisions. They want to do the "right thing," which may not be the same for everyone. Often they ask the genetic professional presenting information, "What would you do?" Regardless of the specific genetic issue and the condition at hand, the patient and family members directly involved must ultimately make decisions that feel right for them.

Certified Genetic Counselor

The most familiar genetic professional who performs genetic counseling is a certified genetic counselor. A **certified genetic counselor (CGC)** is a genetics professional who has a master's degree in genetic counseling from a graduate program accredited by the American Board of Genetic Counselors (ABGC), which is part of the National Society of Genetic Counselors. This profession was first recognized in 1969. Currently, there are 18 accredited genetic counseling programs in the United States, as well as additional programs in Canada and other countries around the world.

The preparation for becoming a genetic counselor starts with a baccalaureate degree from an accredited undergraduate institution. Although the degree can be in any undergraduate major, most genetic counseling graduate programs have admission requirements that include prerequisites of specific biological sciences, advanced mathematics, basic genetics, and behavioral sciences. Graduate courses for the specialty commonly include all aspects of genetics (population and quantitative genetics, molecular genetics, cytogenetics, biochemical genetics), embryology and human development, psychosocial development, counseling, ethics, assessment, crisis counseling, social and legal issues, and case management techniques. Most programs also include extensive laboratory methods courses, not because a CGC is expected to perform these tests as part of his or her role but to ensure that the counselor has adequate background to help clients understand testing procedures and results. Students are engaged in supervised counseling sessions throughout the graduate program.

After successful completion of a master's degree in genetic counseling from a program accredited by the ABGC, the person must pass the certification examination to become a certified genetics counselor (CGC), who is both professionally and legally qualified to perform genetic counseling. In addition to the initial certification, genetic counselors must recertify every 5 years either by taking the certification examination or by participating in appropriate continuing education activities.

The scope of practice for a CGC focuses on three general areas: providing expertise in genetics, communicating directly with and counseling patients and families at potential risk for genetic problems, and ensuring that counseling services are delivered in a manner that is consistent with professional ethics and values. States vary on the extent of CGC practice with regard to ordering tests and performing physical assessment. At all times, a CGC is a client advocate and performs his or her professional duties in a nondirective manner.

Genetic counselors are members of the health-care team who together provide information and support to individuals and families who have an identified genetic problem or are at increased genetic risk for a variety of genetic disorders. Some genetic counselors specialize within the profession. For example, one genetic counselor may work exclusively in prenatal counseling, whereas another might specialize in oncology and cancer risk. Regardless of the area of specialization, the genetic counselor provides information about specific disorders, testing, inheritance patterns, the risk for recurrence, management options, and appropriate referrals.

Clinical Geneticist

Only a physician who graduated from an accredited school/college of medicine, successfully completed a medical board examination, and is eligible for licensure can become a clinical geneticist. The individual must have completed training in a clinical specialty residency such as pediatrics, internal medicine, obstetrics-gynecology, or another relevant specialty, although board certification in the specialty is not necessary. To then become a **clinical geneticist,** the minimum genetic education required is a clinical genetics fellowship in a program accredited by the American Board of Medical Genetics. Most programs are 3 years in length and offer a well-rounded experience that includes formal genetic courses and seminars, direct clinical care, and research.

Responsibilities of a clinical geneticist include diagnosing, clinically managing, and counseling patients with a wide variety of genetic disorders. They may work in a specialty setting or as part of a referral center for genetic disorders. Many clinical geneticists also choose to take additional training and become certified in another aspect of genetics, such as cytogenetics, molecular genetics, or biochemical genetics. For example, a clinical geneticist who specializes in working with patients and families affected by lysosomal storage disorders (see Chapter 8) often also certifies in biochemical genetics.

Initial certification for clinical genetics is valid for 10 years. Clinical geneticists can recertify by examination during the 8th, 9th, or 10th year, and they must demonstrate that they have maintained competence in the field by completing a minimum of 250 hours of continuing education credits in the specialty that has been approved by the ABMG. Most often, these professionals use the online review modules every 2 to 3 years that have been developed by the ABMG.

Clinical Laboratory Geneticist

A **clinical laboratory geneticist** is either a physician with a medical degree (i.e., an MD or DO) or is a scientist with a PhD degree in genetics or biological science. Some clinical laboratory geneticists may have both a medical degree and a PhD. Specialty training for certification is an additional 24-month fellowship in an American Board of Medical Genetics (ABMG)–approved program. These individuals can then be certified by examination through the ABMG in at least one of three subspecialties: cytogenetics, molecular genetics, or biochemical genetics. Just as for a clinical geneticist, initial certification for clinical laboratory geneticists is valid for 10 years. Clinical laboratory geneticists can recertify by examination during the 8th, 9th, or 10th year and must demonstrate that they have maintained competence in the field by completing a minimum of 250 hours of continuing education credits in the specialty that has been approved by the ABMG. Most often, these professionals use the online review modules every 2 to 3 years that have been developed by the ABMG.

The primary role of a clinical laboratory geneticist is to oversee and work in laboratories that perform diagnostic genetic tests. They develop and implement new tests, provide quality assurance of routine tests, interpret test results, and communicate these results to health-care professionals and other genetics professionals. In general, the clinical laboratory geneticist does not participate in the direct care or counseling of patients and families but assists other professionals to provide accurate information and explanations.

Medical Geneticist

In spite of the term *medical* in the title of **medical geneticist,** this individual is not a physician. A medical geneticist has a doctorate (PhD), most commonly in population genetics or epidemiology. As of 2008, this genetic specialty is no longer regulated by the ABMG, although some medical geneticists still have valid certification. These individuals often work along with certified genetic counselors to provide accurate recurrence risk information for affected families. In addition, medical geneticists often teach in academic institutions.

Research Geneticist

A **research geneticist** has a doctorate (PhD) in genetics or relevant biological science and has completed at least one 2- to 4-year postdoctoral program of specialized laboratory training in genetics. The focus of this career is in laboratory or "bench" research to identify exact pathological mechanisms that result from various genetic disorders and to develop possible therapeutic approaches, including gene therapy, to reduce the effects of the pathological mechanisms.

Generally, research geneticists have a minimal role in the genetic counseling process. They may work with a clinical geneticist or a certified genetic counselor to provide the scientific details associated with a specific disorder or explain how a new or experimental therapy may affect the disorder.

Nurse Genetic Professionals

Two levels of genetic professional specialty training and certification are available for licensed registered nurses: the Advanced Practice Nurse in Genetics (APNG) and the Genetics Clinical Nurse (GNC). Certification is currently offered through a professional portfolio review process, rather than by examination, through the Genetic Nursing Credentialing Committee (GNCC). This credential is valid for 5 years.

Advanced Practice Nurse in Genetics

The minimum requirements for the APNG include a master's degree in nursing from an accredited program that includes 50 hours of genetic content (in the past 5 years) acquired through academic courses or continuing education, and 300 hours of supervised genetic practicum experience as a clinical genetic nurse with greater than a 50% genetic practice component. The person must be currently licensed to practice in at least one state and have performance verification from an employer, supervisor, or professional colleague with whom the individual has practiced for the most recent 2 years. Other minimum criteria for certification include completion of logs of 50 cases within 5 years of the application and four written case studies that reflect the standards of clinical genetics nursing practice developed by the International Society of Nurses in Genetics (ISONG). The person must have demonstrated evidence of effective teaching of patients and families and must have participated in the education of nurses, other professionals, consumers, and community groups. Additional proof of achievement in genetics that is considered as part of the professional portfolio review may include abstracts, abbreviated reports, lists of publications, and related materials.

The APNG may work in conjunction with other genetic professionals or in some states may maintain an independent practice and caseload for genetic counseling. Other specific functions include facilitating genetic testing and interpreting genetic test results and laboratory reports (ISONG, 2010). Most APNGs specialize within an area of genetics, such as oncology, specific inborn errors of metabolism, or cystic fibrosis. In addition to counseling, the APNG performs physical assessments and may assist in clinical management. In some states, he or she may order tests and prescribe pharmacological therapy or medical foods.

Genetics Clinical Nurse (GCN)

Certification as a GCN is also performed through a professional portfolio review process by the Genetic Nursing Credentialing Committee (GNCC) rather than by examination. Minimum criteria include that the applicant be a currently licensed registered nurse with a bachelor's degree in nursing from an accredited program. He or she must have at least 5 years of experience as a clinical nurse with greater than a 50% genetic practice component. Other minimum criteria for certification include completion of logs of 50 cases within 5 years of the application and four written case studies that reflect the standards of clinical genetics nursing practice developed by the ISONG. The applicant must have completed at least 45 contact hours of genetic content from academic course work or continuing education within the most recent 3 years. Performance verification from an employer, supervisor, or professional colleague with whom the individual has practiced for the most recent 2 years is required, as is evidence of patient and family teaching and participation in providing genetics-related in-service education. In addition, abstracts, abbreviated reports, lists of publications, and related materials may be recognized as evidence of commitment to and practice of genetics.

The GCN works directly with patients and families and provides some level of genetic counseling. As part of the health-care team and genetic disorder management team, GCN role functions include obtaining a detailed family history and constructing a pedigree, assessing and analyzing hereditary and nonhereditary disease risk factors, identifying potential genetic conditions or genetic predisposition to disease, providing genetic information and psychosocial support to individuals and families, and providing nursing care for patients and families at risk for or affected by diseases with a genetic component (ISONG, 2010). He or she is not an independent practitioner and neither prescribes medications nor orders tests (unless working under the license of a physician or nurse practitioner).

The Role of the General Nurse in Genomic Care

Registered nurses who have not undergone additional education and credentialing in genetics are not genetic professionals but have important roles in genomic care. They are often the health-care professional who has the most interaction with patients. In addition, most patients feel comfortable with nurses and may be willing to share more information or ask more questions of nurses than other health-care professionals. As a result, nurses are in a position to identify a patient or family who may have an increased genetic risk for a health problem. Whenever a nurse performs a patient assessment, the "red flags" of genetic risk and potential need for genetic referral discussed in Chapter 6 should be kept in mind.

The nurse may be the health-care professional who first verifies information to bring a genetic problem to light. For example, during an assessment, a 48-year-old patient reveals that his 55-year-old brother has severe emphysema even though he has never smoked. The patient indicates that he is worried that he, too, might develop the disease. Not only should the nurse know that emphysema in a nonsmoker is rare but also recognize that this patient's expression of concern is a perfect opportunity to obtain specific assessment information. The nurse might then ask, "Did either of your parents, aunts or uncles, or grandparents have emphysema or any other respiratory problems?" Be aware of other cues that may indicate the patient is interested in or concerned about a possible increased genetic risk for any health problem. Such cues may include statements or questions similar to these:

- Do you think there is any possibility that I have passed this problem on to my children?
- Because there are other people in my family with this disease, is something wrong with my genes?
- I have heard that all diseases are genetic. Is this true?
- Can we test my genes?

For this patient who is concerned about a possible genetic issue with his family and emphysema, in addition to asking more about his family history, what other responsibilities do you have? Is this considered "genetic counseling"? Major responsibilities for genomic care by a registered nurse include providing accurate information, ensuring that a referral to an appropriate level of genetic professional occurs, serving as a patient advocate, and maintaining confidentiality. Although each responsibility is presented separately, you may need to perform them all simultaneously.

Providing Accurate Information

Provide as much accurate information as you can in a given situation. You are not a genetic expert and are not expected to be the final or definitive source of information for the patient about the issue of concern. Work with the patient to develop his or her family history as a pedigree that includes at least three generations (see Chapter 6). Using the patient just described, you might respond to him by saying, "Yes, emphysema can have a genetic influence, and more information about your family is needed before anyone could determine whether this is a possibility for you." Another question to ask is, "Have you mentioned your brother's health to your physician?" Although most physicians also are not genetic professionals, it is always helpful to let him or her know about a patient's concerns and any information that supports the concern. Remind the patient that you are not a geneticist but that you can help him find accurate and helpful information about the specific topic in the form of written materials and legitimate Web sites.

Ensuring Appropriate Referral

Providing genomic care is a team effort. By bringing the physician into the picture, you are already beginning the referral process. However, your responsibility may not end at this time. Many physicians, although not genetic experts, may have clinical knowledge of genetic risks for common disorders within their specialty. In the case of the patient concerned about his brother's emphysema, his physician may have been unaware of the brother's health status and, with your communication of this information, may then investigate the problem more deeply, keeping the possibility of genetic testing or referral in mind.

But what about a situation in which the physician either disregards your information or says that it is not important? For example, a 31-year-old woman who is being seen for infertility tells you that her mother, her sister, and her older brother have all had breast cancer by the time they were 40 years old. She then asks, "Do you think I should have genetic testing?" When you report this information to the patient's physician, the response is, "She worries about everything. Don't put anything else into her head." What is your responsibility here?

First, express to the physician that though the patient may have other unfounded concerns, this issue is a well-documented genetic "red flag" with health and practice (and legal) implications. If the physician is not interested in making a referral, be sure to document the patient's concerns in the medical record. If you have generated a pedigree in conjunction with the patient, also place that in the medical record and make a copy for the patient. Tell the patient that you are not a genetic professional but that you will help her find someone who can provide more information about this special issue. Possible resources include the hospital's breast center (which may have a genetic counselor), a breast or gynecological advanced practice nurse, or the local unit of the American Cancer Society. Providing this type of information is within your scope of practice as a registered nurse.

Serving as a Patient Advocate

The situation described in the section "Ensuring Appropriate Referral" demonstrates an aspect of advocating for a patient. Other ways to advocate for the patient as part of genomic care is to make certain that the patient understands any provided genetic information. Communication between the patient and whoever is providing the genetic information must be clear. Determine the patient's cognitive ability and education level. Also check whether the patient is under the influence of any drugs that could interfere with comprehension. Work with the genetic professional to provide information in terms the patient understands. Determine whether the patient can see and hear clearly and understands the language being used.

If possible, and if the patient desires, be present with the patient during any discussion with a genetic professional. Look for patient cues to indicate understanding, and ask the patient to describe what has been said in his or her own words.

An important issue to consider is whether the patient is being coerced to have genetic testing by a relative or even another health-care professional. Remind the patient that he or she has the right to refuse to undergo genetic testing and must make the decision based on his or her belief about whether such testing would be beneficial or harmful.

Maintaining Confidentiality

Just as with all other patient information, genetic information must be kept confidential, even the decision of whether to have a specific genetic test. This is even more important because genetic information reveals issues that affect not only the patient, but also his or her family members. Ensure that any conversations you have with the patient about his or her health problem and family history take place privately (unless the patient requests otherwise). The patient has the right to determine who may be a part of the discussion and can decide to keep the information from his or her physician, family members, or anyone else. If you are present during a discussion between the patient and a genetic professional, do not disclose information, formally or informally, without the patient's permission.

If genetic testing is performed, results are usually received by the genetic professional involved with the patient's case. Even at this point in the process, the patient has the right to choose not to be told the results of the test and can decide not to share the information. Chapters 14 and 17 present more information on the legal, social, and ethical issues surrounding genetic testing.

Summary

Genetic counseling is a process that often involves many team members and occurs in multiple sessions. Most health-care professionals have little, if any, formal education in genetics and are not genetic experts. Thus, they are not genetic professionals and are not qualified to provide final, definitive information to patients and families at increased genetic risk for health problems. All health-care professionals have the responsibility to assess genetic factors that influence the health status of any patient within their care.

GENE GEMS

- All health-care professionals are expected to have basic competencies in genetics, but without additional education and credentialing, they are not considered "genetic professionals."
- All health-care professionals have the responsibility to assess genetic factors that influence the health status of any patient within their care.
- To be a genetic professional, an individual must have an advanced degree in a genetics field from a program that has been accredited by either the American Board of Medical Genetics or the American Board of Genetic Counselors or have completed a residency program accredited by the American Society of Medical Genetics. The person must also have current certification by one of these two accrediting bodies.
- Providing information or performing genetic counseling, regardless of the title or level of the genetic or health-care professional, should always be done in a nondirective manner.
- An advanced practice nurse can be certified as a genetic professional by the Genetic Nursing Credentialing Commission and can perform independent nursing and counseling practice.
- A registered nurse with a valid license may be certified as a genetic professional through the Genetic Nursing Credentialing Commission and perform actions that include obtaining a detailed family history and constructing a pedigree, assessing and analyzing hereditary and nonhereditary disease risk factors, identifying potential genetic conditions or genetic predisposition to disease, providing genetic information and psychosocial support to individuals and families, and providing nursing care for patients and families at risk for or affected by diseases with a genetic component.
- Determine whether any information obtained during patient assessment constitutes a "red flag" for genetic risk.
- Organize data obtained by patient history assessment into a three-generation family pedigree.
- Be sure to check the accuracy of any genetic information you provide to a patient or family.
- Maintain confidentiality regarding any patient data, testing, or decisions.
- Work with other members of the health-care team to determine what type of genetic professional or level of genetic counseling may be most appropriate for a specific patient or family thought to have an increased genetic risk for a health problem.
- Keep in mind that the patient has the right to choose or refuse to have genetic testing and that he or she alone determines whether any of the information is shared with anyone.
- Determine whether the patient understands the genetic information provided to him or her.

Self-Assessment Questions

1. Which statement made by a genetic professional to a man who does not want to know the results of his cytogenetic test (which shows he has a balanced translocation of chromosome 13 and 21) best demonstrates a nondirective approach?
   a. "The results will be available in the future should you change your mind."
   b. "It is important that you know these results before you decide to have children."
   c. "By choosing not to know the results, you will derive no benefit from this test."
   d. "You have a right to make that decision, but it is not being fair to your family."

2. A 1-month-old infant has just been diagnosed with the inherited lysosomal storage disorder of Gaucher disease. Which genetic professional, together with a pediatrician, can best direct this infant's care?
   a. Medical geneticist
   b. Certified genetic counselor
   c. Clinical geneticist
   d. Research geneticist

3. Which activity would a general registered nurse be expected to perform as part of genomic care?
   a. Calculating recurrence risk for parents who have just had a child with nondisjunction Down syndrome
   b. Informing a patient that his test results are positive for a genetic disorder
   c. Obtaining an accurate family history and physical assessment data
   d. Requesting a consultation visit from a clinical geneticist

References

American College of Medical Genetics. (2011). Retrieved February 2011 from www.acmg.net//AM/Template.cfm?Section=Home3.

International Society of Nurses in Genetics (ISONG). (2010). Retrieved February 2011 from www.isong.org/ISONG_professional_practice.php.

National Society of Genetic Counselors. (2006). New definition of genetic counseling. Retrieved February 2011 from www.nsgc.org.

Self-Assessment Answers

1. a 2. c 3. c

Global Genomic Issues

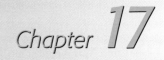
Financial, Ethical, Legal, and Social Considerations

Learning Outcomes

1. Use genetic terminology associated with financial, ethical, legal, and social issues.
2. Describe the history of genetic discrimination.
3. Explain how the Genetic Information and Nondiscrimination Act protects consumers from genetic discrimination in employment and insurance coverage.
4. Compare the professional's "duty to warn" with the consumer's "right to privacy."
5. Discuss the implications of gene patenting for future research and genetic testing.
6. Describe three ways in which financial, ethical, legal, and social issues affect the genetic health of patients.

KEY TERMS

Autonomy

Beneficence

Duty to warn

Ethical, legal, and social issues (ELSI)

Eugenics

Genetic information

Genetic Information and Nondiscrimination Act (GINA)

Intellectual property

Patents

Right to privacy

Introduction

Genetic information is different from other kinds of health information. Of course, all health information should be protected and remain confidential. However, genetic information is even more sensitive. It is typically shared within families, and it provides information about the person being tested and about his or her family members. For example, let's say you are caring for a patient named Jim whose paternal grandfather has Huntington disease (HD). Jim's father does not want to be tested; he would rather not know whether HD was in his future. Jim chooses to have predictive genetic testing to see if he carries the allele for HD, and he tests positive. Now we know something not only about Jim, but also about his father.

Jim's father is almost certainly positive for the allele that causes HD. This devastating disease is in his future (unless he dies from something else first). Even if Jim plans not to tell his father about the genetic test results, the knowledge that his father is also positive could put a significant strain on their relationship. Was it ethical for Jim to be tested when genetic testing could reveal information his father did not want to know? What happens when Jim's "right to know" interferes with his father's "right not to know"? As you can see, the ethical dilemmas that surround genetics can be very challenging. We will discuss some of these issues and circle back to this hypothetical case later on in the chapter.

Ethical Goals of Clinical Genetics

Genetics professionals are trained to provide genetic information in a nondirective and supportive way that allows patients and their families to make informed decisions that are best suited to their needs and values. Respecting patient **autonomy** is an important guiding principle. Counselors provide information to patients and their families that will help them identify their own perspectives on any issue. For example, the counselor may have strong personal feelings about the wisdom of bringing a disabled child into the world. However, when she or he is working with a couple who have just received the results of a prenatal test that indicates that their child will have a significant disability, the counselor must put his or her personal feelings aside and provide the couple with all the information and support they need to make their own decision (Wilson, 2000). There is more information about the role of the genetics professional in Chapter 16.

Genetic Discrimination

Advances in genetic testing and genetic health care promise to make things better for most people seeking treatment for many diseases. However, many Americans report that they are afraid of having genetic testing done because they do not want to be victims of genetic discrimination (NHGRI, 2010b). They are afraid that they will lose their health insurance or have to pay much higher premiums if their insurance companies find out that they are at increased genetic risk for a major health problem. They are also afraid that they might lose their jobs and not be hirable if their genetic risk is documented on their health records. Fortunately, we have relatively new legislation designed to protect people from discrimination in employment and/or insurance coverage based on their genetic information. We will discuss the Genetic Information and Nondiscrimination Act (GINA) in a later section. This law is important in fighting both actual genetic discrimination and reducing the public's fear that they might become victims of genetic discrimination.

Advances in genetic knowledge have brought with them brand-new ethical concerns and puzzles. Fortunately, when the Human Genome Project began, the U.S. Department of Energy (DOE) and the National Institutes of Health (NIH) designated 3% to 5% of their annual budget toward studying the **ethical, legal, and social issues** (ELSI) of the newly available genetic knowledge. This funded the largest bioethics program in the world. The acronym *ELSI* was used to designate this program. More recently, some people have added financial issues to the list to better reflect the societal issues involved. Now the acronym *FELSI* reflects the concern about the financial, ethical, legal, and social issues confronting patients.

Eugenics and Preimplantation Genetic Diagnosis

One of the fears genetics advances bring to mind surrounds the technological ability to produce "designer babies." Much of this fear probably comes from memories of Nazi Germany's efforts to "purify" the human population, which was an appalling chapter in human history. However, efforts to breed superior human beings were not limited to the actions of Nazi Germany. Between the years of

1910 and 1940, there was a strong movement in support of eugenics in both the United States and the United Kingdom. **Eugenics** can be defined as working to improve humankind by selectively breeding people who have genes that society would consider "good" and not allowing reproduction of people with genes that society would consider "bad." Some people during that time supported euthanasia and others suggested genocide, but sterilization of people considered "socially inadequate" had widespread support beginning in the 1920s. By 1924, more than 3000 people had been involuntarily sterilized (Dolan, n.d.). Read more about the American Eugenics Movement at www.eugenicsarchive.org/eugenics/. You will find many disturbing images and much unsettling information. The fear of something like this movement happening again makes people wary of the new ability to choose to implant selected embryos and reject embryos that do not meet specifications. It is important that we remember our history and guard against making decisions that affect the moral structure of our culture.

Preimplantation genetic diagnosis (PGD) was discussed in Chapter 14. The procedure has been around for some time. The first successful use of PGD took place in 1988. In this process, genetic testing is done on an embryo produced through the process of in vitro fertilization. The fertilized egg is allowed to divide until it gets to the 6- or 10-cell stage (blastomere). At this point, one or two cells can be removed without damaging the embryo. Those cells can be tested to see if they contain a genetic abnormality of concern to the parents. The parents can then choose to have any unaffected embryos transferred to the uterus in the hope that it will become implanted and mature into a healthy baby (Basille et al., 2009). This is a very exciting technology that can reduce inherited genetic disease. However, it is very expensive and brings with it major concerns about the ethical use of such a technology. For example, it makes sense to find out if an embryo is male or female if the mother is a carrier of an X-linked recessive disease. There is a 50% risk of being affected for every male child this mother conceives. These parents may prefer to have a female child, with only a 50% risk of being a carrier and virtually no risk of being affected. Testing the embryo for sex determination may be less expensive than testing for particular gene mutations that cause disease. But is it ethical to test embryos for sex determination if a couple has four girls and just wants to have a boy?

There are many additional concerns about this procedure. First of all, what happens to the "unsuitable" embryos? These may be considered "defective" and simply discarded. Many people are concerned with the message this action sends to people living with disability. What is the value of their lives to society when embryos carrying similar traits are thrown away? As you might imagine, people within the disabilities community are very concerned about this process and its ability to reinforce social biases regarding disability. Current estimates report that between 60% and 80% of fetuses diagnosed with Down syndrome are selectively aborted (Stainton, 2007). Some see the use of technology to eliminate or reduce the number of people with disabilities as the ultimate expression of prejudice, and point out that many people with disabilities are productive members of society (Stainton, 2007). It is an ongoing debate that will no doubt continue to grow as reproductive technologies advance. We might consider PGD a very early form of genetic discrimination.

History of Genetic Discrimination

We discussed the fear that many people have of being discriminated against based on their genetic information. It is important to look briefly at the history of genetic discrimination to get a sense of how this problem affects the decisions patients make and how these decisions might be protected.

Several landmark cases set the stage for the development of legislation that addresses genetic discrimination. One case involved the Burlington Northern Santa Fe (BNSF) Railroad. In 2001, the United States Equal Employment Opportunity Commission (EEOC) filed a lawsuit against the BNSF for testing its employees for a genetic predisposition to hereditary neuropathy with liability to pressure palsies

(HNLPP)—without their consent. HNLPP is a rare condition that causes several symptoms, including carpal tunnel syndrome. The railroad wanted to find out if the employees, who were claiming disability from repetitive stress injuries, were genetically predisposed to having carpal tunnel syndrome. The hope was to demonstrate that some claims of work-related carpal tunnel syndrome were not occupational injuries at all but the result of an underlying genetic problem. The doctors employed by the BNSF were also told to screen workers for medical conditions such as diabetes and alcoholism, also without their consent. No mention of genetic testing was made, and an employee who refused to be examined was told he could be terminated. The lawsuit filed by the EEOC was based on the Americans with Disabilities Act, because at that time there was no federal legislation that directly protected people from genetic discrimination. The EEOC claimed that the medical and genetic tests being done were not related to the employee's ability to do the work. Decisions about employment that were based on the results of these tests would be evidence of illegal discrimination based on alleged disability. The EEOC won the case without any difficulty (NHGRI, 2010a).

Many more examples of genetic discrimination are presented by the Council for Responsible Genetics (CRG, 2010). One woman who was diagnosed with hereditary hemochromatosis lost her health insurance, even though she showed no clinical signs of the disease. In another case, a family lost health insurance for their son with fragile X syndrome because the insurance company said that fragile X was a preexisting condition. One man was denied employment for a position with the government based on genetic test results that indicated he carried one copy of the gene variant that causes Gaucher disease. He had no clinical signs of the disease; he was an unaffected carrier for this recessive trait. It is highly likely that there are hundreds more cases that have not been publicized. However, uncovering these cases is difficult because many people do not want others to know about the genetic risk factors in their families. Having actual numbers of cases would be very useful. Unfortunately, much of the information we have now is anecdotal and highly subjective (NHGRI, 2010a).

Legislation to Prevent Genetic Discrimination

On May 21, 2008, the **Genetic Information and Nondiscrimination Act (GINA)** was signed into law by President George W. Bush. This was the result of a 13-year-long effort on the part of the genetics community to get federal legislation that protects genetic information. The bill was passed unanimously by the Senate and by a vote of 414 to 1 in the House of Representatives. Prior to the passage of this law, some protection against discrimination was provided by state laws (some states had laws providing more protection than others) and by the Health Insurance Portability and Accountability Act (HIPAA). The passage of GINA provided federal protection against genetic discrimination in employment and insurance to almost all Americans. The exceptions are people serving in the military, veterans receiving their health care through the Veteran's Administration, and people receiving their health care from the Indian Health Service. These groups are protected by other mechanisms (Coalition, n.d.).

GINA contains two parts. Title I of GINA went into effect on May 21, 2009. This provision makes it illegal for health insurers to use a client's genetic information to make decisions about their eligibility for insurance, the size of their premiums, or the extent of their coverage. Health insurers also cannot use genetic information as evidence of a preexisting condition, and they cannot require that a client have genetic testing. The final regulations for Title II went into effect in January 2011. Title II makes it illegal for employers to use genetic information to make decisions about hiring, promoting, or terminating employees (Coalition, n.d.).

GINA clearly explains what is meant by *genetic information*. **Genetic information** includes the results of one's own genetic tests and those of his or her family members all the way out to fourth-degree relatives (e.g., your great-great-grandparents or your grandnephews and grandnieces). Any clinical signs of a disease in a family member are also protected, so your employer has no legal right to know if you have a parent or grandparent who has Huntington disease. Information about whether you or any of your family members have requested genetic services, such as participating in a research study that included genetic testing, seeking genetic counseling, or attending genetic education programs is also protected (Coalition, n.d.; NHGRI, 2010b).

There is much excellent information on GINA available from reputable Web sites such as www.genome. gov/27535101. It is important that all health-care professionals become familiar with the provisions of this law. Patients worry about their insurance and employment risks should their genetic information be disclosed. As mentioned earlier, many people choose not to have genetic tests that will benefit them or their family members because of the fear of genetic discrimination. You cannot assure them that they will not be discriminated against; however, federal legislation is now in place that protects the use of their genetic information in health insurance and employment decisions.

Duty to Warn Versus the Right to Privacy

As health-care professionals, we often have access to genetic information that could benefit or harm a patient or his or her family members. Sometimes that information has been found incidentally. For example, suppose a female patient is being tested for cardiovascular risk and the clinician finds out that she has the *APOE* genotype that places her at high risk for not only cardiovascular disease, but also for Alzheimer disease. Should she be told that she has an increased risk of getting Alzheimer disease, which could cause her psychological harm? Does she have the right to know? Do you have the **duty to warn** her about this risk? In other words, is it the responsibility of the health-care provider to tell a patient's family members about their genetic risk?

What would you do if your patient tested positive for a mutation that greatly increased his risk of hereditary nonpolyposis colon cancer (HNPCC)? He learned about this from his primary care physician and was told that his children should also be tested because they are at risk as well. What if he tells you that he has no intention of informing his daughter that she is also at risk and the reason why is "none of your business"? Which is more important, his **right to privacy** or your duty to warn his daughter of her risk? If the daughter knows of her risk, she can get the recommended screening and/or choose to have genetic testing herself. What happens if the daughter develops colon cancer and then takes legal action against her father's health-care providers for not warning her? Will she be successful?

Your duty to keep your patient's genetic information confidential is usually seen as stronger than the right of his or her family members to be warned that they are at risk. You are familiar with the importance of maintaining confidentiality of health-care information, which is protected by the privacy rule of the Health Insurance Portability and Accountability Act (HIPAA) of 1996 (P.L.104-191; DHHS, no date). However, as health-care professionals, you also have a duty to abide by the ethical principle of **beneficence.** You want to do good for others. You want to make decisions based on what will benefit your patients and their families. You also need to adhere to the ethical principle of patient autonomy. You need to respect the rights and wishes of your patients. An ethical problem arises when these two important ethical principles contradict each other. It is best for the patient's daughter to know that she is at genetic risk. However, respecting her father's autonomy requires that she not be told.

Some experts say that clinicians have a professional relationship only with their patients and not with their family members, so there is no duty to warn family members of genetic risk. The courts have disagreed on this. Each of these cases has involved the actions (or inactions) of physicians rather than those of other health-care professionals. However, you can still learn much about the complexity of this issue by reviewing these legal decisions.

In the case of _Pate v. Threlkel_, a physician was sued because he had not warned his patient's daughter that she was at genetic risk for thyroid cancer. The daughter developed advanced thyroid cancer 3 years after her mother was diagnosed. The daughter claimed that she would have been diagnosed sooner if she had been warned that she was at risk. The Supreme Court of Florida agreed that the daughter should have been warned and that the physician was obligated to inform the mother that her family members should be warned. The court's decision did recognize that it would be difficult for the physician to directly warn the family members and that his duty to warn would have been satisfied by telling his patient to warn her family members (Offit et al., 2004).

In another case (_Safer v. Estate of Pack_), a New Jersey court made a different decision. Thirty years after her father died, a woman sued the estate of her father's physician for failing to warn her that she was at genetic risk for her father's disease. The father died of familial adenomatous polyposis, a condition that results in hundreds or thousands of colon polyps developing in childhood. Cancer usually results by age 40. The treatment was removal of the colon (prophylactic colectomy) sometime in the teen years, although now disease management may include treatment with anti-inflammatory drugs. The daughter was diagnosed with both polyposis and metastatic colon cancer and claimed that if she had known of her genetic risk, she could have benefited from careful monitoring and early diagnosis. This court decided that simply telling the patient that his family is at risk does not meet the _duty to warn_ requirement and that the physician must take "reasonable steps" to ensure that the risk is communicated to all immediate family members (Offit et al., 2004).

Another important case focuses on the need to inform families of the genetic risk to future pregnancies. In _Molloy v. Meier_, the Minnesota Supreme Court ruled that a physician should have performed a diagnostic genetic test on a child with cognitive impairment to see if that child had a genetic condition. It was established that this family's first child had fragile X syndrome only after a sibling was born who clearly had fragile X. The parents claimed that they would have chosen not to have another child if they had known their first child had fragile X, and other children would be at risk for the same condition. They claimed the physician should have tested their first child so they would have had this information (Offit et al., 2004).

In the United Kingdom, the General Medical Council recommended that physicians disclose genetic information without a patient's consent when it will benefit a family member. This disclosure should occur _only_ after the patient has been told of the importance of warning his or her family members and has refused to do so. The council's decision was based on the need to protect families and the need for physicians to have guidance about what to do if a family member is at genetic risk for something treatable, such as breast or colon cancer. However, it is still controversial (Dyer, 2009).

Most recommendations of professional and governmental organizations try to balance the principles of maximizing benefit and minimizing harm, even if the harm is only psychological. Some organizations recommend that a physician disclose protected genetic information to family members directly, if the patient agrees. However, most recommendations do not support direct contact between the physician and the family members. It is always better if the patient is the one telling his or her relatives so no private information is being disclosed by the health-care provider. One problem arises when the patient says he or she will tell the family members but never does so (Godard et al., 2006). This can be a problem for the family members but is not typically considered the responsibility of the health-care provider. We hope that with new federal legislation in place to protect consumers from genetic discrimination, family members will be more willing to share their relevant genetic information with at-risk family members.

In the mid to late '90s, the Institute of Medicine and a Presidential Commission provided guidance to health-care providers in the United States about when it is acceptable to disclose private health-care information. These times include when it is very likely that harm will result if the information is not disclosed and the harm from not disclosing the information would be greater than the harm of disclosing it (Offit et al., 2004). Most organizations recommend that each case be looked at individually and decisions about whether or not to disclose genetic information be made considering the unique aspects of each case (ASHG, 1998).

Intellectual Property Rights and Gene Patents

The commercialization of genetic testing has brought with it controversy about who owns human genetic information. It is certainly important for scientists to protect their **intellectual property**, the creative products that they develop using their intellects. The government permits people to **patent** the output of their creative work as long as the invention is new, useful, and not obvious to others working in the same area. Physical phenomena, such as gravity or changes in the weather, cannot be patented. This becomes a bit more complicated when we look at scientific advances. For example, a particular microorganism that exists in nature cannot be patented. However, if a scientist genetically alters that microorganism to make it disease-resistant, the newly developed microorganism can be patented (Chuang and Lau, 2010).

Now it becomes even more complicated. The U.S. Patent and Trademark Office has agreed to patent isolated sequences of the human genome. They reasoned that isolating a sequence of DNA from the genome requires considerable human intervention and is therefore patentable, but is it really a new thing? So far almost 20% of the human genome has been patented, and there have been approximately 40,000 DNA-related patents filed (Chuang and Lau, 2010). What does this mean for those of us caring for patients? It turns out that it means a lot. When genes are patented, genetic testing for specific gene variants then becomes proprietary: It becomes something that is the intellectual property of the company or scientist who holds the patent. They have the right to exclude other people from using it or marketing it without their permission, and they have the right to charge whatever they want to grant permission for its use by others.

The case that has brought this issue to the forefront involves the company Myriad Genetics. Myriad is a biotechnology company that holds the gene patent for the gene variants that predispose people to familial breast cancer. They hold the patents on isolated forms of the genes *BRCA1* and *BRCA2*. Remember, we all have copies of *BRCA1* and *BRCA2*. People are genetically predisposed to breast and ovarian cancer when they carry disease-causing mutations in these genes. Because Myriad holds the patent for these two genes, they have control over how and when they are used for research, and they can control the cost of genetic testing for gene mutations. This is highly controversial.

A lawsuit was filed by the American Civil Liberties Union and the Public Patent Foundation claiming that these gene patents held by Myriad were not valid. In March of 2010, a U.S. Federal District Court decided that patenting isolated human gene sequences should not be permitted. The court stated that the isolated DNA sequences were not patentable because they did not differ significantly from the gene sequences that exist by nature in the human genome. In July 2011 the U.S Court of Appeals for the Federal Circuit ruled that Myriad did in fact have the right to patent these two isolated human genes. Of course, this was also controversial and legal action will probably continue. This decision has major implications for biotechnology companies and the future of genetic research and genetic testing. It is expected that the U.S. Supreme Court will have to provide the final determination in this case (Chuang and Lau, 2010).

The American Society of Human Genetics issued a statement in April of 2010 saying that they understand the importance of intellectual property rights and scientific advancement. However, they believe that it is essential that patients not suffer. They could not condone patients having limited access to genetic testing or having to pay excessively high fees for genetic tests because one company holds exclusive rights to an isolated segment of DNA (ASHG, 2010). This issue is further complicated by the rapid advances in genetic testing technologies and the likelihood that whole genome testing will become more common in the future. Many labs are capable of doing this kind of testing now, and the impact of single companies holding patents to segments of the genome means those labs would not be able to market whole genome tests. It seems unlikely that gene patents in their present form will continue, and perhaps some middle ground will be found that will allow scientists and the companies that employ them to benefit from their creative work without penalizing patients in the process.

Summary

There are many legal and ethical issues that have surfaced along with advancements in our knowledge of genetics and genomics. We are confronted with conflicts and controversies that no one imagined. It is likely that the future will provide us with even more controversies that we cannot foresee at this time. Options for reproductive decision-making have changed with the development of advanced reproductive technologies, such as preimplantation genetic diagnosis. Legislation to prevent genetic discrimination in employment and insurance is now in place in the United States; we will see how well it protects our patients and their families. The advances in biotechnology have resulted in controversial decisions about whether genes can be patented. All of these issues have an important impact on the patients for whom we provide care. It is important to know that research into the financial, legal, ethical, and social implications of genetic advances is continuing and will help us understand the best ways to manage these problems.

And what about Jim, who tested positive for the HD disease gene mutation, which means that his father, who did not want to know his mutation status, is also positive for the gene mutation? This situation presents a major problem for genetics professionals and underscores the importance of families having good genetic counseling prior to the completion of any genetic test. The best-case scenario would be for Jim and his father to sit down with a genetic counselor and discuss all the possible outcomes of Jim's genetic test before Jim was tested. The family can then decide what is best for them and what actions Jim should take after he learns his results. Genetic counselors are skilled in helping families work through such dilemmas about sharing genetic information. As with so many issues, advanced planning and open communication can help to reduce the risk of problems for all family members.

GENE GEMS

- Genetic information is different from other kinds of health information because it involves family members as well as patients.
- Respecting autonomy is an important guiding principle in caring for a patient's or family's genetic health.
- Many Americans report that they are afraid of having genetic testing done because they do not want to be victims of genetic discrimination.
- Between 3% and 5% of the annual budget of the Human Genome Project was designated to studying the ethical, legal, and social implications of genetic knowledge.
- The American Eugenics Movement sought to eliminate "defective" people from the reproducing population.

- Fears of the widespread resurgence of eugenics makes some people wary of using advanced reproductive technologies.
- Preimplantation genetic diagnosis allows parents to screen in vitro fertilized embryos for specific genetic traits (or sex) and implant those that are less likely to carry the disease.
- On May 21, 2008, the Genetic Information and Nondiscrimination Act (GINA) was signed into law by President George W. Bush.
- GINA provides protection against genetic discrimination in employment and health insurance.
- Sometimes the health-care professional's duty to warn family members of genetic risk is in conflict with the obligation to maintain the privacy of a patient's health-care information.
- Even though the legal cases presented involved only physicians, the government and professional organization recommendations that resulted from them are important for all health-care professionals.
- Some companies have patented sections of the human genome, claiming this was their intellectual property.
- When genes are patented, the company that holds the patent can restrict research using those genes and can charge excessively high rates for genetic tests.
- In March of 2010, a U.S. Federal District Court decided that patenting isolated human gene sequences should not be permitted. However, further litigation will probably follow.

Self-Assessment Questions

1. You are caring for a college professor who has been offered testing for her family's mutation in *BRCA1*. She expresses fear of genetic discrimination as a reason for refusing genetic testing. What do you tell her?
   a. "There is no need to be concerned about genetic discrimination."
   b. "I appreciate your concern, but there is no way your insurance company or employer will ever be able to get your genetic testing results."
   c. "There is now federal legislation banning genetic discrimination, and in addition we will do everything we can to keep your results confidential."
   d. "There have been no instances of documented genetic discrimination in insurance or employment. This concern is overblown."

2. Which statement describes a consequence of federal legislation enacted in 2008 entitled "Genetic Information Nondiscrimination Act"?
   a. It requires that health-care providers begin keeping genetic information confidential.
   b. It prohibits for-profit direct-to-consumer DNA testing companies from offering genetic tests.
   c. It discourages individuals from using genetic testing and counseling.
   d. It prohibits discrimination regarding health insurance coverage and employment on the basis of an individual's genetic information.

Continued

3. What is true regarding the health-care provider's duty to warn a patient's family members when genetic disease is diagnosed?
   a. Past legal decisions make it clear that health-care providers should inform a patient's family members when they are at genetic risk.
   b. Past legal decisions make it clear that health-care providers should not inform a patient's family members when they are at genetic risk.
   c. There is sometimes a conflict between the health-care provider's duty to warn family members of their genetic risk and their obligation to keep their patients' genetic information private.
   d. Recommendations for the disclosure of genetic information to family members is covered under the Genetic Information and Nondiscrimination Act.

4. Preimplantation genetic diagnosis provides parents with which options?
   a. The ability to screen normally fertilized embryos for genetic traits after the first trimester
   b. The ability to select embryos for implantation that test negative for a familial disease mutation
   c. The opportunity to determine how many children they will conceive
   d. The ability to guarantee that they will have a healthy baby

5. What is a major public health problem related to gene patents?
   a. Patented genes can be used to create "designer babies."
   b. When one company holds the patent for a gene, genetic testing can be excessively expensive.
   c. The results of research using that gene cannot be published.
   d. That gene must be eliminated from any genetic testing that is marketed directly to consumers.

CASE STUDY

You are a nurse caring for a patient who has been diagnosed with terminal colon cancer. His daughter Elizabeth approaches you during your shift and says that she is afraid that she is also at genetic risk for colon cancer because she knows that it often runs in families. She wants to have genetic testing done and has read on the Internet that the test will be less expensive if she knows the specific mutation carried by her father. The problem is that her father does not know that his colon cancer might be inherited and that his children might be at risk. Elizabeth does not want to tell her father and ask his permission to have the genetic test done. She is afraid that he will feel guilty, and she wants to spare him this pain. Elizabeth asks if you would please take a cheek swab from her father so that she can send it off for testing. She is afraid that if she tries to do it herself, she will do it wrong and she knows how important this is.

1. What is the ethical dilemma in this case?

2. What assumptions is Elizabeth making? Are you concerned about the source of her information?

3. Which ethical principles are important in deciding the best action(s) to take?

4. What factors make this situation unique?

5. Who might you consult to get support in this situation?

References

ASHG. (1998). ASHG statement. Professional disclosure of familial genetic information. The American Society of Human Genetics Social Issues Subcommittee on Familial Disclosure. *American Journal of Human Genetics, 62*(2), 474–483.

ASHG. (2010). Guiding principles on protection of intellectual property patenting and licensing in the genetic testing arena. Retrieved January 8, 2011.

Basille, C., Frydman, R., El Aly, A., et al. (2009). Preimplantation genetic diagnosis: State of the art. *European Journal of Obstetrics, Gynecology, and Reproductive Biology, 145*(1), 9–13.

Chuang, C. S., and Lau, D. T. (2010). Patenting human genes: The Myriad controversy. *Clinical Therapeutics, 32*(12), 2054–2056.

Coalition, F. G. F. (n.d.). What does GINA mean? A guide to the Genetic Information Nondiscrimination Act. Retrieved December 20, 2010, from www.geneticfairness.org/act.html.

CRG, C. f. R. G. (2010). Genetic testing, privacy and discrimination. Retrieved December 20, 2010, from www.councilforresponsiblegenetics.org/.

DHHS. (No date). The Health Insurance Portability and Accountability Act of 1996 (HIPAA) Privacy and Security Rules. Retrieved January 5, 2011, from www.hhs.gov/ocr/privacy/.

Dolan, D. L. C. (n.d.). Image Archive on the American Eugenics Movement. Retrieved December 20, 2010, from www.eugenicsarchive.org/eugenics/.

Dyer, C. (2009). Doctors may share genetic information to help patients' relatives. *British Medical Journal, 339*, b4031.

Godard, B., Hurlimann, T., Letendre, M., and Egalite, N. (2006). Guidelines for disclosing genetic information to family members: From development to use. *Familial Cancer, 5*(1), 103–116.

NHGRI. (2010a). Cases of genetic discrimination. Retrieved December 20, 2010, from www.genome.gov/pfv.cfm?pageID=12513976.

NHGRI. (2010b). Genetic discrimination. Retrieved December 16, 2010, from www.genome.gov/10002077.

Offit, K., Groeger, E., Turner, S., Wadsworth, E. A., and Weiser, M. A. (2004). The "duty to warn" a patient's family members about hereditary disease risks. *Journal of the American Medical Association, 292*(12), 1469–1473.

Stainton, T. (2007). Missing the forest for the trees? A disability rights take on genetics. *Journal on Developmental Disabilities, 13*(2), 89–92.

Wilson, G. N. Clinical genetics. New York: Wiley & Sons, 2000.

Self-Assessment Answers

1. c **2.** d **3.** c **4.** b **5.** b

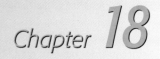

Chapter 18

Genetic and Genomic Variation

Learning Outcomes

1. Use terminology associated with genomic variation.
2. Distinguish between genetic drift and founder effects.
3. Describe what happens in a population bottleneck.
4. Apply aspects of population genetics to explain genetic variation in human populations.
5. Explain how geography can have an impact on the transmission of heritable traits.
6. Describe current ideas about the biological basis of "race" and "ethnicity."

KEY TERMS

Assortative mating

Ethnicity

Evolution

Founder effect

Gene pool

Genetic anthropology

Genetic drift

Haplotypes

Hardy-Weinberg Principle

Heterozygosity

Human genetic variation

Natural selection

Population bottleneck

Population genetics

Race

Introduction

Humans are a very homogenous group. People are 99.9% genetically alike. When you think about the entire genome (remember that the human genome contains approximately 3 billion base pairs), it is amazing that people are so similar. However, that 0.1% difference is important and has both health-related and social-cultural consequences. People vary in their individual DNA sequences by copy numbers, polymorphisms, and the presence or absence of chemical additions that result in differing levels of gene expression *(epigenetics)*. There are about 10 million single nucleotide polymorphisms (SNPs) with a frequency greater than 1% in human populations (NHGRI, 2010). That is a lot of variation for only a 0.1% difference.

Scientists believe that humans have so little genetic diversity because all are descended from the same female African ancestor, who lived about 140,000 years ago. All men are descended from the same male ancestor who lived in Africa about 60,000 years ago (DOE, 2010; Tishkoff and Verrelli, 2003). Humans appear to have migrated out of Africa to southern Asia, China, and Europe about 65,000 years ago (DOE, 2010).

353

When we pass DNA down through the generations, there is a lot of mixing of genetic information. Earlier in this text, you read about some factors that increase our genetic diversity, including Mendel's principle of independent assortment of alleles during meiosis and crossing over of segments of homologous chromosomes, which also occurs during meiosis (Chapter 3). However, there are pieces of genetic material that are passed from generation to generation with very little change. These include the mitochondrial DNA, which is passed from mother to all her children, and the Y chromosome, which is passed from father to son. Small changes to these genetic materials are inherited, and eventually people from the same region end up with common markers that allow us to determine the geographical origin of people's ancestors (DOE, 2010).

Many people are interested in learning about their very distant relatives. The study of **genetic anthropology** uses a combination of genetic information and physical evidence, such as the fossil record, to learn more about our history as a species. In 2006, the National Geographic Society began the Genographic Project with the goal of assembling DNA from more than 100,000 people and creating the largest DNA database in the world. They wanted to get samples from all major populations living on the earth and catalogue genetic similarities and differences. **Human genetic variation** is the phrase used to describe the genetic differences that can be found within and between groups of people. This database is considered "open source," meaning that it is available to interested people everywhere (DOE, 2010). Another way that scientists are working to document human genetic variation is by assembling a map of human haplotypes.

Haplotypes

We all have groups of genes (or SNPs or markers) that tend to be inherited together. These are called **haplotypes,** and one way to think about them is as genetic "neighborhoods." A gene does not exist in isolation. It is always on a chromosome near other genes and intergenic regions. The International HapMap Project was completed in 2005 and provides a catalogue, or map, of common patterns of human genetic variation. This project makes it easier for scientists to study the differences in the risk of disease and the response to drugs found in different human populations (NHGRI, 2010). The HapMap Project is an international collaboration of scientists from the United States, Japan, the United Kingdom, Canada, China, and Nigeria (DOE, 2010).

Population Genetics

In most of this text, we have been discussing the impact of genetics on the health of individuals and their families. However, it is important to remember that people and families exist as parts of larger groups, or populations. Those groups share things in common, such as culture, heritage, customs, and often a higher risk for certain diseases.

The field of **population genetics** examines the ways in which allele frequencies change in human populations over time, including those events that keep the frequencies the same and those events that change them. A species with many different alleles (versions of a gene) will have far more genetic diversity than a species with a small number of alleles for each gene.

Disease Risk and the Geographic Origin of Ancestors

We also see rates of disease risk that vary by the geographical origin of ancestors. For example, why is hemophilia A rare and sickle cell disease so common among people of African descent? Why is there a higher-than-average risk of Huntington disease among Afrikaners, the descendents of Dutch settlers from South Africa? These apparent mysteries have simple genetic explanations, and we have to look at more than individuals and families to answer them. We need to look more broadly at large populations, migration patterns, and the results of foundational ideas, such as **natural selection (the notion that organisms that are best suited to the environment will survive to reproduce and pass on their genetic characteristics)**. Scientists are very interested in how and why the frequencies of different traits change in populations.

When we look at disease risk, some different versions of a gene can be helpful and some can be harmful. For example, we discussed sickle cell disease (SCD) in the chapter on childhood diseases (Chapter 9). Remember that being homozygous for the mutation that causes SCD means you will have the signs and symptoms of SCD. However, being heterozygous confers protection against malaria without most of the problematic manifestations of SCD. If we look at this trait from a population level, the mutation is helpful. Of course, when we are working with an individual patient affected by SCD, it does not seem helpful. Looking at risk or benefit from a population-wide perspective is very different from looking at risk or benefit for one individual.

Unlike the situation with carriers of SCD, as far as we know, people of African descent do not get any advantage from being heterozygous for the mutation that causes hemophilia A, so it makes sense that the hemophilia A mutation would be much less common than the SCD mutation in this group. It will be interesting to see what happens to the frequency of the SCD allele in future generations of African Americans. They are rarely exposed to malaria. In addition, interbreeding between people whose ancestors came from Africa and those whose ancestors came from other regions of the world, such as Europe or northern Asia, should also have an impact on the persistence of the SCD allele in the general population. The SCD carrier rate is much lower in populations that come from regions where malaria is not common.

Allele Frequencies

So, how different are we? At the DNA level, there is one sequence variation for every 200 to 500 nucleotides. Those stretches of DNA that do not code for proteins have even greater variation than our protein-coding regions. These changes underlie our ability to adapt to extreme environments and have been essential to our evolution as a species (Wilson, 2000). Human genetic variation is a good thing, and it is very relevant to planning appropriate health care for our patients. For example, some couples of Ashkenazi Jewish background may choose to have carrier testing before they conceive children, because carrier rates for certain recessive diseases are relatively high in this population (see Chapters 8 and 14).

Many laboratories offer an Ashkenazi Jewish Panel that provides individuals and couples with genetic testing to determine whether they are carriers for diseases that are common among people of Ashkenazi Jewish ancestry. If both partners are carriers of one copy of a mutant gene that results in a disease such as Tay-Sachs, they could choose to have preimplantation genetic diagnosis in order to screen out affected embryos. They could also choose to not have children (the risk of having an affected child if both parents are heterozygous would be 25% with each pregnancy), or they could choose to prepare for the possible birth of a disabled child. The ability to provide anticipatory guidance could improve the outcome for any couple in this situation.

Changes in the Gene Pool

One way to define **evolution** is a change in the genetically inherited frequencies of alleles over time. This reflects changes in the **gene pool**, or the sum total of all the alleles for all the genes in a given population. For example, on a very simple scale, we can see the evolution from one generation to another. If we say that 86% of a population has at least one copy of the "A" allele for a particular gene, then 14% of the population has at least one copy of a different allele for that gene, which we will call "a." Now we will fast-forward a few generations and look at the population's genotypes again. At this new point in time, 90% of the population has at least one copy of the "A" allele and only 10% of the population has the "a" version. We can look at these numbers and see evolution favoring the increasing frequency of the "A" allele and the decreasing frequency of the "a" allele.

Maybe having more copies of the "A" allele means that you are more resistant to getting diabetes mellitus type 2. That would be a very positive change in this population's gene pool. One thing we know is that if 95% of all alleles in a population are "A," most people will be homozygous AA. **Heterozygosity,** or the proportion of a population that is heterozygous at a particular locus, will be very low. Very few people would be Aa at that gene location. There are not very many "a" alleles available. Even fewer people would be aa. So how do you figure out the allele frequency in a population?

Hardy-Weinberg Equilibrium

In the early 1900s, two scientists, a mathematician from England named Godfrey Hardy and a medical doctor from Germany named Wilhelm Weinberg, independently developed ideas about how allele frequencies change in populations. They determined that allele frequencies would remain the same if certain criteria were met. Of course, these criteria are never met in human populations, so we continue to evolve! If allele frequencies were to remain stable, the population would be in **Hardy-Weinberg equilibrium.** We will discuss a few of the requirements for Hardy-Weinberg equilibrium here. See Table 18–1 for a list of the criteria for maintaining Hardy-Weinberg equilibrium. None of them are much fun.

The first criterion a population must meet to remain in Hardy-Weinberg equilibrium is that everyone and all their descendents must stay in the same geographic region. No migration is allowed. When we migrate, we take our genetic traits with us. If only a few of us leave our native land, then future populations in this new place will be more like the small group that migrated than they will be like the original population. This is called the founder effect.

Founder effect occurs when a small group of people leave a larger population and settle somewhere else. For example, in 1652, one shipload of Dutch settlers migrated to South Africa. It happened that one of the immigrants carried the gene mutation that causes Huntington disease (HD), which, you will recall, is an autosomal dominant condition with age-related penetrance. Symptoms of HD do not

---

TABLE 18–1

Requirements for Populations to Stay in Hardy-Weinberg Equilibrium

1. No one migrates.
2. People mate randomly.
3. The population is extremely large.
4. Everyone has children.
5. There are no mutations.

Source: Pierce, B. Transmission and population genetics, 2nd ed., New York: W. H. Freeman, 2009.

usually appear before a person is 35 to 50 years old. By that time, most people have already had children. If a parent is an affected heterozygote, each child has a 50% risk of inheriting the disease-causing allele and getting HD. Once the HD allele is in a population, it often continues to be transmitted. Today, the incidence of HD is much higher in the Afrikaner people than in the original Dutch population their ancestors left behind. Most Afrikaner people with HD today are descendents of this first Dutch immigrant (Ridley, 2003).

In order to maintain Hardy-Weinberg equilibrium, everyone in the population must *mate randomly* (not selecting partners based on similar or different characteristics). There would be no picking your mate based on any particular characteristics. You cannot mate preferentially with someone who likes the same things you like. You cannot mate with someone who enjoys science-fiction movies if you enjoy science-fiction movies. You also cannot choose to mate with someone who is different from you. You cannot select a person who likes to cook because you hate to cook. When you purposefully select your mate based on similar or dissimilar traits, that is called **assortative mating**, and it keeps your population from achieving Hardy-Weinberg equilibrium.

If you practice *random mating*, which is required by the Hardy-Weinberg principle, you could not pick your partner because she or he was attractive or intelligent, or even fun to be with. That is not random mating, and choosing your partner based on particular attributes will increase the likelihood that those traits will increase in frequency in the population. This is particularly true if lots of other people in your population like the same traits. Of course, the terms *random* and *assortative mating* are usually applied to vegetables and laboratory animals, not people.

Probably the most difficult criterion to meet of all the unmeetable Hardy-Weinberg criteria is that the DNA of people within the population must not mutate. Genetic diversity depends on changes in genotypes occurring periodically. This helps us to adapt to environmental changes. It also changes the frequency of alleles in a given population. When you are changing the frequency of alleles, you are ruining your Hardy-Weinberg equilibrium. Of course, no one said that staying in Hardy-Weinberg equilibrium was a good thing for a population.

Hardy and Weinberg also developed an equation that could be used to track the genotype frequencies in a given population and monitor changes over time. The Hardy-Weinberg equation is depicted in Table 18–2. Knowing this may not help you care for a sick patient; however, it helps scientists keep track of how populations change, and it helps clinicians appreciate why people with ancestors from the same geographic region share traits (and risk for certain diseases).

Genetic Drift and Population Bottlenecks

Populations can change and become less diverse because of the process called *genetic drift*. **Genetic drift** is the process by which allele frequencies decline because of what population geneticists call *sampling error*. In every generation, some individuals reproduce and others do not. Some parents have lots of children, and others have only one or two. Future generations are more likely to possess the traits of people who have more children. This will happen whether or not these traits have any survival advantage. The illustration in Figure 18–1 (see next page) provides an example of genetic drift using marbles instead of people.

In the illustration, 10 marbles are randomly drawn from a bag that contains two different colors of marbles, A and B. Future marble bags are restocked in proportion to the marbles drawn from the previous bag. The bag on the left side has been restocked with 60 marbles of color A and 40 marbles of color B, to make a bag with a total of 100 marbles. Someone draws marbles randomly from the bag and gets eight color A marbles and two color B marbles. The next bag is restocked with marbles in the proportion of 8:2 (80 A marbles and 20 B marbles). Now 10 marbles are randomly drawn again. This time

---

TABLE 18–2

Development of the Hardy-Weinberg Equation

p = the frequency of the dominant allele.

Let's call this allele B. How many B alleles are there in a given population? Well, there are all of the alleles in people who are homozygous dominant (BB) and half of the alleles in people who are heterozygous (Bb); p represents all of these together.

p = BB + ½ Bb
q = the frequency of the recessive allele.

Let's call this allele b. How many b alleles are there in a given population? Well, there are all of the alleles in people who are homozygous recessive (bb) and half of the alleles in people who are heterozygous (Bb); q represents all of these together.

q = bb + ½ Bb
$p + q = 1$

The sum of the frequencies of all alleles must be 100%, so if there are only two alleles in the population, we can say that:

$p = 1 - q$

Now if we do just a tiny bit of algebra, we say that the chances of all possible combinations of alleles in a population are:

$(p + q)^2 = 1$ OR $p^2 + 2pq + q^2 = 1$

The frequencies of the three possible genotypes are indicated by the terms of the equation, technically called a *binomial expansion*. SO . . .

p^2 = the predicted frequency of the homozygous dominant genotype (BB)
$2pq$ = the predicted frequency of heterozygous genotype (Bb)
q^2 = the predicted frequency of homozygous recessive genotype (bb)

Source: Pierce, B. Transmission and population genetics, 2nd ed., New York: W. H. Freeman, 2009.

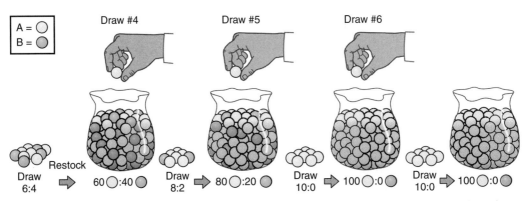

Figure 18–1. Genetic drift. (Image used with permission from the University of California Museum of Paleontology and their "Understanding Evolution" Web site www.evolution.berkeley.edu)

the sample contains 10 A marbles and no B marbles. The next bag is restocked with 100 A marbles. Future marble "generations" will contain only color A marbles. Now, let's apply this idea to human populations. If the genetic trait represented by B "drifted" out of the population, we would have less genetic diversity. If A was a trait that protected us from a particular disease, then our population would be less vulnerable to that disease. These genetic changes are not influenced by natural selection—they are simply the result of random changes in the frequency of a trait in a population (Museum, no date).

A more dramatic way that populations change is by undergoing a population bottleneck (Fig. 18–2). In a **population bottleneck,** some event happens that severely reduces the number of individuals in a population. Only those individuals who survive this event will be able to reproduce, so only their traits will be passed on to future generations. Population bottlenecks can greatly limit genetic diversity in the surviving populations.

In Figure 18–2, in the bag on the left, there are three different colors of marbles; there are 28 of color A, 40 of color B, and 32 of color C. Now someone draws 10 marbles randomly. The draw includes two of color A, five of color B, and three of color C. These proportions are roughly the same as those of the original population (28:40:32). The marbles are then restocked in the new proportions, so the generation 2 bag contains 20 marbles of color A, 50 marbles of color B, and 30 marbles of color C. If we were talking about people instead of marbles, we would say that the smaller population reproduced.

An unusually small number of marbles (only three) is drawn from the generation 2 bag. In this draw, we have no marbles of color A, two marbles of color B, and three marbles of color C. We have encountered a population bottleneck. Now the entire population contains no marbles of color A. It has been eliminated from the population. No future generations of marbles "reproduced" from this small group will have the color A. That "genetic trait" has been eliminated from the population. In generation 4, there are no marbles with this color (Museum, no date).

One example of a population bottleneck can be seen in the history of the northern elephant seal. During the 1890s, these seals were hunted to near extinction. By some estimates, only 20 individuals remained. Since that time, these seals have reproduced, and the population is currently thought to include more than 30,000 seals. What do you expect was the outcome of this population bottleneck? If we compare genetic diversity in the northern elephant seal to genetic diversity in the southern elephant seal, a population that did not experience a bottleneck, the difference is clear: The southern elephant seals are much more diverse genetically than the northern seals, because all the northern seals surviving today are descended from the very small population that survived the bottleneck (Museum, no date).

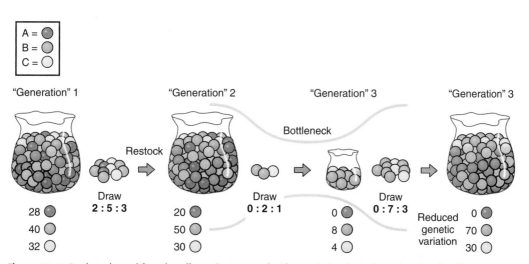

Figure 18–2. Bottlenecks and founder effects. (Image used with permission from the University of California Museum of Paleontology and their "Understanding Evolution" Web site www.evolution.berkeley.edu)

We can see similar patterns if we look at human history. Earlier in this chapter, we discussed the prevalence of certain diseases among people of Ashkenazi Jewish ancestry. These include diseases such as breast cancer caused by mutations in the genes *BRCA1* and *BRCA2,* as well as a number of lysosomal storage diseases, such as Gaucher disease or Tay-Sachs. Although these ideas are controversial, the high prevalence of these diseases among this population may be the result of a combination of founder effects and population bottlenecks (Tishkoff and Verrelli, 2003). Evidence from mitochondrial DNA support that there was a population bottleneck among Ashkenazi Jews about 100 generations ago, which was followed by an increased rate of growth (Behar et al., 2004). This could explain the prevalence of these diseases among this population.

It can be helpful to know the geographic origin of a person's ancestors because we share many traits in common by descent, and populations that have been geographically close will be more likely to share the impact of founder effects, genetic drift, and population bottlenecks. Things become a bit more difficult when we try to put people in clearly bounded categories, such as race and ethnicity, based on the physical traits they may share.

Race, Ethnicity, and Human Genetic Variation

Race and *ethnicity* are somewhat controversial terms with different definitions, depending on the context. In this section, we will present some of the ideas about genetics and race and ethnicity that are of interest to people working in health care. We are not offering a comprehensive discussion of this complicated topic. However, it is important for those developing an understanding of genetics to see how human genetic variation fits in with our social and cultural ideas about population similarities and differences.

Race is often used to categorize people into groups that share common geographical background, ancestry, and physical features. However, the racial categories are overlapping and do not reflect the continuous distribution of genetic variation. While population groups share some traits in common, there are no sharp boundaries between groups (Royal and Dunston, 2004). Self-identified race is often associated with the geographic origin of one's ancestors. Therefore, people who identify themselves as belonging to a particular race are likely to share some traits in common. However, we must remember that there are lots of nongenetic factors that contribute to our ideas of what race is and that many people can trace their ancestors to several different geographic regions (Collins, 2004).

Certainly, there are genes that are associated with various physical traits, such as skin color or hair texture. However, there is no reliable way that we can use the genes associated with these traits to separate people into unique groups. People whose ancestors came from the same geographic region share some alleles in common; however, there is no particular allele that is found in all members of a given population and not found in other populations as well. If we look at genetic diversity of our species, the genetic differences among individuals in the social-cultural groups called *races* are much smaller than the genetic differences within each of these "races" (DOE, 2010).

Ethnicity is a quality claimed by a group of people who identify with each other and believe they share a common cultural heritage. When we look at recent history, we can see variations in ethnicities that have resulted from human migration patterns, the impact of mutations, and small subgroups settling in isolated areas. These are some of the factors in population genetics (founder effects, genetic drift) that we previously discussed. When we look over a much longer period of history, we can see changes that reflect natural selection and adaptation to variations in climate and availability of food sources (Wilson, 2000).

Some experts have suggested that it is time for a new way of thinking about human genetic variation. Results from the Human Genome Project have made it clear that our old conceptions of race and ethnicity are not biologically based but represent geographical and sociocultural divisions at best (Royal and Dunston, 2004). On the other hand, knowing someone's race or ethnicity can be useful in identifying which genetic disorders an individual is more likely to have. For example, people of Celtic background (descended from Irish or Scottish ancestors) are more likely to carry mutations leading to the autosomal recessive disease hemochromatosis.

The terms *race* and *ethnicity* are used in a wide range of settings, including to categorize people in governmental databases. Sometimes these categories can be helpful because we do not have more accurate ways to describe groups of people whose ancestors came from the same geographic region. We know that research studies often compare the effect of a particular drug in one race to the effects of that drug in another race. For example, the American Heart Association recently published a set of recommendations for the management of hypertension in black people based on current research and the consensus of experts. The statement contains useful information for clinicians caring for this population, even though we have no biological way to determine the boundaries of this group (Flack et al., 2010; Keita et al., 2004).

We also know that there are important disparities that can be described by looking at the health care available to those classified as belonging to different races. This is greatly due to social, cultural, and political issues. However, it is useful to be able to identify people who are more likely to experience these disparities, and genetics certainly contributes to the risk of disease and response to treatment. We do not know whether genetics can contribute much to our understanding of health disparities (Collins, 2004).

People argue about whether we should retain the ideas of race and ethnicity or even if self-identified race/ethnicity is useful when we talk about the risk to health (Collins, 2004). It is clear that more studies are needed to help scientists sort out these ideas. These studies must take into consideration both genetics and environment. If we choose to continue to use the terms *race* and *ethnicity*, we must remember that they have significant limitations when we try to apply them strictly to what we now know about human genetic variation.

Francis Collins, the director of the National Institutes of Health and the former director of the Human Genome Project in the United States, agrees that the terms *race* and *ethnicity* are very poorly defined. In addition, these words carry with them ideas about history, culture, and socioeconomic status that are not reflected in genetic variation. What can be determined with some degree of accuracy from looking at someone's genotype is the likely geographical origins of their ancestors—that is, if their ancestors came from the same parts of the world. People whose ancestors came from the same geographical location often share genetic sequences in common and often identify themselves as belonging to the same race. In that sense, there is a connection between biology and race; however, it is a slippery one at best (Collins, 2004).

Summary

The study of human genomic variation is complex. As a species, we are very similar. However, we differ from one another in important ways, including our risk for diseases and our responses to drugs. Efforts to catalogue human genetic diversity have produced much useful information. People have tried to categorize humans into different groups (races and ethnicities) and have assumed that these group differences were based in biology. With the completion of the Human Genome Project, we have learned that these racial and ethnic groups do not have clear biological boundaries. There is a lot of overlap between and among racial and ethnic groups.

Racial and ethnic categories may still be helpful when we look at social, cultural, and political issues, such as health disparities. However, we must be careful not to use these words to imply that everyone in a group is biologically like everyone else in that group. There is a bigger range of genetic difference within groups than there are between groups. There is benefit in understanding how human genetic variation has progressed over time and the factors that have altered the frequencies of alleles in a given population. There is also much more to learn about the ways in which we, as a species, are the same and the ways in which we are different.

GENE GEMS

- Humans are genetically homogenous. We are 99.9% the same at the DNA level.
- The 0.1% genetic differences among humans have both health-related and sociocultural consequences.
- The National Geographic Society began the Genographic Project with the goal of assembling the largest DNA database in the world, which will ultimately contain DNA from more than 100,000 people.
- Humans are descended from the same African ancestor.
- The International HapMap Project provides a map of human genetic variation.
- People have different risks for diseases and tend to respond differently to drugs, depending on the geographical origin of their ancestors.
- Population genetics is the study of the changes in allele frequency in different populations over time.
- The founder effect can result in lack of genetic diversity within an isolated population.
- Genetic drift is a random change in allele frequencies not based on natural selection.
- Population bottlenecks reduce the size of a population and limit the diversity of alleles available to future populations.
- Many factors can cause population bottlenecks, including dramatic climate changes, famine, and sociopolitical events.
- The Hardy-Weinberg equilibrium equation calculates changes in allele frequency over time.
- For a population to remain in Hardy-Weinberg equilibrium, several criteria must be met. These include random mating, no migration, no mutations, and everyone in the population reproducing.
- People of Ashkenazi Jewish ancestry have an increased risk for breast cancer caused by mutations in the genes *BRCA1* and *BRCA2,* as well as for lysosomal storage diseases such as Gaucher disease or Tay-Sachs.
- It is unclear whether genetics can be of any help in explaining health disparities.
- The terms *race* and *ethnicity* are defined differently, depending on context.
- We can see genetic similarities in people whose ancestors came from the same geographic regions.

Self-Assessment Questions

1. What factors could increase genetic diversity in a particular population?
   a. Increased number of haplotypes
   b. Genetic drift
   c. The population effect
   d. The bottleneck effect

2. Why are people of Ashkenazi Jewish descent more likely to be carriers of the mutations that cause Tay-Sachs and Gaucher disease?
   a. The environment of Eastern Europe increased their risk of developing a mutation.
   b. The common diet shared by these people has reduced their genetic diversity.
   c. Founder or bottleneck effects have reduced genetic diversity in this population.
   d. Being heterozygous for these diseases gives the carrier immunity to cholera.

3. What criteria must a population meet in order to stay in Hardy-Weinberg equilibrium?
   a. Random mating, no migration, and no mutation
   b. Founding commonalities and no haplotype differences
   c. Assortative mating, migration, and frequent mutation
   d. Natural selection is sufficient.

4. A small group of people left their homeland and set sail for a tropical island. They settled there and their descendents lived for many generations. Unfortunately, a relatively high proportion of this new population is afflicted with an autosomal dominant disease. What would explain this?
   a. They simply had bad luck.
   b. An unidentified environmental radiation source was on the island.
   c. One of the founders of this population carried the gene mutation with him or her.
   d. Their lack of genetic diversity made them more vulnerable to new mutations.

5. A population of animals called *Hanksters* has white fur. Historic illustrations indicate that, in early times, there were Hanksters with brown and black fur as well as those with white coats. What could have happened to eliminate all but the white-coated Hanksters?
   a. Excessive hunting of brown and black Hanksters for their beautiful coats
   b. A reduction in food supply that killed off only brown and black Hanksters
   c. A climate change that included continual snow, so hunters could not see the white-coated Hanksters
   d. Any of these. Each one could cause a population bottleneck.

CASE STUDY

Jane is a 24-year-old pediatric nurse who identifies herself as African American. Her brother has sickle cell disease (SCD), and she knows that she is a carrier. She understands the genetics of SCD and the risk to her children if she marries someone who is also a carrier. Jane is very active in human rights groups and insists that race is a social and cultural idea with no biological basis. One of Jane's coworkers is a member of the same human rights group, but he sees race differently. He tells Jane that he believes that there are biological determinants of race and points out physical features that many African Americans share.

1. How can ideas about the geographic origin of one's ancestors help Jane and her friend come to terms with their differences of opinion?

2. What concepts from population genetics could you use to help explain physical differences that people attribute to race?

3. Is there value in retaining categories such as "race" and "ethnicity"?

4. How could Jane's knowledge about SCD help her and her coworker understand human genetic variation?

References

Behar, D. M., Hammer, M. F., et al. (2004). MtDNA evidence for a genetic bottleneck in the early history of the Ashkenazi Jewish population. *European Journal of Human Genetics, 12*(5), 355–364.

Collins, F. S. (2004). What we do and don't know about "race," "ethnicity," genetics and health at the dawn of the genome era. *Nature Genetics, 36*(11 Suppl): S13–15.

DOE. (2010). Genetic anthropology, ancestry, and ancient human migration. Retrieved January 25, 2011, from www.ornl.gov/sci/techresources/Human_Genome/elsi/humanmigration.shtml.

Flack, J. M., Sica D. A., et al. (2010). Management of high blood pressure in blacks: An update of the International Society on Hypertension in Blacks consensus statement. *Hypertension, 56*(5), 780–800.

Keita, S. O., Kittles, R. A., et al. (2004). Conceptualizing human variation. *Nature Genetics, 36*(11 Suppl), S17–20.

Museum. (No date). Evolution 101. Retrieved January 21, 2011, from http://evolution.berkeley.edu/evosite/evo101/index.shtml.

NHGRI. (2010). About the International HapMap Project. Retrieved January 22, 2011, from www.genome.gov/11511175.

Pierce, B. Transmission and population genetics, 2nd ed. New York: W. H. Freeman, 2009.

Ridley, M. Evolution. Hoboken, NJ: Wiley-Blackwell, 2003.

Royal, C. D., and Dunston, G. M. (2004). Changing the paradigm from "race" to human genome variation. *Nature Genetics, 36*(11 Suppl), S5–7.

Tishkoff, S. A., and Verrelli B. C. (2003). Patterns of human genetic diversity: Implications for human evolutionary history and disease. *Annual Review of Genomics and Human Genetics, 4*, 293–340.

Wilson, G. N. Clinical genetics. New York: Wiley & Sons, 2000.

Self-Assessment Answers

1. a **2.** c **3.** a **4.** c **5.** d

Genetic Competencies Identified by the American Association of Colleges of Nursing

The American Association of Colleges of Nursing (AACN) is an organization that is responsible for accrediting schools and colleges of nursing with programs leading to a bachelor of science in nursing (BSN) degree. This organization has published program content and outcome expectations for baccalaureate-level nursing education in the document *The Essentials of Baccalaureate Education for Professional Nursing Practice*. The most recent revision of this document was published in 2008 and contains nine identified essential content areas. Within each essential content area, specific learning outcomes are presented together with sample content.

Revision of the document is based on the rationale of "strong forces influencing the role of nurses" and "scientific advances, particularly in the area of genetics and genomics" (p. 6).

Genetic/genomic competence is now an expectation for professional nurses. Of the nine content areas identified in the AACN essentials document, the three relevant for genetics/genomics are presented below.

Essential I: Liberal Education for Baccalaureate Generalist Nursing Practice

This document defines a liberal education to include both the sciences and the arts. The four science categories listed as essential include the physical sciences (e.g., physics and chemistry), the life sciences (e.g., biology and genetics), the mathematical sciences, and the social sciences (e.g., psychology and sociology).

Essential VII: Clinical Prevention and Population Health (pp. 23–26)

Thirteen outcomes are listed for this essential. The first two are related to genetics/genomics.

1. Assess protective and predictive factors, including genetics, which influence the health of individuals, families, groups, communities, and populations.
2. Conduct a health history, including environmental exposure and a family history that recognizes genetic risks, to identify current and future health problems.

The specific sample genetic/genomic content associated with this essential includes:

- Genetics and genomics
- Screening
- Pedigree from a three-generation family history using standardized symbols and terminology

Essential IX: Baccalaureate Generalist Nursing Practice (pp. 29–33)

Twenty-two outcomes are listed for this essential, and the second one is specific for genetics/genomics: Recognize the relationship of genetics and genomics to health, prevention, screening, diagnosis, prognostics, selection of treatment, and monitoring of treatment effectiveness, using a constructed pedigree from collected family history information as well as standardized symbols and terminology.

The specific sample genetic/genomic content associated with this essential includes:

- Genetics and genomics
- Pharmacology/pharmacogenetics

American Association of Colleges of Nursing. The essentials of baccalaureate education for nursing practice. Washington, DC: Author, 2008.

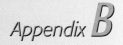

Core Competencies From the National Coalition for Health Professional Education in Genetics (NCHPEG)

Core Competencies for All Health-Care Professionals (2007)

Baseline Competencies

At a minimum, each health-care professional should be able to:

a. examine one's competence of practice on a regular basis, identifying areas of strength and areas where professional development related to genetics and genomics would be beneficial.
b. understand that health-related genetic information can have important social and psychological implications for individuals and families.
c. know how and when to make a referral to a genetics professional.

1. Knowledge

All health professionals should understand:

1.1. basic human genetics terminology.
1.2. the basic patterns of biological inheritance and variation, both within families and within populations.
1.3. how identification of disease-associated genetic variations facilitates development of prevention, diagnosis, and treatment options.
1.4. the importance of family history (minimum three generations) in assessing predisposition to disease.
1.5. the interaction of genetic, environmental, and behavioral factors in predisposition to disease, onset of disease, response to treatment, and maintenance of health.
1.6. the difference between clinical diagnosis of disease and identification of genetic predisposition to disease (genetic variation is not strictly correlated with disease manifestation).
1.7. the various factors that influence the client's ability to use genetic information and services; for example, ethnicity, culture, related health beliefs, ability to pay, and health literacy.
1.8. the potential physical and/or psychosocial benefits, limitations, and risks of genetic information for individuals, family members, and communities.
1.9. the resources available to assist clients seeking genetic information or services, including the types of genetics professionals available and their diverse responsibilities.
1.10. the ethical, legal, and social issues related to genetic testing and recording of genetic information (e.g., privacy, the potential for genetic discrimination in health insurance and employment).
1.11. one's professional role in the referral to or provision of genetics services and in follow-up for those services.

2. Skills

All health professionals should be able to:

2.1. gather genetic family history information, including at minimum a three-generation history.

2.2. identify and refer clients who might benefit from genetic services or from consultation with other professionals for management of issues related to a genetic diagnosis.

2.3. explain effectively the reasons for and benefits of genetic services.

2.4. use information technology to obtain credible, current information about genetics.

2.5. assure that the informed-consent process for genetic testing includes appropriate information about the potential risks, benefits, and limitations of the test in question.

3. Attitudes

All health professionals should:

3.1. appreciate the sensitivity of genetic information and the need for privacy and confidentiality.

3.2. seek coordination and collaboration with an interdisciplinary team of health professionals.

Competencies that delineate the components of the genetic-counseling process are not expected of all health-care professionals. Health professionals should, however, be able to facilitate the genetic-counseling process and prepare clients and families for what to expect, communicate relevant information to the genetics team, and follow up with the client after genetic services have been provided. Those health professionals who choose to provide genetic-counseling services to their clients should be able to perform all components of the process, as delineated at http://abgc.iamonline.com/english/View.asp?x=1529.

National Coalition for Health Professional Education in Genetics (NCHPEG). (2007). Core competencies for all health care professionals, 3rd ed. www.nchpeg.org/index.php?option=com_content&view=article&id=94&Itemid=84. Accessed on February 23, 2011.

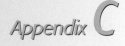

Essentials for Genetic and Genomic Nursing: Competencies, Curricula Guidelines, and Outcome Indicators, Second Edition

Background and Context of the Competencies

Genetic and genomic science is redefining the understanding of the continuum of human health and illness. Therefore, recognition of genomics as a central science for health professional knowledge is essential. Because all diseases and conditions have a genetic or genomic component, options for care for all persons will increasingly include genetic and genomic information along the pathways of prevention, screening, diagnostics, prognostics, selection of treatment, and monitoring of treatment effectiveness. The clinical application of genetic and genomic knowledge has major implications for the entire nursing profession regardless of academic preparation, role, or practice setting.

The public will increasingly expect that the registered nurse (RN) will use genetic and genomic information and technology when providing care. These expectations have direct implications for RN preparatory curricula, as well as for the 2.9 million practicing nurses. The rate of progress for applying a genomic approach throughout the continuum of care depends not only on technological advances, but also on nursing expertise. In its report on genetics and nursing in 2000, an expert Health Resources and Services Administration (HRSA) panel emphasized the importance of integrating genetics content into nursing curricula to provide an adequately prepared nursing workforce now and for the future. To care for persons, families, communities, and/or populations throughout the life span, registered nurses will need to demonstrate proficiency with incorporating genetic and genomic information into their practice. For example:

- Understand the genetic and genomic basis of health and/or an illness for which the person is seeking care and the variables that impact his or her response.
- Recognize a newborn at risk for morbidity or mortality resulting from genetic metabolism errors.
- Identify an asymptomatic adolescent who is at high risk for hereditary colon cancer.
- Identify a couple at risk for having a child with a genetic condition.
- Guide interventions for the prevention of cardiovascular disease in young adults.
- Facilitate drug selection or dosage in treatment of an adult with cancer based on molecular markers.
- Promote informed consent that includes the risks, benefits, and limitations of participation in genetic research.
- Assist anyone having questions about genetic and genomic information or services.
- Identify Caucasians of Northern European descent (a population at risk for hemachromatosis) who have joint disease, severe and continuing fatigue, heart disease, elevated liver enzymes, impotence, and diabetes, because they are candidates for hemochromatosis *HFE* genetic testing.

Purpose

The primary purpose of this document is to define essential genetic and genomic competencies for all registered nurses. This document is intended to guide nurse educators in the design and implementation of learning experiences that help students, learners, and practicing nurses achieve these genetic and genomic competencies. These competencies are not intended to replace or re-create existing standards of practice but are intended to incorporate the genetic and genomic perspective into all nursing education and practice. The goal is to prepare the nursing workforce to deliver competent genetic- and genomic-focused nursing care.

Applicability

The genetic and genomic competencies are integral to the practice of all registered nurses regardless of academic preparation, practice setting, role, or specialty.

Definitions

The first two definitions of two central and somewhat overlapping terms remain a work in progress, because the new knowledge produced by genome research will create an ongoing need to assess and revise our understanding of the influence of both genetic and genomic factors for health outcomes. For the purpose of this document, both genetic and genomic information will be used as the context for defining required competencies.

- *Genetics*—Study of individual genes and their impact on relatively rare single-gene disorders.
- *Genomics*—Study of all the genes in the human genome together, including their interactions with each other, the environment, and the influence of other psychosocial and cultural factors.

The rest of the key definitions are more established but are offered to clarify the use in this report of what can have more general meanings:

- *Clients*—Recipients of health care may include persons, families, communities, and/or populations from any race, ethnicity, ancestry, culture, or religious background. The term *clients* will be used throughout the document to reflect the focus of nursing care.
- *Pedigree*—A graphic illustration of a family health history using standardized symbols.
- *Resources*—A collection of genetic and genomic tools and sites for health-care referrals for delivery of nursing care.
- *Services*—The delivery of genetic and genomic health care.
- *Technology*—The use of tools and/or machines to perform tasks; in this case, the identification and assessment of genetic and genomic information (e.g., the use of microarray technology to assess the genetic features of a specific tumor).

Outcome Indicators Example Page

Domain: Professional Practice
Essential Competency: Nursing Assessment:
Applying/Integrating Genetic and Genomic Knowledge

Demonstrates an understanding of the relationship of genetics and genomics to health, prevention, screening, diagnostics, prognostics, selection of treatment, and monitoring of treatment effectiveness.

Specific Areas of Knowledge

Relationship of genetics and genomics to health, prevention, screening, diagnostics, prognostics, selection of treatment, and monitoring of treatment effectiveness.

Relationship of genetics and genomics to normal physiology and pathophysiology, including:

Basics of gene function and genetic mutations in individual and populations:

- Germline mutations, somatic mutations, polymorphisms
- Selected mutations associated with single-gene disorders, chronic disease
- Concept of genotype/phenotype
- Selected genotype predictors for disease prognosis and treatment

Basic Principles of Pharmacogenetics and Pharmacogenomics

- Polymorphisms and drug metabolism
- Selected examples (e.g., warfarin and CYP polymorphisms)

Patterns of disease associated with single-gene and multifactorial inheritance.

Clinical Performance Indicators

Collect a client's personal and three-generation family health history to assess for genomic factors that impact the client's health.

Identify potentially significant information from a family history.

Identify clients who might benefit from referral to genetics specialists and/or information resources.

Facilitate appropriate referral to genetic specialists, accurately documenting and communicating relevant history and clinical data.

Describe a typical client journey that might be experienced in the process of genetic counseling.

Describe genetic/genomic factors that contribute to variability of response to pharmacologic agents.

Incorporate genetic and genomic health assessment data into routinely collected biopsychosocial and environmental assessments of health and illness parameters in client, using culturally sensitive approaches.

Identify resources available to assist clients seeking genetic and genomic information or services, including the types of services available.

Consensus Panel on Genetic/Genomic Nursing Competencies. *Essentials of genetic and genomic nursing: Competencies, curricula guidelines, and outcome indicators,* 2nd ed. Silver Spring, MD: American Nurses Association, 2009.

Glossary

Absorption	The entering of a drug from its route of administration into the bloodstream.
Achondroplasia	A monogenic disorder of human dwarfism that occurs as a result of a mutation in the gene that codes for the fibroblast growth factor receptor 3 (*FGFR 3*).
Acquired disease	A disease that did not appear at birth. Some acquired diseases are not present in other family members.
Adenosine triphosphate (ATP)	The high-energy chemical that is a very common source of energy used to drive cellular actions and reactions.
Agonist	A drug that binds tightly and functionally to a cell receptor, increasing the expected function of the cell (tissue or organ).
Allele	An alternative or variable form of a gene at a specific chromosome location.
Alzheimer disease (AD)	The most common cause of dementia among the elderly.
Anaplastic	A cellular appearance or morphology that is without a specific shape or differentiation (usually small and round with a large nuclear-to-cytoplasmic ratio).
Aneuploid	A cell's nucleus that contains either more chromosomes than normal diploid number for the species or less chromosomes than the normal diploid number for the species.
Antagonist	A drug that binds incorrectly (nonfunctionally) to a cell receptor, acting in opposition to a natural agonist, and inhibiting the expected cell function by preventing receptor interaction with agonist substances.
Anticodon	The tRNA complementary code for an amino acid codon.
Apoptosis	Programmed cell death (cellular suicide).
Arrhythmogenic right ventricular dysplasia/ cardiomyopathy (ARVD/C)	A structural alteration in the heart muscle that makes the heart much more likely to experience ventricular tachycardia.
Associations	Multiple anomalies that often occur together but are not known to be either syndromes or sequences.
Assortative mating	Selecting a mate based on whether you have characteristics that are similar to or dissimilar from them.
Asthma	A chronic disease of the airways that is characterized by intermittent reversible airflow obstruction.
Autism	A behavioral pattern in which a person has difficulty with social interactions and the development of language, often accompanied by a narrow range of repetitive behaviors and interests.

Autism spectrum disorders (ASD)	Developmental problems that seem like autism but do not meet the threshold for diagnosis as a pervasive developmental disorder.
Autoimmune disease	A condition of immune excess in which components of a person's immune system no longer recognize the person's own cells, tissues, and organs as "self," and attack them as if they were invading organisms.
Autonomy	The ethical principle of respecting a person's right to make his or her own choices.
Autosomes	The 22 pairs of human chromosomes that do not code for the sexual differentiation of the individual.
Balanced translocation	A chromosomal translocation in which the right amount of DNA is present (no more and no less) but is not located in its customary place.
Base pairs	Nucleotides (one purine and one pyrimidine) that pair up loosely together when DNA is double-stranded.
Bases	The four nucleoproteins that form the essential nitrogen-containing components of DNA (adenine, cytosine, guanine, thymine).
Behavioral genetics	The study of the way our genomes influence our behaviors.
Behavioral phenotype	Demonstrating the behaviors commonly associated with a particular disorder.
Beneficence	The ethical principle of making decisions based on what is considered "good" or of the most benefit to others.
Benign tumor	A type of neoplastic cell growth that is usually harmless.
Bioavailability	The amount of an administered drug dose that actually reaches the bloodstream, regardless of the method of administration.
Biologically plausible	A situation in which it seems likely that a gene that has been associated with a disorder could be involved, given the function of the protein the gene encodes.
Bipotential gonad	The early embryonic tissue that has the potential to develop into a testis or an ovary, depending on which hormones and other factors influence it.
Brachydactyly	Fingers or toes that are unusually short compared to the palm of the hand or the foot.
Cancer	Unregulated cell growth that has no useful purpose, is invasive, and that would lead to death without intervention. Also known as *malignancy*.
Canthus	The angle that is formed by the meeting of the upper and lower eyelids. The inner canthus is closest to the nose and the outer canthus is closest to the ears.
Carcinogen	Any substance or event that can damage a normal cell's DNA and lead to cancer development.
Cardiomyopathy	A primary disease of the heart muscle.
Carrier	A person who is heterozygous for an autosomal recessive gene allele and does not fully express the trait or disorder but can transmit the allele to his or her children.
Carrier test	A genetic test done in persons who are not affected by, but suspect they have genetic risk for, a condition they could pass on to their children.
Cell adhesion molecules	A family of cell surface proteins that allow normal cells to adhere tightly together and not migrate out of a specific tissue or organ. Also known as *CAMs*.

Centromere	The pinched area of a chromosome where the two chromatids are connected.
Certified genetic counselor (CGC)	A genetics professional who has a master's degree in genetic counseling from a graduate program accredited by the American Board of Genetic Counselors (ABGC).
Channelopathy	A disorder caused by a variation in a gene coding for an ion channel.
Chromatid	The longitudinal half of a metaphase chromosome (split through the centromere), including its p arm and q arm.
Chromosome	A temporary but consistent state of condensed DNA structure formed for the purpose of cell division.
Classic hemophilia	A monogenic disorder in which the production of blood-clotting factor VIII is either absent or greatly below normal.
Cleft lip/palate	A malformation caused by the failure of lip and/or palate tissues to fuse during development.
Clinical geneticist	A physician who first completes residency training in pediatrics, obstetrics, internal medicine, or another related medical specialty and then is board certified by the American Board of Medical Genetics (ABMG) after completing a 3-year residency in an ABMG-approved clinical genetics program.
Clinical laboratory geneticist	A doctorally prepared individual who has completed a 24-month specialty fellowship in cytogenetics, molecular genetics, or biochemical genetics and is certified in one of these subspecialties by the American Board of Medical Genetics (ABMG).
Clinodactyly	A laterally curved digit.
Codominant expression	A single gene trait in which two different dominant gene alleles are both expressed equally.
Codominant trait	A single gene trait in which two different dominant gene alleles are both expressed equally.
Codon	A specific RNA base sequence containing the complementary code to each amino acid's DNA triplet.
Collagen	A group of glycoprotein fibers that forms the major component of the connective tissue found in nearly all body tissues.
Complementary pairs	Nitrogenous bases that normally pair using hydrogen bonds. Adenine and thymine are a complementary pair, and cytosine and guanine are the other complementary pair.
Complex traits	Traits that are caused by several genes working together (polygenic) and/or a combination of genes and environment. (Also known as *multifactorial traits and diseases*.)
Congenital anomalies	Defects that are present at birth.
Contact inhibition of mitosis	The inhibition of normal cells to undergo mitosis when membranes are completely contacted with the membranes of other cells.
Copy number variants (CNVs)	Variations in stretches of DNA found throughout the genome. These are often either deletions or duplications.
Craniofacial anomalies	Variations from the usual formation of the skull and face.

Craniosynostosis	A distortion in the shape of the skull that occurs when more than one of the cranial sutures fuses together earlier than it should.
Cyclins	A family of proteins that, when active, stimulates the cell to move through the cell cycle and complete cell division.
Cystic fibrosis (CF)	A monogenic disorder with autosomal recessive expression in which the *CTFR* gene has one or more mutations that result in problems with the transmembrane transport of chloride.
Cytogenetic test	A "chromosome study" that looks for variations in the number and structure of chromosomes from a cell's nucleus.
Cytokinesis	The separating of a cell at the M phase of the cell cycle into two new cells that each have a complete set of chromosomes.
De novo mutation	A new mutation that has not been found in the family members of the proband.
Deformation	A defect in the shape or form of a body part that is due to compression from mechanical forces.
Deoxyribonucleic acid (DNA)	The basic genetic chemical structure, containing gene coding regions and noncoding regions, that can be compacted into a chromosome form.
Diagnostic test	A test done to confirm or refute a particular diagnosis in a symptomatic person.
Differentiation	The process by which a cell leaves the pluripotent stage and acquires the maturational features and functions of a specific cell type.
Diploid chromosome number	The complete set of chromosome pairs found in all of an individual's somatic cells (23 pairs [2N] of human chromosomes, 46 chromosomes altogether).
Direct-to-consumer (DTC) genetic testing	Genetic testing that is offered directly to individuals. There is typically no input, recommendation, or follow-up by a genetics professional.
Disruption	A defect in the shape or form of a body part that is due to a disturbance in the normal developmental process.
DNA antisense strand	The single strand of DNA exactly opposite the sense strand that contains the complementary base sequence to the gene, not the actual gene itself. Same as antisense DNA.
DNA coding region	An area of DNA that contains many genes that generally have the same base sequences from one person to another.
DNA noncoding region	A section of DNA containing multiple repeat sequences that is not composed of genes and does not code for specific proteins.
DNA replication	A duplication or reproduction of one cell's DNA during cell division resulting in two identical sets of DNA.
DNA sense strand	One strand of double-stranded DNA that contains the actual gene coding sequence for the protein to be synthesized. Same as sense DNA.
DNA sequencing	Testing that consists of analyzing and reporting the order of bases in a stretch of DNA. It is the most specific and accurate test for base sequence variation.
DNA triplet	The exact three nucleotide base sequences that code for a specific amino acid.
Dominant trait	A single gene trait that is expressed regardless of whether the two gene alleles are identical (homozygous) or different (heterozygous).

Duchenne muscular dystrophy (DMD)	A monogenic disorder of progressive muscle weakness caused by any one of a variety of mutations in an allele of the *DMD* gene, which codes for the protein dystrophin.
Duty to warn	The ethical obligation of a health-care professional to inform a patient or his/her family members they are at risk for a disease.
Dysmorphology	The study of congenital anomalies in the anatomical form or body parts of a person, or abnormal patterns of development.
Dysplasia	An alteration in the size, shape, and organization of cells.
Dystrophin	A structural protein that functions to maintain the integrity of skeletal, cardiac, and smooth muscles.
Ehlers-Danlos syndrome	A group of different inherited disorders that occur as a result of mutations in collagen formation or modification.
Elimination	The inactivation and final removal of drugs from the body.
ELSI	The portion of the Human Genome Project that focuses on the ethical, legal, and social issues that come with advances in genetics.
Enterohepatic circulation	A circulatory detour in which venous blood drained from the entire gastrointestinal tract enters liver circulation before entering systemic circulation.
Enzyme	A biological catalyst that causes a biochemical reaction to occur or increases the rate of a biochemical reaction within a cell, body tissue, or organ.
Enzyme replacement therapy (ERT)	The actual replacement of a missing or malfunctioning enzyme with one that has been generated artificially.
Epicanthic folds	A fold of skin that partially or completely covers the inner canthus of the eye.
Epigenome	Biochemical factors that alter gene expression but do not involve changes in the underlying DNA sequence.
Epistasis	The process of gene-to-gene interaction.
Ethnicity	Quality claimed by a group of people who identify with each other and believe that they share a common cultural heritage.
Eugenics	A program to "improve" the human race by the selective breeding of people considered to have "good genes."
Euploid	A cell nucleus containing the normal diploid number of chromosomes for the species.
Evolution founder effect	Changes in allele frequency in a population over time. The reduction in genetic variability that comes from the separation of a population subgroup and the reproduction of that less diverse subgroup.
Executive functions	Those behavioral functions associated with prefrontal lobe brain activity, including problem-solving, impulse control, planning, and goal-directed actions.
Exons	The sectional parts of DNA within a gene-coding region that actually belong in the gene-coding sequence for a specific protein.
Expressivity	The degree of trait expression a person has when a dominant gene is present.
Externalizing psychopathology	The idea that conduct disorders, such as antisocial personality disorder and addictive behaviors, share both common and unique causes.

F generations	The succeeding generations of offspring or progeny produced from the parental generation. Each succeeding generation is designated by a numeric subscript (F_1, F_2, F_3, etc.).
Fabry disease	An X-linked recessive genetic lysosomal storage disease in which there is a deficiency of the enzyme alpha-galactosidase A (also known as *ceramide trihexosidase*), which results in the accumulation of globotriaosylceramide (GL-3) within the lysosomes of many tissues and organs.
Factor V Leiden	A genetic disorder that results in increased risk for blood clots.
Familial cancer	Cancer that occurs at a higher-than-expected frequency within a kindred but does not demonstrate any observable pattern of inheritance.
Familial dilated cardiomyopathy (DCM)	A genetic disease that results in weakening and distending of the heart muscle, leading to ineffective pumping.
Familial hypercholesterolemia (FH)	A single-gene disorder that follows an autosomal dominant transmission pattern and causes very high blood cholesterol levels, which greatly increases a person's risk of myocardial infarction.
Familial hypertrophic cardiomyopathy (HCM)	A genetic disease that results in a thickening of the heart muscle wall and possible obstruction to outflow of blood from the ventricle.
Fertilization	The union of one mature haploid sperm with one mature haploid ovum to form a diploid zygote.
Fibrillin	A glycoprotein that assembles into long strands of microfibrils and is an essential component of specific connective tissues, especially those that respond by stretching when a force is applied.
First-pass loss	The rapid liver metabolism and elimination of enteral drugs that are absorbed into the enterohepatic circulation before entering systemic circulation.
Fluorescent in situ hybridization (FISH)	A test that creates a fluorescently dyed segment of nucleic acids that bind to complementary regions on DNA or mRNA.
Frameshift mutations	Disruptions of the DNA reading frame as a result of having a whole base or group of bases added or deleted.
Frontal bossing	An unusual forehead with bilateral bulging of the frontal bone prominences.
Gametes	Mature, haploid, specialized germ cells (ova and sperm) capable of fertilization into a zygote.
Gametogenesis	The conversion of diploid germ cells into haploid gametes that are capable of uniting at conception to start a new person.
Gaucher disease	An autosomal recessive genetic lysosomal storage disease in which there is a deficiency of the enzyme beta-glucosidase, which results in the accumulation of glucosylceramide (also called *glucocerebroside*) in macrophages and some other mononuclear white blood cells.
Gene	A specific set of instructions cells use to produce a specific protein.
Gene expression	The activation of a gene leading to the transcription, translation, and synthesis of a specific protein.
Gene locus	Specific chromosome location of an individual gene.

Gene pool	The combination of all the alleles in all the genes in all the people in a given population.
Genetic anthropology	The study of human ancestry and migration patterns using a combination of DNA and physical evidence.
Genetic counseling	The process of helping people understand and adapt to the medical, psychological, and familial implications of genetic contribution to disease occurrence or recurrence.
Genetic drift	Changes in allele frequency in a population that are due to chance.
Genetic heterogeneity	The situation in which several different genes can independently cause disease.
Genetic information	The information protected under GINA. This includes a person's genetic test results and the genetic test results of his or her family members.
Genetic resistance	Having one or more gene variations that are protective and decrease the risk for disease development or expression.
Genetic susceptibility	Having one or more gene variations that increase the risk for disease expression.
Genetic test	The analysis of DNA, RNA, chromosomes, proteins, and protein metabolites to identify heritable genotypes, mutations, phenotypes, or karyotypes.
Genetics	The study of the general mechanisms of heredity and the variation of inherited traits.
Genome	The complete set of genes for the species.
Genome-wide association study (GWAS)	A test that looks for areas of the genome associated with a certain disease by comparing the genomes of affected and unaffected populations.
Genomic care	Ensuring that the influence of a person's genetic history on health and disease is considered as part of general assessment information for all patients and families.
Genomic imprinting	An epigenetic event in which a gene (or gene allele) is inactivated by means other than mutation so that the DNA sequence of the gene remains normal but its expression is inhibited.
Genomics	The study of the function of all the nucleotide sequences present within the entire genome of a species, including genes and nongene areas of the DNA.
Genotype	The exact allele pair composition present for any given single-gene trait.
Germline mutation	A mutation that occurs in germ cells (sperm or ova) and can be passed on to one's children at conception.
Gestalt	The overall impression of a person's appearance.
Gestational diabetes mellitus (GDM)	A disorder involving elevated blood sugar levels that is diagnosed as diabetes mellitus during pregnancy.
GINA	The Genetic Information and Nondiscrimination Act, signed into U.S. law on May 21, 2008.
Haploid chromosome number	A set of chromosomes in a germ cell's nucleus that consist of only half of each chromosome pair, 23 chromosomes (1N).
Haplotypes	Groups of genes that tend to be inherited together.

Hardy-Weinberg equilibrium	The idea that the frequency of alleles (and genotypes) in a population will remain the same as long as certain population criteria are met. It is demonstrated by the equation: $p^2 + 2pq + q^2 = 1$.
Hemizygosity	The expression in males of recessive single alleles on the X chromosome as if they were all dominant.
Hereditary hemochromatosis (*HFE*-HHC)	An autosomal-recessive disease that results in excessive absorption of dietary iron by the gastric mucosa.
Heteroplasmy	A condition in which a newly produced daughter cell inherits mitochondria with a mixture of normal mtDNA and mutated mtDNA.
Heterozygosity	The proportion of a population who are heterozygous at a particular locus. If 98% of all alleles in a population are A, then heterozygosity will be low.
Heterozygous	Having two different gene alleles for a specific single-gene trait.
Histones	Globular protein balls that allow DNA to supercoil and compress tightly into dense chromosome structures without damaging or disorganizing the order of base pairs.
Homoplasmy	A condition in which a newly produced daughter cell inherits mitochondria that have either all normal mtDNA or all mutated mtDNA.
Homozygous	Having two identical gene alleles for a specific single-gene trait.
Human genetic variation	The genetic diversity within and between groups of people.
Human leukocyte antigens (HLA)	Unique identifiers on the surface of most body cells.
Hunter syndrome	An X-linked recessive genetic lysosomal storage disease in which there is a deficiency of the enzyme iduronate sulfatase, which results in the accumulation of mucopolysaccharides (MPSs) within the lysosomes of many tissues and organs. (Also known as mucopolysaccharidosis II.)
Hurler syndrome	An autosomal recessive genetic lysosomal storage disease in which there is a deficiency of the enzyme alpha L-iduronidase, which results in the accumulation of mucopolysaccharides (MPSs) in the lysosomes of most cells. (Also known as mucopolysaccharidosis I.)
Hyperaminoacidemia	Any one of several metabolic disorders in which one particular amino acid accumulates in the blood to toxic levels.
Hyperglycemia	An elevated blood glucose level.
Hyperplasia	Mitotic cell growth in which the tissue/organ increases in size by increasing the number of cells within it.
Hypertelorism	Eyes that are widely spaced apart.
Hypertrophy	The increase in tissue size from the expansion of the size of each individual cell rather than by the generation of new cells that increase the number of cells in the tissue.
Hypoteliorism	Eyes that are closely spaced together.
Inherited cancer	Cancer that occurs with an observable autosomal-dominant pattern of inheritance among much-younger-than-expected individuals in a kindred.

Initiation	The first and irreversible step in malignant transformation that involves damage to a cell's DNA, especially in suppressor genes, which leads to the reduced expression of suppressor genes and the enhanced expression of oncogenes.
Insulitis	An infiltration of the islet cells by white blood cells following a viral infection, resulting in inflammation and destruction of these cells.
Intellectual property	Creative innovations and inventions that belong to the creator or inventor.
Intended action	The desired and expected change in the function of one or more tissues or organs as a result of drug therapy. Same as therapeutic effect.
Introns	The sectional parts of DNA within a gene-coding region that do not belong to the gene-coding sequence of the protein being synthesized.
Jervell and Lange-Nielsen syndrome	A phenotype of LQTS that is transmitted as an autosomal recessive trait and includes sensorineural deafness.
Karyotype	An organized arrangement of all the chromosomes within one cell during the metaphase section of mitosis.
Kindred	Extended family relationships over several generations. Same as kinship.
Knockout mice	Mice that are bred, using genetic engineering, with one or several genes "turned off" (knocked out).
Latency period	The time between the initiation of a cell and the development of an identifiable tumor.
Liability model	An estimate of the risk of experiencing a complex disease based on the number of risk alleles in a kindred.
Lip pits	A depression in the lower lip that is usually lateral to the midline.
Long fingers/toes	Fingers or toes that are unusually long compared to the size of the palm or the foot.
Long QT syndrome (LQTS)	A congenital or acquired disorder in which the phenotype shows lengthening of the refractory period of the cardiac cycle and vulnerability to a potentially lethal ventricular arrhythmia.
Low-set ears	The upper ears insert into the scalp below an imaginary horizontal line drawn through the inner canthi of the eyes and going back to the ears.
Lysosomal storage disease	A disorder in which the enzyme within lysosomes is defective or deficient, causing the buildup of a precursor substance that becomes toxic to the cell.
Lysosomes	Intracellular vesicles that contain many enzymes whose function is to degrade the protein and lipid by-products of metabolism.
Macrocephaly	An unusually large head in proportion to the body.
Major anomaly	A significant abnormality for which surgery would often be recommended to treat a significant impairment of physical function or appearance.
Malformation	A defect in the shape or form of a body part that is caused by an abnormal developmental process.
Malignant transformation	The many-stepped process by which a normal cell changes into a cancer cell. Also known as carcinogenesis and oncogenesis.

Marfan syndrome (MFS)	An inherited, genetic, connective tissue disorder in which the gene for the glycoprotein fibrillin is mutated.
Maturity-onset diabetes of the young (MODY)	A single-gene disorder that causes hyperglycemia, usually before the age of 25.
Medical geneticist	A genetic professional with a doctorate (PhD), most commonly in population genetics or epidemiology.
Meiosis	The process of chromosomal reduction cell divisions required during gametogenesis to ensure that gametes are haploid.
Meiotic cell division	A special type of cell division in which the chromosome number per cell is reduced to half.
Mendelian inheritance	The patterns of inheritance for monogenic traits as first recognized by Gregor Mendel in the 19th century.
Metabolism	Chemical reactions in the body that change the chemical shape, size, content, and activity of the drug.
Metastasis	The spread of cancer cells to other body areas, where they may grow and damage additional tissues and organs, often leading to death.
Microcephaly	An unusually small head in proportion to the body.
Micrognathia	A smaller-than-normal length and width of the lower jaw.
MicroRNA	A small noncoding piece of RNA that regulates gene expression at the mRNA level by inhibiting the translation and promoting the degradation of specific (targeted) cytoplasmic mRNA molecules.
Midface hypoplasia	A disproportionately small central face, including the upper jaw, cheeks, and eye region, as compared to the rest of the face.
Minimum effective concentration (MEC)	The lowest blood or tissue drug level required to cause the intended action.
Minor anomaly	A variation in a body part that may be helpful with diagnosis but is not a threat to the person's well-being (e.g., low-set ears).
Mitochondria	Organelles within a cell's cytoplasm that are responsible for most of the generation of the high-energy chemical adenosine triphosphate (ATP).
Mitosis	A duplication cell division that results in two new cells that are identical both to each other and to the original cell (parent cell) that began the mitosis.
Modifier genes	Genes that are not the primary cause of the disorder, but their variants alter the phenotype.
Monogenic trait	A trait whose expression is determined by the input of the two alleles of a single gene. Same as single-gene trait.
Monosomy	Inheritance of only one chromosome of a pair instead of two.
Mosaicism	The condition in which two (or more) different karyotypes are consistently present in one individual.
Multiple sclerosis (MS)	A progressive autoimmune disorder that results in damage to the myelin sheath of the neurons in the central nervous system.

Mutagen	Any substance or event that can inflict temporary or permanent changes in the normal DNA sequence.
Mutation	An alteration in the base sequence of DNA or RNA.
Natural selection	The process by which genetic traits become more or less common based on the survival advantage they provide.
Neoplasia	New cell growth not needed for normal development or the replacement of dead and damaged tissues. It can be benign or malignant.
Newborn screening	A test done shortly after birth to identify those infants at high risk of diseases for which immediate treatment or intervention is available.
Nondirective	Providing genetic information and counseling and presenting all facts and available options in a way that neither promotes nor excludes any decision or action (within legal boundaries).
Nondisjunction	Failure of a chromosome pair to separate during meiosis so that one of the two new cells is missing a chromosome and the other new cell has both chromosomes of the pair from the same parent.
Nucleokinesis	The process occurring in the M phase of cell division in which each chromosome is pulled apart so that the two sets of chromosomes are separated within the single large cell.
Nucleoside	A nitrogenous base of adenine, guanine, cytosine, or thymine attached to a five-sided sugar (ribose sugar).
Nucleotide	A nitrogenous base attached to a five-sided sugar and connected to a phosphate group.
Oligohydramnios	Not having enough amniotic fluid.
Oncogenes	A large group of genes that produce proteins that promote entering and completing the cell cycle. Also known as promitotic genes.
Oogenesis	The process of forming oocytes from precursor germ cells.
Osteogenesis imperfecta (OI)	A group of genetic disorders in which collagen formation is impaired, resulting in bones that fracture easily.
Oxidative phosphorylation	The metabolic pathway in mitochondria responsible for the efficient generation of ATP under conditions in which oxygen and hydrogen ions are plentiful.
Palpebral fissure	The outlined space between the eyelids of each eye.
p arm	The segment of a chromosome above the centromere (short arm).
Patents	Government protection that gives the owner exclusive rights to keep others from making or using whatever is patented.
Pedigree	A pictorial or graphic illustration of family members' places within a kindred and their history for a specific trait or health problem over several generations.
Penetrance	How often, within a population, a gene is expressed when it is present.
P_1 generation	The parental generation of a family or group being observed for a specific trait or traits.
Pharmacodynamics	Body responses induced by a drug, including mechanism of action, desired effects, and side effects.

Pharmacogenetics	The use of single-gene information in the study of drug development and drug therapy.
Pharmacogenomics	The use of genome-wide information in drug development and drug therapy.
Pharmacokinetics	The actions of the body that change the physical and chemical properties of a drug.
Phenotype	The observed expression of any given single-gene trait.
Phenylketonuria (PKU)	An autosomal recessive genetic disorder in which the enzyme phenylalanine hydroxylase (PAH) is deficient and the amino acid phenylalanine cannot be enzymatically converted to tyrosine, resulting in an excess of phenylalanine and a deficiency of tyrosine.
Philtrum	The groove or depression that lies in the midline between the upper lip and the nose.
Phosphorylation	A chemical reaction in which a phosphate group is added to another chemical through the action of a tyrosine kinase enzyme. The result of phosphorylation is activation of the chemical.
Plagiocephaly	Asymmetrical distortion of the cranium.
Pleiotropy	An effect in which a single-gene disorder results in problems expressed in many tissues and functions.
Ploidy	The actual number of chromosomes present in a single cell's nucleus at mitosis.
Pluripotent cell	An undifferentiated early embryonic cell that, under the right conditions, can become any human body cell.
Point mutations	Substitutions of one base for another and can occur in DNA or RNA.
Polydactyly	Having an extra finger or toe.
Polygenic	Traits, characteristics, or structures that involve the input of more than one gene.
Polymerase chain reaction (PCR)	A process used to amplify (greatly increase the quantity of) tiny amounts of DNA for examination.
Population bottleneck	The situation that occurs when some event severely reduces the number of individuals in a population. Only the traits of those individuals who survive will be passed on to future generations.
Population genetics	The study of the changes in the frequency of alleles, and the mechanisms for those changes, based on alterations in populations.
Post-transcriptional modification	A process that eliminates the introns before the mRNA can be translated and used to direct the precise synthesis of the protein coded for by the gene.
Post-translational modification	Further processing of a newly translated primary protein structure into its secondary and tertiary structures (and sometimes even a quaternary structure) needed to make it fully functional.
Predictive test	A genetic test designed for asymptomatic persons wanting to know about their risk of getting a genetic disease in the future.
Predispositional test	A predictive test that, when positive, means the person being tested has a higher likelihood of getting the disease in the future than the general population.

Preimplantation genetic diagnosis (PGD)	A procedure done in conjunction with in vitro fertilization (IVF), in which six to eight cell embryos are tested for specific genetic variants. Embryos that test negative can be used for IVF.
Prenatal test	A test done during pregnancy to determine if the fetus carries a gene variant.
Presbycusis	Age-related hearing loss.
Presymptomatic test	A predictive test that, when positive, means that the individual *will* get the disease at some point in his or her life as long as he or she does not die earlier from some other means.
Primary tumor	The original tissue location in which normal cells develop into cancer.
Private mutations	Mutations that are very uncommon; frequently, they are found in only one family.
Proband	The person within a family who brought the potential genetic issue to the attention of a health-care professional.
Prodrug	A drug that is ingested as an inactive parent compound and must undergo first-stage metabolism to become active.
Progression	The continuing genetic changes that occur in cancer cells that alter their physical, biochemical, and metabolic processes and confer survival advantages to these cells.
Promotion	A step in cancer development that enhances the growth potential of a cell that has been initiated.
Protein synthesis	The selective activation of a gene, resulting in its transcription and translation into the production of the appropriate protein.
Proteome	The DNA that codes for the complete set of all proteins that a person can make.
Proteomics	The study of how protein genes are selectively expressed, how they are modified after expression, and how they interact with each other.
Ptosis	Drooping eyelids.
Punnett squares	Diagrams that are used to determine the risk of offspring being affected when the mode of transmission and the parents' carrier status are known.
q arm	The segment of a chromosome below the centromere (long arm).
Race	A controversial term that denotes a group of people classified as sharing a common geographical background, ancestry, and physical features.
Receptors	Sites on a cell surface or within a cell where naturally occurring substances can bind and control cell function.
Recessive trait	A single gene trait that is expressed only when both gene alleles for the trait are identical (homozygous).
Reciprocal translocation	A specific type of balanced translocation in which segments of two nonhomologous chromosomes break and are equally exchanged.
Recurrence risk	The risk of another child in a family being affected when one child is already affected.
Regression to the mean	Extremes of a condition or trait tend to become more average over time in successive generations.
Replication segregation	The random sorting of newly synthesized mitochondria to new daughter cells.

Research geneticist	A doctorally prepared (PhD) individual with postdoctoral training in laboratory genetics whose role is the performance of laboratory or "bench" research to identify exact pathologic mechanisms that result from various genetic disorders and to develop possible therapeutic approaches to reduce the effects of the pathologic mechanisms.
Retrognathia	A backward positioning of the lower jaw.
Rheumatoid arthritis	An autoimmune disorder that results in inflammation of the joints and the tissues surrounding them.
Ribonucleic acid (RNA)	A single strand of nitrogenous bases (adenine, guanine, cytosine, and uracil) constructed during transcription from a segment of DNA containing the gene for a specific protein.
Ribosome	A cytoplasmic adapter molecule containing a complex of proteins and RNA that essentially decodes the mRNA to place the proper individual amino acid into the peptide chain during protein synthesis.
Right to privacy	The ethical obligation of health-care professionals to not disclose a patient's private health-care information.
Risk alleles	Gene variants that confer increased risk for a particular trait or disorder.
Risk stratification	The process of identifying whether a person is at a high, moderate, or low risk of developing a genetic disorder.
Robertsonian translocation	A specific type of balanced translocation created by the fusion of the entire long arms of two acrocentric chromosomes (which include chromosome numbers 13, 14, 15, 21, and 22).
Romano-Ward syndrome	A phenotype of LQTS that is transmitted as an autosomal dominant trait and is not accompanied by deafness.
Self-tolerance	The ability of the immune system to recognize and not attack the body's own cells and tissues.
Sequence	A group of anomalies that are thought to follow in a chain, from a single cause.
Sex chromosomes	The pair of chromosomes that code for the sexual differentiation of the individual.
Sex reversal	A condition in which sex genotype and phenotype are mismatched, with phenotypic women having a 46,XY karyotype and phenotypic men having a 46,XX karyotype.
Sickle cell crisis	An acute period of low-oxygen tension in which extensive tissue hypoxia/anoxia, cell sickling, and blood flow obstruction occur, leading to severe pain.
Sickle cell disease (SCD)	A monogenetic disorder caused by a single nucleotide polymorphism in both alleles of the *HBB* gene that results in the abnormal formation of the beta chain of hemoglobin (beta globin).
Sickle cell trait	A monogenic disorder caused by a single nucleotide polymorphism in only one allele of the *HBB* gene that results in red blood cells having only 50% or less of abnormal hemoglobin molecules.
Side effects	Drug effects that are not the main purpose of the intended action.

Signal transduction	A set of communication system chains that allows information about events, conditions, and substances external to the cell to reach the nucleus and influence whether the cell then divides, undergoes apoptosis, or performs its differentiated functions.
Single-gene trait	A trait whose expression is determined by the input of the two alleles of a single gene. Same as a *monogenic trait.*
Single nucleotide polymorphism (SNP)	A type of point mutation commonly inherited in a gene that alters gene activity in a certain percentage of the general population.
Somatic mutation	A mutation that occurs after conception in general body cells (somatic cells) and cannot be passed on to one's children.
Spermatogenesis	The process of converting diploid spermatogonia into mature haploid sperm.
Sporadic cancer	A cancer that occurs usually as a result of environmental exposure and does not have any observable pattern of inheritance within a kindred.
Suppressor genes	A set of master control genes that produce proteins that restrict a cell from entering the cell cycle and that inhibit movement of a cell from one phase to the next within the cell cycle. Some products of these genes also trigger apoptosis.
Syndactyly	A condition in which two or more of the fingers or toes are joined together at either the soft tissue or bone level.
Syndrome	A collection of anomalies that are related, most often with a known cause.
Systemic lupus erythematosus (SLE)	An autoimmune disorder that affects multiple systems, including the skin, joints, and kidneys.
Targets	Cells with receptor sites that can bind with specific drugs and have a change in their functional activity as a result of drug binding.
Tay-Sachs disease	An autosomal recessive genetic lysosomal storage disorder in which there is a deficiency of the enzyme beta-hexosaminidase A, which results in the accumulation of GM2-ganglioside in brain cells.
Teratogen	A drug, chemical, or condition that can alter the development of an embryo or fetus, resulting in a birth defect.
Therapeutic effect	The desired and expected change in the function of one or more tissues or organs as a result of drug therapy. Same as intended action.
Threshold	The theoretical point at which genetic liability (number of risk alleles) is great enough that the disorder is likely to be expressed.
Thrombophilia	A disorder that increases the risk of blood clots.
Transcription	The process of making a strand of RNA that is complementary to the DNA sequence that contains the gene for the protein needed.
Transcription factors	A variety of promitotic substances that enter a cell nucleus and signal to the cell that specific gene transcription or mitosis is needed.
Transfer RNA (tRNA)	Specialized carrier and transfer molecules that can move an amino acid into position to be incorporated into a growing peptide chain during protein synthesis.
Translation	The process of using a mature mRNA molecule as the directions for proper placement of amino acids in the correct sequence to synthesize a protein.

Translocation	A chromosomal abnormality in which all or part of a chromosome is transferred to another nonhomologous chromosome.
Transmission	The term used to describe how a trait is inherited (passed) from one human generation to the next.
Triploidy	The inheritance of an extra copy of each chromosome, resulting in an individual who has 69 chromosomes per cell instead of 46.
Trisomy	The inheritance of an extra copy of one chromosome from one parent so that the cells contain three copies of that chromosome instead of just two.
Twin concordance	The percentage of time a person is likely to be affected if his or her twin is affected. Concordance can be reported for monozygotic or dizygotic twins.
Type 1 diabetes mellitus	An autoimmune, metabolic, endocrine disorder in which insulin-producing cells in the pancreas have been destroyed and the person no longer synthesizes insulin.
Tyrosine kinases (TKs)	A family of enzymes that function to activate other substances through the process of phosphorylation.
Unbalanced translocation	The inheritance from one parent of more or less than one copy of a chromosome or part of a chromosome.
Uniparental disomy (UPD)	A condition in which both chromosomes of a pair in a child came from just one parent.
Uracil	A pyrimidine base nearly identical to thymine that is used in place of thymine in RNA synthesis.
von Willebrand disease (VWD)	A monogenic disorder in which the affected person produces less than normal amounts of von Willebrand factor (vWf).
Zygote	The single diploid cell formed from fertilization that is capable of developing into a multicelled embryo.

Index

Note: Page numbers followed by "f" and "t" indicate figures and tables, respectively.